evolve

W9-DBO-743

To access your Student Resources, visit:

http://evolve.elsevier.com/KeeMarshall/clinical

Evolve® Student Resources for *Kee: Clinical Calculations with Applications to General and Specialty Areas* offer the following features:

Student Resources

- **WebLinks**
  An exciting resource that lets you link to hundreds of websites carefully chosen to supplement the content of your textbook. The WebLinks are regularly updated with new ones added as they develop.

- **Sign-up for Nurse Advise-ERR™–a Medication Safety Alert!® from the Institute for Safe Medication Practices**
  Published monthly by the internationally recognized Institute for Safe Medication Practices (ISMP) and distributed free to students and instructors by Elsevier, Nurse Advise-ERR™ provides tips for safe medication practice and up-to-date information on preventing medication errors.

Master Drug Calculations
in an EXCITING New Way!

Ideal for diverse learning styles and circumstances, **Drug Calculations Online** takes learning to new places! Designed to accompany **Clinical Calculations, 5th Edition**, this unique, innovative, and affordable new online course supplement includes numerous practice problems and interactive activities, so you have ample opportunities for application and practice.

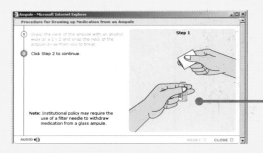

Drug Calculations Online has all of the tools you need for a complete learning experience!

- **Animations are used throughout the course** to demonstrate various concepts related to drug administration.

- Content includes **all four major drug calculation methods** (ratio & proportion, formula, fractional equation, and dimensional analysis) to expose you to all calculation methods, so you can apply the method that works best for you.

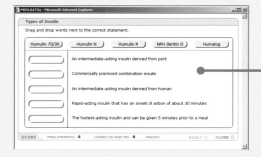

- All of the practice problems include tutorials for each of the four drug calculation methods, providing **step-by-step solutions for the problem**.

- **Voice-overs** enhance the step-by-step explanation of math skills and drug calculation methods, in addition to livening up the discussion.

- **Quizzes within each module** allow you to test your knowledge of all major topics covered in that particular section.

- **Interactive self-assessment activities** are incorporated to allow you to apply your knowledge in context, especially helpful in light of the fact that the NCLEX® examination also has these types of questions.

- And much, much more!

You'll also receive a **User's Guide** that provides you with a unique access code, a description of the types of activities provided, technical instruction, and support to get you started on this one-of-a-kind learning experience!

For a preview of this powerful study tool, go to
http://evolve.elsevier.com/keemarshall/clinical

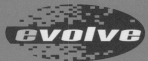

Clinical Calculations

With Applications to General and Specialty Areas

FIFTH EDITION

Joyce LeFever Kee, RN, MS

Associate Professor Emerita
College of Health and Nursing Sciences
University of Delaware
Newark, Delaware

Sally M. Marshall, RN, MSN

Nursing Service
Department of Veterans Affairs
Regional Office and Medical Center
Wilmington, Delaware

SAUNDERS
An Imprint of Elsevier

SAUNDERS
An Imprint of Elsevier

11830 Westline Industrial Drive
St. Louis, Missouri 63146

CLINICAL CALCULATIONS WITH APPLICATIONS TO GENERAL
AND SPECIALTY AREAS, FIFTH EDITION
Copyright © 2004, Elsevier (USA). All rights reserved.

NOTICE

Nursing is an ever-changing field. Standard safety precautions must be followed, but as new research and clinical experience broaden our knowledge, changes in treatment and drug therapy may become necessary or appropriate. Readers are advised to check the most current product information provided by the manufacturer of each drug to be administered to verify the recommended dose, the method and duration of administration, and contraindications. It is the responsibility of the treating physician, relying on experience and knowledge of the patient, to determine dosages and the best treatment for each individual patient. Neither the publisher nor the author assumes any liability for any injury and/or damage to persons or property arising from this publication.

Previous editions copyrighted 2000, 1996, 1992, 1988

ISBN-13: 978-1-4160-3177-2
ISBN-10: 1-4160-3177-4

Executive Vice President, Nursing and Health Professions: Sally Schrefer
Senior Editor: Yvonne Alexopoulos
Developmental Editor: Danielle M. Frazier
Publishing Services Manager: Catherine Jackson
Senior Project Manager: Jeff Patterson
Designer: Teresa McBryan

Printed in the United States of America

Last digit is the print number: 9 8 7 6 5 4 3 2

To my grandchildren
Christopher, Brenda, Jessica, and Kimberly
Joyce Kee

To my mother
and to my children, Drew and Sarah
Sally Marshall

To our nursing colleagues

Reviewers

Rhonda Armstrong, RN, MSN
Instructor
Nursing Department
Hinds Community College
Jackson, Mississippi

Sara L. Clutter, RN, MSN
Assistant Professor
Nursing Department
Waynesburg College
Waynesburg, Pennsylvania

Kathleen Kline Matzinger, RN, BSN
Learning Lab Coordinator
Nursing Education
Pennsylvania College of Technology
Williamsport, Pennsylvania

Catherine Renz, BSN, MEd
Instructor
Nursing Department
Iowa Western Community College
Council Bluffs, Iowa

Sandra C. Wardell, RN, BSN, MEd
Professor
Nursing Department
Orange County Community College
Middletown, New York

Preface to the Instructor

INTRODUCTION

Clinical Calculations with Applications to General and Specialty Areas arose from the need to bridge the learning gap between education and practice. We believe that this bridge is needed for the student to understand the wide range of clinical calculations used in nursing practice. This book provides a comprehensive application of calculations in nursing practice.

Clinical Calculations has been expanded in this fifth edition on topics in several areas to show the interrelationship between calculation and drug administration, such as in the use of the latest equipment (insulin pump, patient-controlled analgesia pumps, multi-channel infusion pumps), various new syringes (prefilled syringes, insulin and tuberculin syringes), various methods of calculating body surface area, and more. This text also provides the six methods for calculating drug dosages—basic formula, ratio and proportion, fractional equation, dimensional analysis, body weight, and body surface area.

Clinical Calculations is unique in that it has problems not only for the general patient areas but also for the specialty units—pediatrics, critical care, pediatric critical care, labor and delivery, and community. This text is useful for nurses in all levels of nursing education who are learning for the first time how to calculate dosage problems and for beginning practitioners in specialty areas. It also can be used in nursing refresher courses, inservice programs, hospital units, home health care, and other places of nursing practice.

This book is divided into five parts. Part I is the basic math review, written concisely for nursing students to review Roman numerals, fractions, decimals, percentages, and ratio and proportion. A post-math review test follows. The post-math test can be taken first, and if the student has a score of 90% or higher, the basic review section can be omitted. Part II covers metric, apothecary, and household systems used in drug calculations; conversion of units; reading drug labels, drug orders, and abbreviations; and methods of calculations. We suggest that you assign Parts I and II, which cover delivery of medication, prior to the class. Part III covers calculation of drug and fluid dosages for oral, injectable, and intravenous administration. Clinical drug calculations for specialty areas are found in Part IV. This part includes pediatrics, critical care for adults and children, labor and delivery, and community. Part V contains the Post-Test for students to test their competency in mastering oral, injectable, intravenous, and pediatric drug calculations. A passing grade is 88%.

Appendix A includes guidelines for administrations of medications (oral, injectable, and intravenous), and Appendix B contains nomograms.

Each chapter has a content list, objectives, introduction, and numerous practice problems. The practice problems are related to clinical drug problems that are currently used in clinical settings. Illustrations such as tablets, capsules, medicine cup, syringes, ampules, vials, intravenous bag and bottle, IV tubing, electronic IV devices, intramuscular injection sites, central venous sites, and many others are provided throughout the text.

Calculators may be used in solving dosage problems. Many institutions have calculators available. The nurse should work the problem without a calculator and then check the answer with a calculator.

FEATURES OF THE FIFTH EDITION

- Problems using the newest drug labels are provided in most chapters.
- Six methods for calculating drug dosages have been divided into two chapters. Chapter 5 gives four methods—basic formula, ratio and proportion, fractional equations, and dimensional analysis. Chapter 6 contains two individual methods for calculating drug doses—body weight and body surface area.
- Additional dimensional analysis has been added to the examples of drug dosing and to the answers to practice problems in most of the chapters.
- Additional drug problems have been added throughout.
- More emphasis is placed on the metric system than on the apothecary system.
- Several chapters have nomograms for adults and children.
- Explanation of the bar code and the computer-based medication administration system is provided.
- Use of fingertip units for cream applications is illustrated.
- Explanations are provided for the use of the insulin pump, insulin pen injectors, intranasal insulin jet injectors, and the patient-controlled analgesic pump.
- Illustrations of new types of syringes, safety needle shield, various insulin and tuberculin syringes, and needleless syringes are provided.
- Illustrations of pumps are provided, including insulin, enteral infusion, and various intravenous infusion pumps (single and multi-channel, patient-controlled analgesia, and syringe).
- Coverage of direct intravenous injection (IV push or IV bolus) is provided with practice problems in Chapter 9.
- Coverage of home infusion therapy is provided with practice problems.

ANCILLARIES

Instructor's Manual and Test Bank for Clinical Calculations with Applications to General and Specialty Areas, Fifth Edition, is specifically geared toward this edition and includes the following:
- Teaching strategies
- Three different course outlines for teaching calculation of drug dosage: (1) as a separate course, (2) as part of a pharmacology course, or (3) integrated into

the nursing curriculum and covered in the skill laboratory and clinical courses

- A Basic Math Test for the instructor to administer to the students early in the course to evaluate basic math skills
- Test Bank with about 300 drug calculation problems covering general and specialty areas

This resource is also available on CD-ROM and online. To use this great resource online, visit the **Evolve** website at http://evolve.elsevier.com/KeeMarshall/clinical/.

Romans & Daugherty Dosages and Solutions CTB (Version II) is a generic computerized test bank (CD-ROM) that has been completely updated and is provided as a gratis item to instructors upon adoption of this book. It contains over 700 questions on general math, converting within systems of measurement, oral dosages, parenteral dosages, flow rates, pediatric dosages, IV calculations, and more. This CTB is also available online at the **Evolve** website at http://evolve.elsevier.com/KeeMarshall/clinical/.

Daugherty & Romans Dosages and Solutions CD-ROM Companion (Version II) is an updated student tutorial. It is a user-friendly, interactive program that includes an extensive menu of various topic areas within dosages and solutions. This CD is packaged with the book and provides hundreds of practice problems in the ratio and proportion, formula, dimensional analysis, and fractional equation methods. Engaging animations allow the user to complete interactive exercises and practice problems. This CD also includes a comprehensive post-test.

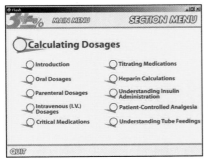

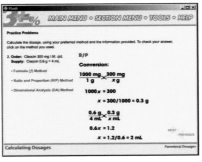

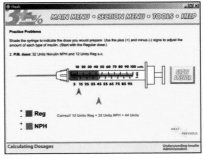

Preface to the Student

Clinical Calculations with Applications to General and Specialty Areas, Fifth Edition, can be used as a self-instructional mathematics and dosage calculation review tool.

Part I, Basic Math Review, is a review of math concepts usually taught in middle school. Some of you may need to review Part I as a refresher of basic math and then take the comprehensive math test at the end of the book. Others may choose to take the math test first. If your score on this test is 90% or higher, you should proceed to Part II; if your score is less than 90%, you should review Part I.

Part II, Systems, Conversion, and Methods of Drug Calculation, should be studied before the class related to oral, injectable, and intravenous calculations, which is covered in Part III. In Part II you will learn the various systems of drug administration, conversion within the various systems, charting, drug orders, abbreviations, methods of drug calculation, and alternative methods for drug administration. You can study Part II on your own.

Chapter 5, Methods of Calculation, gives the four methods commonly used to calculate drug dosages. You or the instructor should select one of the four methods to calculate drug dosages. Use that method in all practice problems starting in Chapter 5. This approach will improve your proficiency in the calculation of drug dosages.

Part III, Calculations for Oral, Injectable, and Intravenous Drugs, is usually discussed in class and during a clinical practicum. Before class, you should review the three chapters in Part III. Questions may be addressed and answered during class time. During the class or clinical practicum you may practice drug calculations and the drawing up of drug doses in a syringe.

Part IV, Calculations for Specialty Areas, is usually presented when the topics are discussed in class. You should review this content in these chapters—Pediatrics, Critical Care, Pediatric Critical Care, Labor and Delivery, and Community—before the scheduled class. According to the requirements of your specific nursing program, this content may or may not be covered.

Daugherty & Romans Dosages and Solutions CD-ROM Companion (Version II) is also included with this text. This updated student tutorial is a user-friendly, interactive program that includes an extensive menu of various topic areas within dosages and solutions. This CD-ROM is packaged with the book and provides hundreds of practice problems in the ratio and proportion, formula, dimensional analysis, and fractional equation methods. Engaging animations allow the user to complete interactive exercises and practice problems. This CD-ROM also includes a comprehensive post-test.

 Look for this icon in each chapter. It will refer you to the Daugherty & Romans Dosages and Solutions CD-ROM Companion (Version II) for additional practice problems.

Acknowledgments

We wish to extend our sincere appreciation to the individuals who have helped with this fifth edition: Dr. Ha B. Hua, Pharm D, Clinical Pharmacist, Veterans Administration Medical Center, Wilmington, Delaware; Katherine E. Carr, RN, BSN, Patient Care Coordinator, Christiana Care Center, Newark, Delaware; Susan Douglas, RN, St. Francis Hospital—Newborn Nursery, Wilmington, Delaware; Karen Rockhill, RN, Oncology Clinical Nurse Specialist, Veterans Administration Medical Center, Wilmington, Delaware; and Drew Marshall for his typing assistance. We also thank Don Passidomo, Head Librarian at the Veterans Administration Medical Center, for his research assistance.

We extend our sincere thanks to the companies and publishers who gave us permission to use photographs, illustrations, and other materials in the text. These include:

American Association of Critical Care Nursing
Baxter Healthcare
Becton Dickinson & Company
Ciba-Geigy Pharmaceuticals
F.A. Davis
Mini MED, Inc.
Oncology Nursing Press, Inc.
Prentice Hall Health

Our deepest appreciation goes to the following drug companies:

Abbott Laboratories
American Regent
    Luitold Pharmaceuticals
Bayer Corporation
Bristol-Myers Squibb
    Apothecon
    Mead Johnson Pharmaceuticals
    Squibb Diagnostic Division
Du Pont Merck Pharmaceutical
Eli Lilly and Company
Elkins-Sinn, Incorporated
    A subsidiary of A.H. Robins, Wyeth-Ayerst
    Laboratories, Cherry Hill, New Jersey

GlaxoWellcome
Marion Merrell Dow, Incorporated
McNeil Consumer Products Company
Merck & Company
Mylan Pharmaceuticals
Ortho McNeil Pharmaceutical
Parke-Davis
Pfizer Laboratories
SmithKline Beecham Pharmaceuticals
Warner-Lambert Consumer Health Products
Wyeth-Ayerst Laboratories

Joyce LeFever Kee
Sally M. Marshall

Contents

PART I   BASIC MATH REVIEW, 1

NUMBER SYSTEMS, 3
    Arabic System, 3
    Roman System, 3
    Conversion of Systems, 3
FRACTIONS, 4
    Proper, Improper, and Mixed Fractions, 5
    Multiplying Fractions, 5
    Dividing Fractions, 6
    Decimal Fractions, 6
DECIMALS, 7
    Multiplying Decimals, 8
    Dividing Decimals, 8
RATIO AND PROPORTION, 9
PERCENTAGE, 10
POST-MATH TEST, 12
    Roman and Arabic Numerals, 13
    Fractions, 13
    Decimals, 14
    Ratio and Proportion, 15
    Percentage, 15

PART II   SYSTEMS, CONVERSION, AND METHODS OF DRUG CALCULATION, 17

CHAPTER 1   Systems Used for Drug Administration, 19

METRIC SYSTEM, 20
    Conversion within the Metric System, 22
APOTHECARY SYSTEM, 25
    Conversion within the Apothecary System, 26
HOUSEHOLD SYSTEM, 28
    Conversion within the Household System, 28
SUMMARY PRACTICE PROBLEMS, 31

CHAPTER 2 Conversion within the Metric, Apothecary, and Household Systems, 33

UNITS, MILLIEQUIVALENTS, AND PERCENTS, 34
METRIC, APOTHECARY, AND HOUSEHOLD EQUIVALENTS, 35
    Conversion in Metric and Apothecary Systems by WEIGHT, 35
    Conversion in Metric, Apothecary, Household Systems by LIQUID VOLUME, 38
SUMMARY PRACTICE PROBLEMS, 41
    Weight: Metric and Apothecary Converions, 41
    Volume: Metric, Apothecary, and Household Conversion, 42

CHAPTER 3 Interpretation of Drug Labels, Drug Orders, Bar Codes, Charting, "5 Rights," and Abbreviations, 45

INTERPRETING DRUG LABELS, 46
    Military Time versus Traditional (Universal) Time, 50
DRUG DIFFERENTIATION, 50
    Drug Orders, 52
    Computer-Based Medication Administration, 55
    Bar Code, 56
    Charting Medications, 57
    Methods of Drug Distribution, 58
THE "5 RIGHTS" IN DRUG ADMINISTRATION, 59
ABBREVIATIONS, 62
    Drug Form, 62
    Drug Measurements, 62
    Routes of Drug Administration, 63
    Times of Drug Administration, 63

CHAPTER 4 Alternative Methods for Drug Administration, 67

TRANSDERMAL PATCH, 68
INHALATION, 69
NASAL SPRAY AND DROPS, 71
EYE DROPS AND OINTMENT, 73
EAR DROPS, 74
PHARYNGEAL SPRAY, MOUTHWASH, AND LOZENGE, 75
TOPICAL PREPARATIONS: LOTION, CREAM, AND OINTMENT, 76
RECTAL SUPPOSITORY, 77
VAGINAL SUPPOSITORY, CREAM, AND OINTMENT, 78

CHAPTER 5 **Methods of Calculation**, 79

DRUG CALCULATION, 80
  Method 1: Basic Formula, 80
  Method 2: Ratio and Proportion, 82
  Method 3: Fractional Equation, 84
  Method 4: Dimensional Analysis, 86
SUMMARY PRACTICE PROBLEMS, 88
  Additional Dimensional Analysis (Factor Labeling), 92

CHAPTER 6 **Methods of Calculation for Individualized Drug Dosing**, 97

CALCULATION FOR INDIVIDUALIZED DRUG DOSING, 98
  Body Weight, 98
  Body Surface Area, 99
SUMMARY PRACTICE PROBLEMS, 103

PART III **CALCULATIONS FOR ORAL, INJECTABLE, AND INTRAVENOUS DRUGS**, 111

CHAPTER 7 **Oral and Enteral Preparations with Clinical Applications**, 113

TABLETS AND CAPSULES, 114
  Calculation of Tablets and Capsules, 115
LIQUIDS, 118
  Calculation of Liquid Medications, 118
SUBLINGUAL TABLETS, 120
  Calculation of Sublingual Medications, 120
ENTERAL NUTRITION AND DRUG ADMINISTRATION, 131
  Enteral Feedings, 131
  Enteral Medications, 134

CHAPTER 8 **Injectable Preparations with Clinical Applications**, 147

INJECTABLE PREPARATIONS, 148
  Vials and Ampules, 148
  Syringes, 149
  Needles, 152
INTRADERMAL INJECTIONS, 155
SUBCUTANEOUS INJECTIONS, 155
  Calculations for Subcutaneous Injections, 156

INSULIN INJECTIONS, 159
TYPES OF INSULIN, 159
MIXING INSULINS, 161
   Insulin Pen Injectors, 163
   Intranasal Insulin, 163
   Insulin Jet Injectors, 164
   Insulin Pumps, 164
INTRAMUSCULAR INJECTIONS, 165
   Drug Solutions for Injection, 166
   Reconstitution of Powdered Drugs, 168
MIXING OF INJECTABLE DRUGS, 170

CHAPTER 9 Intravenous Preparations with Clinical Applications, 191

INTRAVENOUS ACCESS SITES, 192
   Intermittent Infusion Devices, 194
DIRECT INTRAVENOUS INJECTIONS, 194
CONTINUOUS INTRAVENOUS ADMINISTRATION, 199
   Intravenous Sets, 200
CALCULATION OF INTRAVENOUS FLOW RATE, 201
   Safety Considerations, 203
   Mixing Drugs Used for Continuous Intravenous Administration, 203
INTERMITTENT INTRAVENOUS ADMINISTRATION, 208
   Secondary Intravenous Sets, 208
   Electronic Intravenous Delivery Devices, 209
FLOW RATES FOR IV PUMPS, 211
   Calculating Flow Rates for Intravenous Drugs and Electrolytes, 212

PART IV CALCULATIONS FOR SPECIALTY AREAS, 229

CHAPTER 10 Pediatrics, 231

FACTORS INFLUENCING PEDIATRIC DRUG ADMINISTRATION, 232
   Oral, 232
   Intramuscular, 233
   Intravenous, 233
PEDIATRIC DRUG CALCULATIONS, 234
   Dosage per Kilogram Body Weight, 235
   Dosage per Body Surface Area, 238
PEDIATRIC DOSAGE FROM ADULT DOSAGE, 249
   Body Surface Area Formula, 249
   Age Rules, 250
   Body Weight Rule, 250

CHAPTER 11 Critical Care, 259

CALCULATING AMOUNT OF DRUG OR CONCENTRATION OF A SOLUTION, 260
    Calculating Units per Milliliter, 260
    Calculating Milligrams per Milliliter, 261
    Calculating Micrograms per Milliliter, 261
CALCULATING INFUSION RATE FOR CONCENTRATION AND VOLUME
    PER UNIT TIME, 263
    Concentration and Volume per Hour and Minute with a Drug in Units, 263
    Concentration and Volume per Hour and Minute with a Drug in Milligrams, 264
    Concentration and Volume per Hour and Minute with a Drug in Micrograms, 265
CALCULATING INFUSION RATES OF A DRUG FOR SPECIFIC BODY WEIGHT
    PER UNIT TIME, 267
    Micrograms per Kilogram Body Weight, 268
BASIC FRACTIONAL FORMULA, 269
    Using Basic Formula to Find Volume per Hour or Drops per Minute, 269
    Using Basic Formula to Find Desired Concentration per Minute, 269
    Using Basic Formula to Find Concentration of Solution, 270
TITRATION OF INFUSION RATE, 271
TOTAL AMOUNT OF DRUG INFUSED OVER TIME, 276

CHAPTER 12 Pediatric Critical Care, 293

FACTORS INFLUENCING INTRAVENOUS ADMINISTRATION, 294
CALCULATING ACCURACY OF DILUTION PARAMETERS, 294
SUMMARY PRACTICE PROBLEMS, 297

CHAPTER 13 Labor and Delivery, 301

FACTORS INFLUENCING INTRAVENOUS FLUID AND DRUG MANAGEMENT, 302
TITRATION OF MEDICATIONS WITH MAINTENANCE INTRAVENOUS FLUIDS, 302
    Administration by Concentration, 302
    Administration by Volume, 304
INTRAVENOUS LOADING DOSE, 304
INTRAVENOUS FLUID BOLUS, 306

CHAPTER 14 Community, 311

METRIC TO HOUSEHOLD CONVERSION, 312
PREPARING A SOLUTION OF A DESIRED CONCENTRATION, 314
    Changing a Ratio to Fractions and Percentages, 315
    Calculating a Solution from a Ratio, 316
    Calculating a Solution from a Percentage, 317
PREPARING A WEAKER SOLUTION FROM A STRONGER SOLUTION, 317
GUIDELINES FOR HOME SOLUTIONS, 318
HOME INFUSION THERAPY, 320
    Home Infusion Devices, 320

PART V   POST-TEST: ORAL PREPARATIONS, INJECTABLES, INTRAVENOUS, AND PEDIATRICS, 327

ORAL PREPARATIONS, 329
INJECTABLES, 335
INTRAVENOUS, 340
PEDIATRICS, 343

References, 351

APPENDIX A   Guidelines for Administration of Medications, 353

APPENDIX B   Nomograms, 359

Index, 363

PART I

BASIC MATH REVIEW

OBJECTIVES

- Convert Roman numerals to Arabic numerals.
- Multiply and divide fractions and decimals.
- Solve ratio and proportion problems.
- Change percentages to decimals, fractions, and ratio and proportion.
- Demonstrate an understanding of Roman numerals, fractions, decimals, ratio and proportion, and percentage by passing the math test.

OUTLINE

NUMBER SYSTEMS
    Arabic System
    Roman System
    Conversion of Systems
FRACTIONS
    Proper, Improper, and Mixed
      Fractions
    Multiplying Fractions
    Dividing Fractions
    Decimal Fractions

DECIMALS
    Multiplying Decimals
    Dividing Decimals
RATIO AND PROPORTION
PERCENTAGE
POST-MATH TEST
    Roman and Arabic Numerals
    Fractions
    Decimals
    Ratio and Proportion
    Percentage

The basic math review assists nurses in converting Roman and Arabic numerals, multiplying and dividing fractions and decimals, and solving ratio and proportion problems and percentage problems. Nurses need to master basic math skills to solve drug problems used in the administration of medication.

A math test, found on pages 12 to 16, follows the basic math review. The test may be taken first, and if a score of 90% or greater is achieved, the math review, or Part One, can be omitted. If the test score is less than 90%, the nurse should do the basic math review section. Some nurses may choose to start with Part One and then take the test.

Answers to the Practice Problems are at the end of Part One, before the Post-Math Test

 An additional "Mathematics Review" is available on the CD-ROM.

NUMBER SYSTEMS

Two systems of numbers currently used are Arabic and Roman. Both systems are used in drug administration.

Arabic System

The Arabic system is expressed in numbers: 0, 1, 2, 3, 4, 5, 6, 7, 8, 9. These can be written as whole numbers or with fractions and decimals. This system is commonly used today.

Roman System

Numbers used in the Roman system are designated by selected capital letters, e.g., I, V, X. Roman numbers can be changed to Arabic numbers.

Conversion of Systems

Roman Number	Arabic Number
I	1
V	5
X	10
L	50
C	100

The apothecary system of measurement uses Roman numerals for writing drug dosages. The Roman numerals are written in lower case letters, e.g., i, v, x, xii. The lower case letters can be topped by a horizontal line, e.g., ī, v̄, x̄, x̄ii.

Roman numerals can appear together, such as xv and ix. Reading multiple Roman numerals requires the use of addition and subtraction.

METHOD A

If the first Roman numeral is greater than the following numeral(s), then **ADD.**

EXAMPLES

$$\overline{\text{viii}} = 5 + 3 = 8$$
$$\overline{\text{xv}} = 10 + 5 = 15$$

METHOD B

If the first Roman numeral is less than the following numeral(s), then **SUBTRACT.** Subtract the first numeral from the second (i.e., the smaller from the larger).

EXAMPLES

$$\overline{\text{iv}} = 5 - 1 = 4$$
$$\overline{\text{ix}} = 10 - 1 = 9$$

Some Roman numerals require both addition and subtraction to ascertain their value. Read from left to right.

EXAMPLES

$$\overline{\text{xix}} = 10 + 9 \ (10 - 1) = 19$$
$$\overline{\text{xxxiv}} = 30 \ (10 + 10 + 10) + 4 \ (5 - 1) = 34$$

PRACTICE PROBLEMS | Roman Numerals

Answers can be found on page 11.

1. $\overline{\text{xvi}}$

2. $\overline{\text{xii}}$

3. $\overline{\text{xxiv}}$

4. $\overline{\text{xxxix}}$

5. XLV

6. XC

FRACTIONS

Fractions are expressed as part(s) of a whole or part(s) of a unit. A fraction is composed of two basic numbers: a *numerator* (the top number) and a *denominator* (the bottom number). The denominator indicates the total number of parts.

EXAMPLE

$$\text{Fraction: } \frac{3}{4} \frac{\text{numerator (3 of 4 parts)}}{\text{denominator (4 of 4 parts, or 4 total parts)}}$$

The value of a fraction depends mainly on the denominator. When the denominator increases, for example, from $\frac{1}{10}$ to $\frac{1}{20}$, the value of the fraction decreases, because it takes more parts to make a whole.

EXAMPLE

Which fraction has the greater value: $\frac{1}{4}$ or $\frac{1}{6}$? The denominators are 4 and 6.

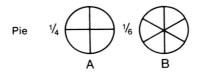

Pie $\frac{1}{4}$ $\frac{1}{6}$

A   B

The larger value is $\frac{1}{4}$, because four parts make the whole, whereas for $\frac{1}{6}$, it takes six parts to make a whole. Therefore $\frac{1}{6}$ has the smaller value.

Proper, Improper, and Mixed Fractions

In a *proper fraction* (simple fraction), the numerator is less than the denominator, e.g., $\frac{1}{2}$, $\frac{2}{3}$, $\frac{3}{4}$, $\frac{2}{6}$. When possible, the fraction should be reduced to its lowest terms, e.g., $\frac{2}{6} = \frac{1}{3}$ (2 goes into 2 and 6).

In an *improper fraction,* the numerator is greater than the denominator, e.g., $\frac{4}{2}$, $\frac{8}{5}$, $\frac{14}{4}$. Reduce improper fractions to whole numbers or mixed numbers, e.g., $\frac{4}{2} = 2$ ($\frac{4}{2}$ means the same as $4 \div 2$); $\frac{8}{5} = 1\frac{3}{5}$ ($8 \div 5$, 5 goes into 8 one time with 3 left over, or $\frac{3}{5}$); and $\frac{14}{4} = 3\frac{2}{4} = 3\frac{1}{2}$ ($14 \div 4$, 4 goes into 14 three times with 2 left over, or $\frac{2}{4}$, which can then be reduced to $\frac{1}{2}$).

A *mixed number* is a whole number and a fraction, e.g., $1\frac{3}{5}$, $3\frac{1}{2}$. Mixed numbers can be changed to improper fractions by multiplying the denominator by the whole number, then adding the numerator, e.g., $1\frac{3}{5} = \frac{8}{5}$ ($5 \times 1 = 5 + 3 = 8$).

The apothecary system uses fractions to indicate drug dosages. Fractions may be added, subtracted, multiplied, or divided. Multiplying fractions and dividing fractions are the two common methods used in solving dosage problems.

Multiplying Fractions

To multiply fractions, multiply the numerators and then the denominators. Reduce the fraction, if possible, to lowest terms.

EXAMPLES

PROBLEM 1: $\dfrac{1}{3} \times \dfrac{3}{5} = \dfrac{\overset{1}{\cancel{3}}}{\underset{5}{\cancel{15}}} = \dfrac{1}{5}$

The answer is $\frac{3}{15}$, which can be reduced to $\frac{1}{5}$. The number that goes into both 3 and 15 is 3. Therefore 3 goes into 3 one time, and 3 goes into 15 five times.

PROBLEM 2: $\dfrac{1}{3} \times 6 = \dfrac{6}{3} = 2$

A whole number can also be written as that number over one $\left(\frac{6}{1}\right)$. Six is divided by 3 ($6 \div 3$); 3 goes into 6 two times.

Dividing Fractions

To divide fractions, invert the *second fraction,* or divisor, and then multiply.

EXAMPLES

PROBLEM 1: $\dfrac{3}{4} \div \dfrac{3}{8}$ (divisor) $= \dfrac{\overset{1}{\cancel{3}}}{\underset{1}{\cancel{4}}} \times \dfrac{\overset{2}{\cancel{8}}}{\underset{1}{\cancel{3}}} = \dfrac{2}{1} = 2$

When dividing, invert the divisor $\frac{3}{8}$ to $\frac{8}{3}$ and multiply. To reduce the fraction to lowest terms, 3 goes into both 3s one time, and 4 goes into 4 and 8 one time and two times, respectively.

PROBLEM 2: $\dfrac{1}{6} \div \dfrac{4}{18} = \dfrac{1}{\underset{1}{\cancel{6}}} \times \dfrac{\overset{3}{\cancel{18}}}{4} = \dfrac{3}{4}$

Six and 18 are reduced, or canceled, to 1 and 3.

Decimal Fractions

Fractions can be changed to decimals. Divide the numerator by the denominator, e.g., $\frac{3}{4} = 4\overline{)3.00}\,$ with quotient 0.75. Therefore $\frac{3}{4}$ is the same as 0.75.

PRACTICE PROBLEMS | | **Fractions**

Answers can be found on page 11.

1. a. Which has the greatest value: $\frac{1}{50}$, $\frac{1}{100}$, or $\frac{1}{150}$? _____

 b. Which has the lowest value: $\frac{1}{50}$, $\frac{1}{100}$, or $\frac{1}{150}$? _____

2. Reduce improper fractions to whole or mixed numbers.

 a. $\frac{12}{4} =$ **c.** $\frac{22}{3} =$

 _____   _____

 b. $\frac{20}{5} =$ **d.** $\frac{32}{6} =$

 _____   _____

3. Multiply fractions.

　　a. $\frac{2}{3} \times \frac{1}{8} =$

　　b. $2\frac{2}{5} \times 3\frac{3}{4} =$
　　　$\frac{12}{5} \times \frac{15}{4} =$

　　c. $\frac{500}{350} \times 5 =$

　　d. $\frac{400,000}{200,000} \times 3 =$

4. Divide fractions.

　　a. $\frac{2}{3} \div 6 =$

　　b. $\frac{1}{4} \div \frac{1}{5} =$

　　c. $\frac{1}{6} \div \frac{1}{8} =$

　　d. $\frac{1}{150} / \frac{1}{100} = (\frac{1}{150} \div \frac{1}{100}) =$

　　e. $\frac{1}{200} \div \frac{1}{300} =$

　　f. $9\frac{3}{5} \div 4 =$
　　　$\frac{48}{5} \div \frac{4}{1} =$

5. Change each fraction to a decimal.

　　a. $\frac{1}{4} =$　　　　**b.** $\frac{1}{10} =$　　　　**c.** $\frac{2}{5} =$

DECIMALS

Decimals consist of (1) whole numbers (numbers to the left of decimal point) and (2) decimal fractions (numbers to the right of decimal point). The number 2468.8642 is an example of the division of units for a whole number with a decimal fraction.

Whole Numbers					Decimal Fractions			
2	4	6	8	•	8	6	4	2
Thousands	Hundreds	Tens	Units		Tenths	Hundredths	Thousandths	Ten Thousandths

Decimal fractions are written in tenths, hundredths, thousandths, and ten-thousandths. Frequently, decimal fractions are used in drug dosing. The metric system is referred to as the *decimal system*. After decimal problems are solved, decimal fractions are rounded off to tenths. If the hundredth column is 5 or greater, the tenth is increased by 1, e.g., 0.67 is rounded up to 0.7 (tenths).

Decimal fractions are an integral part of the metric system. Tenths mean 0.1 or $\frac{1}{10}$, hundredths mean 0.01 or $\frac{1}{100}$, and thousandths mean 0.001 or $\frac{1}{1000}$. When a decimal is changed to a fraction, the denominator is based on the number of digits to the right of the decimal point (0.8 is $\frac{8}{10}$, 0.86 is $\frac{86}{100}$).

EXAMPLES	PROBLEM 1: 0.5 is $\frac{5}{10}$, or 5 tenths.
	PROBLEM 2: 0.55 is $\frac{55}{100}$, or 55 hundredths.
	PROBLEM 3: 0.555 is $\frac{555}{1000}$, or 555 thousandths.

Multiplying Decimals

To multiply decimal numbers, multiply the multiplicand by the multiplier. Count how many numbers (spaces) are to the right of the decimals in the problem. Mark off the number of decimal spaces in the answer (right to left) according to the number of decimal spaces in the problem. Round off in tenths.

EXAMPLE

```
  1.34   multiplicand
  2.3    multiplier
  402
 2680
 3.082   or   3.1 (rounded off in tenths)
```

Answer: 3.1. Because 8 is greater than 5, the "tenth" number is increased by 1.

Dividing Decimals

To divide decimal numbers, move the decimal point in the divisor to the right to make a whole number. The decimal point in the dividend is also moved to the right according to the number of decimal spaces in the divisor.

EXAMPLE

$$\text{Dividend} \div \text{Divisor}$$

$$2.46 \div 1.2 \quad \text{or} \quad \frac{2.46}{1.2} =$$

$$2.05 = 2.1$$

(divisor) $1.2\,\overline{)2.4\,60}$ (dividend)

```
        2 4
          60
          60
           0
```

PRACTICE PROBLEMS III Decimals

Answers can be found on page 12.

1. Multiply decimals.

   a. $6.8 \times 0.123 =$

   b. $52.4 \times 9.345 =$

2. Divide decimals.

   a. $69 \div 3.2 =$

   c. $100 \div 4.5 =$

   b. $6.63 \div 0.23 =$

   d. $125 \div 0.75 =$

3. Change decimals to fractions.

   a. $0.46 =$

   b. $0.05 =$

   c. $0.012 =$

4. Which has the greatest value: 0.46, 0.05, or 0.012? Which has the smallest value? _____

RATIO AND PROPORTION

A *ratio* is the relation between two numbers and is separated by a colon, e.g., 1:2 (1 is to 2). It is another way of expressing a fraction, e.g., $1:2 = \frac{1}{2}$.

Proportion is the relation between two ratios separated by a double colon (::) or equals sign (=).

To solve a ratio and proportion problem, the middle numbers *(means)* are multiplied and the end numbers *(extremes)* are multiplied. To solve for the unknown, which is X, the X goes to the left side and is followed by an equals sign.

EXAMPLES

PROBLEM 1: 1:2::2:X (1 is to 2, as 2 is to X)

means

extremes

$X = 4$ (1 X is the same as X)

Answer: 4 (1:2::2:4)

PROBLEM 2: 4:8 = X:12

$8X = 48$

$X = \frac{48}{8} = 6$

Answer: 6 (4:8 = 6:12)

PROBLEM 3: A ratio and proportion problem may be set up as a fraction.

Ratio and Proportion	Fraction

$$2:3::4:X \qquad \frac{2}{3} = \frac{4}{X} \text{ (cross multiply)}$$

$$2X = 12 \qquad 2X = 12$$
$$X = {}^{12}\!/_2 = 6 \qquad X = 6$$

Answer: 6. Remember to cross-multiply when the problem is set up as a fraction.

PRACTICE PROBLEMS IV Ratio and Proportion

Answers can be found on page 12.

Solve for X.

1. $2:10::5:X$

_____

2. $0.9:100 = X:1000$

_____

3. Change the ratio and proportion to a fraction.
$3:5::X:10$

_____

4. It is 500 miles from Washington, DC, to Boston, MA. Your car averages 22 miles per 1 gallon of gasoline. How many gallons of gasoline will be needed for the trip?

_____

PERCENTAGE

Percent (%) means 100. Two percent (2%) means 2 parts of 100, and 0.9% means 0.9 part (less than 1) of 100. A percent can be expressed as a fraction, a decimal, or a ratio.

EXAMPLE

Percent		Fraction	Decimal	Ratio
60%	=	${}^{60}\!/_{100}$	0.60	$60:100$

Note: *To change a percent to a decimal, move the decimal point two places to the left. In the example, the decimal point comes before the whole number 60.*

PRACTICE PROBLEMS V Percentage

Answers can be found on page 12.

Change percent to fraction, decimal, and ratio.

Percent	Fraction	Decimal	Ratio
1. 2%			
2. 0.33%			
3. 150%			
4. $\frac{1}{2}$% (0.5%)			
5. 0.9%			

ANSWERS

I   Roman Numerals
1. $10 + 5 + 1 = 16$
2. $10 + 2 = 12$
3. $20 (10 + 10) + 4 (5 - 1) = 24$
4. $30 (10 + 10 + 10) + 9 (10 - 1) = 39$
5. $40 (50 - 10) + 5 = 45$
6. $100 - 10 = 90$

II   Fractions
1. a. $\frac{1}{50}$ has the greatest value.   **b.** $\frac{1}{150}$ has the lowest value.
2. a. 3   **c.** $7\frac{1}{3}$
   b. 4   **d.** $5\frac{2}{6}$ or $5\frac{1}{3}$

3. a. $\frac{2}{24} = \frac{1}{12}$

$$\text{c.} \quad \frac{\overset{10}{\cancel{500}}}{\underset{7}{\cancel{350}}} \times 5 = \frac{50}{7} = 7.1$$

$$\text{b.} \quad {}^{12}\!/_{5} \times {}^{15}\!/_{4} = \frac{180}{20} = 9$$

$$\text{d.} \quad \frac{\overset{2}{\cancel{400,000}}}{\underset{1}{\cancel{200,000}}} \times 3 = 6$$

4. a. $\frac{2}{3} \div 6 = \frac{2}{3} \times \frac{1}{6}$
            $= \frac{2}{18} = \frac{1}{9}$

$$\text{d.} \quad \frac{1}{150} \div \frac{1}{100} = \frac{1}{\underset{3}{\cancel{150}}} \times \frac{\overset{2}{\cancel{100}}}{1}$$

   b. $\frac{1}{4} \div \frac{1}{5} =$
      $\frac{1}{4} \times \frac{5}{1} = \frac{5}{4} =$
      $1\frac{1}{4}$, or 1.25

      $= \frac{2}{3}$, or 0.666, or 0.67
   e. $\frac{1}{200} \div \frac{1}{300} = \frac{1}{200} \times \frac{300}{1} =$
      ${}^{300}\!/_{200} = 1\frac{1}{2}$, or 1.5

$$\text{c.} \quad \frac{1}{6} \div \frac{1}{8} = \frac{1}{\underset{3}{\cancel{6}}} \times \frac{\overset{4}{\cancel{8}}}{1} = \frac{4}{3} = 1.33$$

$$\text{f.} \quad {}^{48}\!/_{5} \div {}^{4}\!/_{1} = {}^{48}\!/_{5} \times \frac{1}{4}$$

$$= \frac{48}{20} = 2.4$$

$$\textbf{5. a. } \frac{1}{4} = 4)\overline{1.00}^{\,0.25} \qquad\qquad \textbf{b. } \frac{1}{10} = 10)\overline{1.00}^{\,0.10} \qquad\qquad \textbf{c. } \frac{2}{5} = 5)\overline{2.00}^{\,0.40}$$

III Decimals

1. a. 0.8364, or 0.8

```
    0.123
    6.8
    984
    738
```

    0.8364, or 0.8 (round off in tenths: 3 hundredths is less than 5)

  b. 489.6780, or 489.7 (7 hundredths is greater than 5)

2. a. 21.56, or 21.6 (6 hundredths is greater than 5, so the tenth is increased by one)

  b. 28.826, or 28.8 (2 hundredths is *not* 5 or greater than 5, so the tenth is not changed)

  c. $100 \div 4.5 = 4.5\,)\overline{100.0} = 22.2$, or 22

  d. $125 \div 0.75 = 0.75\,)\overline{125.00} = 166.6$, or 167

3. a. $\frac{46}{100}$ **b.** $\frac{5}{100}$ **c.** $\frac{12}{1000}$

4. 0.46 has the greatest value; 0.012 has the lowest value. Forty-six hundredths is greater than 5 hundredths or 12 thousandths.

IV Ratio and Proportion

1. $2X = 50$
    $X = 25$

2. $100X = 900$
    $X = 9$

3. $\frac{3}{5} = \frac{x}{10} = 5X = 30$
    $X = 6$

4. 1 gal : 22 miles : : X gal : 500
    $22X = 500$
    $X = 22.7$ gal

22.7 gallons of gasoline are needed.

V Percentage

	Percent	Fraction	Decimal	Ratio
1.	2	$\frac{2}{100}$	0.02	2 : 100
2.	0.33	$\frac{0.33}{100}$, or $\frac{33}{10,000}$	0.0033	0.33 : 100, or 33 : 10,000
3.	150	$\frac{150}{100}$	1.50	150 : 100
4.	0.5	$\frac{0.5}{100}$, or $\frac{5}{1000}$	0.005	0.5 : 100, or 5 : 1000
5.	0.9	$\frac{0.9}{100}$, or $\frac{9}{1000}$	0.009	0.9 : 100, or 9 : 1000

POST-MATH TEST

The math test is composed of five sections: Roman and Arabic numerals, fractions, decimals, ratios and proportions, and percentages. There are 60 questions. A passing score is 54 or more correct answers (90%). A nonpassing score is 7 or more incorrect answers. Answers to the Post-Math Test can be found on page 16.

Roman and Arabic Numerals

Convert Roman numerals to Arabic numerals.

1. $\overline{vii}$

4. $\overline{xiv}$

_____

_____

2. $\overline{xi}$

5. xliii, or XLIII

_____

_____

3. $\overline{xvi}$

_____

Convert Arabic numerals to Roman numerals.

6. 4

9. 37

_____

_____

7. 18

10. 62

_____

_____

8. 29

_____

Fractions

Which fraction has the larger value?

11. $\frac{1}{100}$ or $\frac{1}{150}$?

_____

12. $\frac{1}{3}$ or $\frac{1}{2}$?

_____

Reduce improper fractions to whole or mixed numbers.

13. $\frac{45}{9} =$

14. $\frac{74}{3} =$

_____

_____

Change a mixed number to an improper fraction.

15. $5\frac{2}{3} =$

_____

Change fractions to decimals.

16. $\frac{2}{3} =$ **17.** $\frac{1}{12} =$

_____   _____

Multiply fractions.

18. $\frac{7}{8} \times \frac{4}{6} =$ **19.** $2\frac{3}{5} \times \frac{5}{8} =$

_____   _____

Divide fractions.

20. $\frac{1}{2} \div \frac{1}{3} =$ **22.** $\frac{1}{8} \div \frac{1}{12} =$

_____   _____

21. $6\frac{3}{4} \div 3 =$ **23.** $20\frac{3}{4} \div \frac{1}{6} =$

_____   _____

Decimals

Round off decimal numbers to tenths.

24. $0.87 =$ **26.** $0.42 =$

_____   _____

25. $2.56 =$

_____

Change decimals to fractions.

27. $0.68 =$ **29.** $0.012 =$

_____   _____

28. $0.9 =$ **30.** $0.33 =$

_____   _____

Multiply decimals.

31. $0.34 \times 0.6 =$

_____

32. $2.123 \times 0.45 =$

_____

Divide decimals.

33. $3.24 \div 0.3 =$

_____

34. $69.4 \div 0.23 =$

_____

Ratio and Proportion

Change ratios to fractions.

35. $3:4 =$ **37.** $65:90 =$

_____   _____

36. $1:175 =$ **38.** $0.9:100 =$

_____   _____

Solve ratio and proportion problems.

39. $2:3::8:X$

_____

40. $0.5:20::X:100$

_____

41. $3:100 = X:1000$

_____

42. $5:25 = 10:X$

_____

Change ratios and proportions to fractions and solve.

43. $1:2::4:X$

_____

44. $5:50::X:300$

_____

45. $0.9:10 = X:100$

_____

Percentage

Change percents to fractions.

46. $3\% =$ **47.** $27\% =$ **48.** $1.2\% =$ **49.** $5.75\% =$

Change percents to decimals.

50. 8% =	**52.** 0.9% =	**54.** 0.25% =
51. 15% =	**53.** 3.5% =	**55.** 0.45% =

Change percents to ratios.

56. 35% =	**58.** 4% =	**60.** 0.45% =
57. 12.5% =	**59.** 0.9% =	

ANSWERS   POST-MATH TEST

Roman and Arabic Numerals

1. 7	**3.** 16	**5.** 43	**7.** $\overline{\text{xviii}}$	**9.** $\overline{\text{xxxvi}}$
2. 11	**4.** 14	**6.** $\overline{\text{iv}}$	**8.** $\overline{\text{xxix}}$	**10.** LXII

Fractions

11. $\frac{1}{100}$
12. $\frac{1}{2}$
13. 5
14. $24\frac{2}{3}$
15. $\frac{17}{3}$
16. 0.66, or 0.7

17. 0.08

18. $\frac{28}{48}$ or $\frac{7}{12}$

19. $\frac{13}{\cancel{5}_1} \times \frac{\cancel{5}^1}{8} =$
$\frac{13}{8} = 1\frac{5}{8}$

20. $\frac{1}{2} \times \frac{3}{1} =$
$\frac{3}{2} = 1\frac{1}{2}$

21. $\frac{\cancel{27}^9}{4} \times \frac{1}{\cancel{3}_1} =$
$\frac{9}{4} = 2\frac{1}{4}$

22. $\frac{1}{\cancel{8}_2} \times \frac{\cancel{12}^3}{1} =$
$\frac{3}{2} = 1\frac{1}{2}$

23. $\frac{83}{\cancel{4}_2} \times \frac{\cancel{6}^3}{1} =$
$\frac{249}{2} = 124.5$

Decimals

24. 0.9
25. 2.6
26. 0.4

27. $\frac{68}{100}$
28. $\frac{9}{10}$
29. $\frac{12}{1000}$

30. $\frac{33}{100}$
31. 0.204
32. 0.95535,
or 0.96, or 1.0

33. 10.8
34. 301.739, or 301.7

Ratio and Proportion

35. $\frac{3}{4}$
36. $\frac{1}{175}$
37. $\frac{65}{90}$
38. $\frac{9}{1000}$
39. 12
40. 2.5

41. 30
42. 50
43. $\frac{1}{2} \times \frac{4}{x} =$ (cross-multiply)
X = 8

44. $\frac{\cancel{5}_1}{\cancel{50}_{10}} = \frac{X}{300}$
10 X = 300
X = 30

45. $\frac{0.9}{10} = \frac{X}{100}$
10 X = 90
X = 9

Percentage

46. $\frac{3}{100}$
47. $\frac{27}{100}$
48. $\frac{12}{1000}$
49. $\frac{575}{10,000}$
50. 0.08

51. 0.15
52. 0.009
53. 0.035
54. 0.0025
55. 0.0045

56. 35:100
57. 12.5:100, or 125:1000
58. 4:100
59. 0.9:100, or 9:1000
60. 0.45:100, or 45:10,000

PART II

SYSTEMS, CONVERSION, AND METHODS OF DRUG CALCULATION

Systems Used for Drug Administration

OBJECTIVES

- Recognize the system of measurement accepted worldwide and the system of measurement used in home settings.
- List the basic units and subunits of weight, volume, and length of the metric system.
- Explain the rules for changing grams to milligrams and milliliters to liters.
- Give abbreviations for the frequently used metric units and subunits.
- List the basic units in the apothecary system for weight and volume.
- Give the abbreviations for the apothecary and household units of measurement.
- List the basic units of measurement for volume in the household system.
- Convert units of measurement within the metric system, within the apothecary system, and within the household system.

OUTLINE

METRIC SYSTEM
   Conversion within the Metric System
APOTHECARY SYSTEM
   Conversion within the Apothecary System
HOUSEHOLD SYSTEM
   Conversion within the Household System

The three systems used for measuring drugs and solutions are the metric, apothecary, and household systems. The metric system, developed in 1799 in France, is the chosen system for measurements in the majority of European countries. The metric system, also referred to as *the decimal system,* is based on units of 10. Since the enactment of the Metric Conversion Act of 1975, the United States has been moving toward the use of this system. The intention of the act is to adopt the International Metric System worldwide. The metric system is known as the *International System of Units,* abbreviated as SI units. Eventually, it will be the only system used in drug dosing.

The apothecary system dates back to the Middle Ages and has been the system of weights and measurements used in England since the seventeenth century. It was brought to the United States from England. The system is also referred to as *the fractional system* because anything less than one is expressed in fractions. In the United States, the apothecary system is rapidly being phased out and is being replaced by the metric system. You may omit the apothecary system if you desire.

Standard household measurements are used primarily in home settings. With the trend toward home care, conversions to household measurements may gain importance.

Additional information on the metric, apothecary, and household systems is available on the CD-ROM in the "Introducing Drug Measures" section.

METRIC SYSTEM

The metric system is a decimal system based on multiples of 10 and fractions of 10. There are three basic units of measurements. These basic units are as follows:

Gram (g, gm, G, Gm): unit for weight
Liter (l, L): unit for volume or capacity
Meter (m, M): unit for linear measurement or length

Prefixes are used with the basic units to describe whether the units are larger or smaller than the basic unit. The prefixes indicate the size of the unit in multiples of 10. The prefixes for basic units are as follows:

Prefix for Larger Unit		**Prefix for Smaller Unit**	
Kilo	1000 (one thousand)	Deci	0.1 (one-tenth)
Hecto	100 (one hundred)	Centi	0.01 (one-hundredth)
Deka	10 (ten)	Milli	0.001 (one-thousandth)
		Micro	0.000001 (one-millionth)
		Nano	0.000000001 (one-billionth)

Abbreviations of metric units that are frequently written in drug orders are listed in Table 1–1. Lowercase letters are usually used for abbreviations rather than capital letters.

The metric units of weight, volume, and length are given in Table 1–2. Meanings of the prefixes are stated next to the units of weight. Note that the

Table 1-1

Metric Units and Abbreviations

	Names	Abbreviations
Weight	Kilogram	kg, Kg
	Gram	g, gm, G, Gm
	Milligram	mg, mgm
	Microgram	mcg, μg
	Nanogram	ng
Volume	Kiloliter	kl, kL
	Liter	l, L
	Deciliter	dl, dL
	Milliliter	ml, mL
Length	Kilometer	km, Km
	Meter	m, M
	Centimeter	cm
	Millimeter	mm

Table 1-2

Units of Measurement in the Metric System with Their Prefixes

Weight Per Gram	Meaning
1 kilogram (kg) = 1000 grams	One thousand
1 hectogram (hg) = 100 grams	One hundred
1 dekagram (dag) = 10 grams	Ten
1 gram (g) = 1 gram	One
1 decigram (dg) = 0.1 gram ($\frac{1}{10}$)	One tenth
1 centigram (cg) = 0.01 gram ($\frac{1}{100}$)	One hundredth
1 milligram (mg) = 0.001 gram ($\frac{1}{1,000}$)	One thousandth
1 microgram (mcg) = 0.000001 gram ($\frac{1}{1,000,000}$)	One millionth
1 nanogram (ng) = 0.000000001 gram ($\frac{1}{1,000,000,000}$)	One billionth

Volume Per Liter	Length Per Meter
1 kiloliter (kl) = 1000 liters	1 kilometer (km) = 1000 meters
1 hectoliter (hl) = 100 liters	1 hectometer (hm) = 100 meters
1 dekaliter (dal) = 10 liters	1 dekameter (dam) = 10 meters
1 liter (l, L) = 1 liter	**1 metric (m) = 1 meter**
1 deciliter (dl) = 0.1 liter	1 decimeter (dm) = 0.1 meter
1 centiliter (cl) = 0.01 liter	1 centimeter (cm) = 0.01 meter
1 milliliter (ml) = 0.001 liter	1 millimeter (mm) = 0.001 meter

larger units are 1000, 100, and 10 times the basic units (in bold type) and the smaller units differ by factors of 0.1, 0.01, 0.001, 0.000001, and 0.000000001. The size of a basic unit can be changed by multiplying or dividing by 10. Micrograms and nanograms are the exceptions: one (1) milligram = 1000 micrograms, and one (1) microgram = 1000 nanograms. Micrograms and nanograms are changed by 1000 instead of by 10.

Conversion within the Metric System

Drug administration often requires conversion within the metric system to prepare the correct dosage. Two basic methods are given for changing larger to smaller units and smaller to larger units.

METHOD A

To change from a *larger* unit to a *smaller* unit, multiply by 10 for each unit decreased or move the decimal point one space to the right for each unit changed.

When changing three units from larger to smaller, such as from gram to milligram (a change of three units), multiply by 10 three times (or by 1000) or move the decimal point three spaces to the right.

Change 1 gram (g) to milligrams (mg):

a. $1 \times 10 \times 10 \times 10 = 1000$ mg

b. $1 \text{ g} \times 1000 = 1000$ mg

or

c. $1 \text{ g} = 1.000$ mg (1000 mg)

When changing two units, such as kilogram to dekagram (a change of two units from larger to smaller), multiply by 10 twice (or by 100) or move the decimal point two spaces to the right.

Change 2 kilograms (kg) to dekagrams (dag):

a. $2 \times 10 \times 10 = 200$ dag

b. $2 \text{ kg} \times 100 = 200$ dag

or

c. $2 \text{ kg} = 2.00$ dag (200 dag)

When changing one unit, such as liter to deciliter (a change of one unit from larger to smaller), multiply by 10 or move the decimal point one space to the right.

Change 3 liters (L) to deciliters (dl):

a. $3 \times 10 = 30$ dl
b. $3 \text{ L} \times 10 = 30$ dl

or

c. $3 \text{ L} = 3.0$ dl (30 dl)

A micro unit is one thousandth of a milli unit, and a nano unit is one thousandth of a micro unit. To change from a milli unit to a micro unit, multiply by 1000 or move the decimal place three spaces to the right. Changing micro units to nano units involves the same procedure, mulitplying by 1000 or moving the decimal place three spaces to the right.

EXAMPLES   PROBLEM 1: Change 2 grams (g) to milligrams (mg).

$$2 \text{ g} \times 1000 = 2000 \text{ mg}$$

or

$$2 \text{ g} = 2.000 \text{ mg} \ (2000 \text{ mg})$$

PROBLEM 2: Change 10 milligrams (mg) to micrograms (mcg or μg).

10 mg × 1000 = 10,000 mcg (μg)

or

10 mg = 10.000 mcg (10,000 mcg)

PROBLEM 3: Change 4 liters (L) to milliliters (ml).

4 L × 1000 = 4000 ml

or

4 L = 4.000 ml (4000 ml)

PROBLEM 4: Change 2 kilometers (km) to hectometers (hm).

2 km × 10 = 20 hm

or

2 km = 2.0 hm (20 hm)

METHOD B

To change from a *smaller* unit to a *larger* unit, divide by 10 for each unit increased or move the decimal point one space to the left for each unit changed.

When changing three units from smaller to larger, divide by 1000 or move the decimal point three spaces to the left.

Change 1500 milliliters (ml) to liters (L):

a. 1500 ml ÷ 1000 = 1.5 L

or

b. 1500 ml = 1 500. L (1.5 L)

When changing two units from smaller to larger, divide by 100 or move the decimal point two spaces to the left.

Change 400 centimeters (cm) to meters (m):

a. 400 cm ÷ 100 = 4 m

or

b. 400 cm = 4 00. m (4 m)

When changing one unit from smaller to larger, divide by 10 or move the decimal point one space to the left.

Change 150 decigrams (dg) to grams (g):

a. 150 dg ÷ 10 = 15 g

or

b. 150 dg = 15 0. g (15 g)

EXAMPLES   PROBLEM 1: Change 8 grams to kilograms (kg).

8 g ÷ 1000 = 0.008 kg

or

8 g = 008. kg (0.008 kg)

PROBLEM 2: Change 1500 milligrams (mg) to decigrams (dg).

$$1500 \text{ mg} \div 100 = 15 \text{ dg}$$

or

$$1500 \text{ mg} = 15 \underset{\smile}{00}. \text{ dg (15 dg)}$$

PROBLEM 3: Change 750 micrograms (mcg) to milligrams (mg).

$$750 \text{ mcg} \div 1000 = 0.75 \text{ mg}$$

or

$$750 \text{ mcg} = \underset{\smile}{750}. \text{ mg (0.75 mg)}$$

PROBLEM 4: Change 2400 milliliters (ml) to liters (L).

$$2400 \text{ ml} \div 1000 = 2.4 \text{ L}$$

or

$$2400 \text{ ml} = 2 \underset{\smile}{400}. \text{ L (2.4 L)}$$

PRACTICE PROBLEMS | **Metric Conversions**

Answers can be found on page 30.

1. Conversion from larger units to smaller units: *multiply* by 10 for each unit changed (multiply by 10, 100, 1000) or move the decimal point one space to the *right* for each unit changed (move one, two, or three spaces), Method A.

a. 7.5 grams to milligrams

_____

b. 10 milligrams to micrograms

_____

c. 35 kilograms to grams

_____

d. 2.5 liters to milliliters

_____

e. 1.25 liters to milliliters

_____

f. 20 centiliters to milliliters

_____

g. 18 decigrams to milligrams

_____

h. 0.5 kilograms to grams

_____

2. Conversion from smaller units to larger units: *divide* by 10 for each unit changed (divide by 10, 100, 1000) or move the decimal point one space to the *left* for each unit changed (move one, two, or three spaces), Method B.

   a. 500 milligrams to grams

   _____

   b. 7500 micrograms to milligrams

   _____

   c. 250 grams to kilograms

   _____

   d. 4000 milliliters to liters

   _____

   e. 325 milligrams to grams

   _____

   f. 100 milliliters to deciliters

   _____

   g. 2800 milliliters to liters

   _____

   h. 75 millimeters to centimeters

   _____

APOTHECARY SYSTEM

The apothecary system of measurement was the common system used by most practitioners prior to the universal acceptance of the International Metric System. Now all pharmaceuticals are manufactured using the metric system, and the apothecary system is no longer included on any drug labels. All medication should be prescribed and calculated using metric measures, but occasionally the use of the fluid ounce or grains may be found. In those rare circumstances, nurses should have a general understanding of the apothecary system.

The basic unit of weight in the apothecary system is the grain (gr), and the basic unit of fluid volume is the minim (ɱ); these are the smaller units in the apothecary system. As a safety issue, please note that the abbreviation for minim, ɱ, must not be mistaken for milliliter, ml. Larger units of measurement for weight and fluid volume are the dram (dr or ℨ) and the ounce (oz or ℥). In the apothecary system, Roman numerals are written in lowercase letters, e.g., gr x, to express numbers.

Table 1–3 gives the equivalents of units of dry weight (grain, dram, ounce) and units of liquid volume (minim, fluid dram, fluid ounce). The apothecary system uses fluid ounces and fluid drams to differentiate between liquid volume and dry weight. In clinical practice, units of liquid volume are commonly seen as dram and ounce. Often, the term *fluid,* which is the correct la-

Table 1-3

Abbreviations and Units of Measurement in the Apothecary System

Abbreviations

Weight		Liquid Volume	
grain	gr	quart	qt
ounce	oz, ℥	pint	pt
dram*	dr, ʒ	fluid ounce	fl oz, fl ℥
		fluid dram	fl ʒ
		minim†	♍

Basic Equivalent Units

Weight		Liquid Volume†	
Larger units	*Smaller units*	*Larger units*	*Smaller units*
1 ounce	= 480 grains	1 quart	= 2 pints
1 ounce	= 8 drams	1 pint	= 16 fluid ounces
1 dram†	= 60 grains	1 fluid ounce	= 8 fluid drams
		1 fluid dram	= 60 minims
		1 minim†	= 1 drop (gt)

*Drams and minims are rarely used for drug administration; however, know their symbols.
†Liquid volume of basic units is frequently used.
Note: Constant values are the numbers of the smaller equivalent units.

beling of liquid volume, is dropped. However, the proper names for units of dry weight and units of liquid volume are used in this text.

The most common drugs in the past prescribed using the apothecary system designation are listed with their metric equivalent:

Aspirin gr X (650 mg)
Codeine gr ½ (30 mg)
Phenobarbital gr ¼ (15 mg)
Nitroglycerin gr $\frac{1}{150}$ (0.4 mg)

Conversion within the Apothecary System

It is often necessary to change units within the apothecary system. The method applied when changing larger units to smaller units is as follows:

METHOD C

To change a **larger** unit to a **smaller** unit, multiply the constant value found in Table 1–3 by the number of the larger unit.

NOTE

The constant values are the basic equivalent numbers of the smaller units given in Table 1–3. You might want to memorize these equivalents or refer to the table as needed.

EXAMPLES

PROBLEM 1: 2 drams (dr) = _____ grains (gr).
1 dr = 60 gr (60 is the constant value, dry weight)
2 × 60 = 120 gr

PROBLEM 2: 3 pints (pt) = _____ fluid ounces (fl oz or fl ℥).
1 pt = 16 fl oz (16 is the constant value)
3 × 16 = 48 fl oz, fl ℥

PROBLEM 3: 3 fluid ounces (fl ℥) = _____ fluid drams (fl dr or fl ʒ).
1 fl oz = 8 fl dr (8 is the constant value)
3 × 8 = 24 fl dr, fl ʒ

The method applied when changing smaller units to larger units is as follows:

METHOD D

To change a *smaller* unit to a *larger* unit, divide the constant value found in Table 1–3 into the number of the smaller unit.

EXAMPLES

PROBLEM 1: 30 grains (gr) = _____ dram (dr or ʒ).
1 dr = 60 gr (60 is the constant value)
30 ÷ 60 = ½ dr

PROBLEM 2: 80 fluid ounces (fl oz, fl ℥) = _____ pints (pt).
1 pt = 16 fl oz (16 is the constant value)
80 ÷ 16 = 5 pt

PROBLEM 3: 2 fluid drams (fl dr, fl ʒ) = _____ fluid ounces (fl oz, fl ℥).
1 fl oz = 8 fl dr (8 is the constant value)
2 ÷ 8 = ¼ fl oz

PRACTICE PROBLEMS II Apothecary System

Answers can be found on page 31.

1. Give the abbreviations for:

a. grain = _____

b. dram = _____

c. fluid dram = _____

d. drop = _____

e. fluid ounce = _____

f. pint = _____

g. quart = _____

2. Give the equivalent using Method C, changing larger units to smaller units.

a. ʒ v = _____ gr

b. fl ℥ (fl oz) v = _____ fl ʒ (fl dr)

c. qt iii, = _____ pt

d. pt ii = _____ fl ℥ (fl oz)

3. Give the equivalent using Method D, changing smaller units to larger units.

   a. gr 240 = _____ dr or ℨ

   b. ℨ xvi = _____ oz or ℥

   c. fl ℨ (fl dr) xxiv = _____ fl ℥ (fl oz)

   d. ♏ xv = _____ gtt

HOUSEHOLD SYSTEM

The use of household measurements is on the increase because more patients/clients are being cared for in the home. The household system of measurement is not as accurate as the metric system because of a lack of standardization of spoons, cups, and glasses. A teaspoon (t) is considered 5 ml, although it could be anywhere from 4 to 6 ml. Three household teaspoons are equal to one tablespoon (T). A drop size can vary with the size of the lumen of the dropper. Basically, a drop and a minim are considered equal. Again, household measurements must be considered approximate measurements. Some of the household units are the same as the apothecary units, because there is a blend of these two systems.

The community health nurse may use and teach the household units of measurements to patients/clients.

Table 1–4 gives the commonly used units of measurement in the household system. You might want to memorize the equivalents in Table 1–4 or refer to the table as needed.

Conversion within the Household System

For changing larger units to smaller units and smaller units to larger units within the household system, the same methods that applied to the apothecary system can be used. With household measurements, a fluid ounce is usually indicated as an ounce.

Table 1-4

Units of Measurement in the Household System

1 drop (gt)	= 1 minim (♏)
1 teaspoon (t)	= 60 drops (gtt), 5 ml
1 tablespoon (T)	= 3 teaspoons (t)
1 ounce (oz)	= 2 tablespoons (T)
1 coffee cup (c)	= 6 ounces (oz)
1 medium size glass	= 8 ounces (oz)
1 measuring cup	= 8 ounces (oz)

Note: Constant values are the numbers of the smaller equivalent units.

METHOD E

To change a *larger* unit to a *smaller* unit, multiply the constant value found in Table 1–4 by the number of the larger unit.

NOTE

The constant values are the basic equivalent numbers of the smaller units in Table 1–4.

EXAMPLES

PROBLEM 1: 2 medium size glasses = _____ ounces (oz).
1 medium glass = 8 fl oz (8 is the constant value)
$2 \times 8 = 16$ oz

PROBLEM 2: 3 tablespoons (T) = _____ teaspoons (t).
1 T = 3 t (3 is the constant value)
$3 \times 3 = 9$ t

PROBLEM 3: 5 ounces (oz or ℥) = _____ tablespoons (T).
1 oz = 2 T (2 is the constant value)
$5 \times 2 = 10$ T

PROBLEM 4: 2 teaspoons (t) = _____ drops (gtt).
1 t = 60 gtt (60 is the constant value)
$2 \times 60 = 120$ gtt

METHOD F

To change a *smaller* unit to a *larger* unit, divide the constant value found in Table 1–4 into the number of the smaller unit.

EXAMPLES

PROBLEM 1: 120 drops (gtt) = _____ teaspoons (t).
1 t = 60 gtt (60 is the constant value)
$120 \div 60 = 2$ t

PROBLEM 2: 6 teaspoons (t) = _____ tablespoons (T).
1 T = 3 t (3 is the constant value)
$6 \div 3 = 2$ T

PROBLEM 3: 18 ounces (oz) = _____ coffee cups (c).
1 c = 6 oz (6 is the constant value)
$18 \div 6 = 3$ c

PROBLEM 4: 4 tablespoons (T) = _____ ounces (oz).
1 oz = 2 T (2 is the constant value)
$4 \div 2 = 2$ oz

Answers can be found on page 31.

1. Give the equivalents using Method E, changing larger units to smaller units.

   a. 2 glasses = _____ oz

   b. 3 ounces = _____ T

   c. 4 tablespoons = _____ t

   d. 1½ cups = _____ oz

   e. ½ teaspoon = _____ gtt

2. Give the equivalents using Method F, changing smaller units to larger units.

   a. 9 teaspoons = _____ T

   b. 6 tablespoons = _____ oz

   c. 90 drops = _____ t

   d. 12 ounces = _____ c

   e. 24 ounces = _____ medium size glasses

ANSWERS

I   Metric Conversions

1. a. 7.5 g to mg

$7.5 \text{ g} \times 1000 = 7500 \text{ mg}$

or

$7.\underset{\smile}{500}$ mg (7500 mg)

b. 10,000 mcg (µg)

c. 35,000 g

d. 2500 ml

e. 1250 ml

f. 200 ml

g. 1800 mg

h. 500 g

2. a. 500 mg to g

$500 \div 1000 = 0.5 \text{ g}$

or

$500 \text{ mg} = \underset{\smile}{500}. \text{ g} (0.5 \text{ g})$

b. 7.5 mg

c. 0.25 kg

d. 4 L

e. 0.325 g

f. 1 dl

g. 2.8 L

h. 7.5 cm

II Apothecary System

Abbreviations

1. a. grain = gr
 b. dram = dr or ʒ
 c. fluid dram = fl ʒ, fl dr
 d. drop = gt
 e. fluid ounce = fl ℥, fl oz
 f. pint = pt
 g. quart = qt

Equivalents

2. a. ʒ v = _____ gr
 5 × 60 = 300 gr
 b. 40 fl ʒ, fl dr
 c. 6 pt
 d. 32 fl ℥, fl oz

Equivalents

3. a. gr 240 = _____ dr
 240 ÷ 60 = 4 dr or ʒ
 b. 2 oz or ℥
 c. 3 fl ℥, fl oz
 d. 15 gtt

III Household System

1. a. 2 glasses = _____ oz
 2 × 8 = 16 oz
 b. 6 T
 c. 12 t
 d. 9 oz
 e. 30 gtt

2. a. 9 teaspoons = _____ T
 9 ÷ 3 = 3 T
 b. 3 oz
 c. 1½ t
 d. 2 c
 e. 3 glasses

SUMMARY PRACTICE PROBLEMS

Make conversions within the three systems. Answers are on page 32.

1. Metric system

 a. 30 mg = _____ mcg (μg)

 b. 3 g = _____ mg

 c. 6 L = _____ ml

 d. 1.5 kg = _____ g

 e. 10,000 mcg = _____ mg

 f. 500 mg = _____ g

 g. 2500 ml = _____ L

 h. 125 g = _____ kg

 i. 120 mm = _____ cm

 j. 5 m = _____ cm

2. Apothecary system

 a. 90 gr = _____ dr

 b. fl ʒ (fl dr) iv = _____ fl ℥ (fl oz)

 c. fl ℥ (fl oz) iiss = _____ fl ʒ (fl dr)

 d. 8 pt = _____ qt

3. Household system

    a. 12 t = _____ T

    b. 5 glasses = _____ oz

    c. 3 T = _____ t

    d. 2 c = _____ oz

    e. 30 oz = _____ c

    f. 4 oz = _____ T

ANSWERS   SUMMARY PRACTICE PROBLEMS

1. a. 30,000 mcg
  b. 3000 mg
  c. 6000 ml
  d. 1500 g
  e. 10 mg
  f. 0.5 g
  g. 2.5 L
  h. 0.125 kg
  i. 12 cm
  j. 500 cm

2. a. 1.5 ℥
  b. ½ or $\overline{ss}$ fl ℥ (fl oz)
  c. 20 fl ℥ (fl dr)
  d. 4 qt

3. a. 4 T
  b. 40 oz
  c. 9 t
  d. 12 oz
  e. 5 c
  f. 8 T

Conversion within the Metric, Apothecary, and Household Systems

OBJECTIVES

- State rules for converting drug dosage by weight between the apothecary and metric systems.
- Convet grams/milligrams to grains and grains to grams/milligrams.
- Convert drug dosage by weight from one system to another system by using the ratio method.
- State rules for converting drug dosage by volume among the metric, apothecary, and household systems.
- Convert liters/milliliters to ounces/pints and milliliters to drams, tablespoons, and teaspoons.

OUTLINE

UNITS, MILLIEQUIVALENTS, AND PERCENTS

METRIC, APOTHECARY, AND HOUSEHOLD EQUIVALENTS

    Conversion in Metric and Apothecary Systems by WEIGHT

    Conversion in Metric, Apothecary, and Household Systems by LIQUID VOLUME

Today, conversion within the metric system is more common than conversion within the metric-apothecary systems. If the faculty find that the apothecary system is not being used in their institutions, they may wish to omit part of Chapter 2—Metric-Apothecary equivalents and conversion.

Drug doses are usually ordered in metric units (grams, milligrams, liters, and milliliters). Although the apothecary system is being phased out, there are some physicians who still order drug doses by apothecary units. To calculate a drug dose, the same unit of measurement must be used. Therefore the nurse must know the metric and apothecary equivalents either by memorizing a conversion table or by using methods for converting from one system to the other if necessary. After the conversion is made, the dosage problem can be solved. Some authorities state that it is easier to *convert to the unit used on the container (bottle).* If the physician ordered phenobarbital gr ½ and the bottle is labeled 30 mg, then the conversion would be from grains to milligrams.

Metric and apothecary equivalents are approximations, e.g., 1 gram equals 15.432 grains. When values are unequal, they should be rounded off to the nearest whole number (1 gram = 15 grains).

Dosage conversion tables are available in many institutions; however, when you need a conversion table, one might not be available. Nurses should either memorize metric and apothecary equivalents or be able to convert from one system to the other by using calculation methods.

UNITS, MILLIEQUIVALENTS, AND PERCENTS

Units, milliequivalents, and percents are measurements used to indicate the strength or potency of certain drugs. When a drug is developed, its strength is based on either chemical assay or biological assay. Chemical assay denotes strength by weight, e.g., milligrams or grains. Biological assays are used for drugs in which the chemical composition is difficult to determine. Biological assays assess potency by the effect that one unit of the drug can have on a laboratory animal. Units mainly measure the potency of hormones, vitamins, anticoagulants, and some antibiotics. Drugs that were once standardized by units and later synthesized to their chemical composition may still retain units as an indication of potency, e.g., insulin.

Milliequivalents measure the strength of an ion concentration. Ions are given primarily for electrolyte replacement. They are measured in milliequivalents (mEq), one of which is $\frac{1}{1000}$ of the equivalent weight of an ion. Potassium chloride (KCl) is a common electrolyte replacement and is ordered in milliequivalents.

Percents are the concentrations of weight dissolved in a volume and are always expressed as units of mass per units of volume. Common concentrations are g/ml, g/L, and mg/ml. These concentrations, expressed as percentages, are based on the definition of a 1% solution as 1 g of a drug in 100 ml of solution. Dextrose 50% in a 50-ml pre-filled syringe is a concentration of 50 g of dextrose in 100 ml of water. Calcium gluconate 10% in a 30-ml bottle is a concentration of 10 g of calcium gluconate in 100 ml of solution. Proportions can also express concentrations. A solution that is 1:100 has the same concentration as a 1% solution. Epinephrine 1:1000 means that 1 g of epinephrine was dissolved in a 1000-ml solution.

Units, milliequivalents, and percents cannot be directly converted into the metric, apothecary, or household system.

METRIC, APOTHECARY, AND HOUSEHOLD EQUIVALENTS

Knowing how to convert drug doses among the systems of measurement is essential in the clinical setting. In discharge teaching for individuals receiving liquid medication, converting metric to household measurement may be important.

Table 2–1 gives the metric and apothecary equivalents by weight and the metric, apothecary, and household equivalents by volume.

Remember, conversion from one system to another is an approximation. Memorize Table 2–1, refer to Table 2–1, or use the methods that follow in the text for system conversion.

Conversion in Metric and Apothecary Systems by WEIGHT

GRAMS AND GRAINS 1 g = 15 gr

a. To convert grams to grains, *multiply* the number of grams by 15, the constant value.

b. To convert grains to grams, *divide* the number of grains by 15, the constant value.

Table 2-1

Approximate Metric, Apothecary, and Household Equivalents

	Metric System	Apothecary System	Household System
Weight	1 kg; 1000 g	2.2 lb	2.2 lb
	30 g	1 oz	
	15 g	4 dr	
	1 g; 1000 mg*	15 (16) gr	
	0.5 g; 500 mg	7½ gr	
	0.3 g; 300 mg	5 gr	
	0.1 g; 100 mg	1½ gr	
	0.06 g; 60 (65) mg*	1 gr	
	0.03 g; 30 (32) mg	½ gr	
	0.01 g; 10 mg	⅙ gr	
	0.6 mg	$\frac{1}{100}$ gr	
	0.4 mg	$\frac{1}{150}$ gr	
	0.3 mg	$\frac{1}{200}$ gr	
Volume	1 L; 1000 ml (cc)	1 qt; 32 fl oz (fl ℥)	1 qt
	0.5 L; 500 ml	1 pt; 16 fl oz	1 pt
	0.24 L; 240 ml	8 oz	1 glass
	0.18 L; 180 ml	6 oz	1 c
	30 ml	1 oz or 8 dr (fl ℥)	2 T or 6 t
	15 ml	½ oz or 4 dr	1 T
	4-5 ml		1 t
	4 ml	1 dr or 60 minims (♏)	1 t
	1 ml	15 (16) ♏	15-16 gtt
Height	2.54 cm	1 inch	1 inch
Distance	25.4 mm	1 inch	1 inch

*Equivalents commonly used for computing conversion problems by ratio.
Note: ½ may be written as s̄s̄.

EXAMPLES | PROBLEM 1: Change 2 grams to grains.

$$2 \times 15 = 30 \text{ gr (grains)}$$

PROBLEM 2: Change 60 grains to grams.

$$60 \div 15 = 4 \text{ g (grams)}$$

GRAINS AND MILLIGRAMS 1 gr = 60 mg

a. To convert grains to milligrams, *multiply* the number of grains by 60, the constant value.

b. To convert milligrams to grains, *divide* the number of milligrams by 60, the constant value.

EXAMPLES | PROBLEM 1: Change 3 grains to milligrams

$$3 \times 60 = 180 \text{ mg (milligrams)}$$

PROBLEM 2: Change 300 milligrams to grains.

Note: *325 milligrams may be ordered instead of 300. Round off to the whole number. One grain is equivalent to 60, 64, or 65 milligrams. In this situation, you may want to divide by 65 instead of rounding off to the whole number.*

$$300 \div 60 = 5 \text{ gr (grains)}$$

or

$$325 \div 65 = 5 \text{ gr}$$

or

$$325 \div 60 = 5.43 \text{ gr, or } 5 \text{ gr (0.43 is less than 0.5)}$$

RATIO AND PROPORTION

Multiply the means (numbers that are closest to each other) by the extremes (numbers that are farthest from each other). You are solving for X, so X goes first.

If it is difficult for you to recall these methods, then use the ratio and proportion method to convert from one system to another.

you must MEMORIZE

Metric Equivalence:

1 gram (g) = 1000 milligrams (mg)

1 milligram (mg) = 1000 micrograms (mcg or µg)

Metric-Apothecary Equivalence:

1 gram (g) = 15 grains (gr)

1 grain (gr) = 60 milligrams (mg)

EXAMPLES

PROBLEM 1: Convert 2.5 grams to grains.

Known   Desired
g: gr:: g :gr
1:15::2.5:X

means

extremes

X = 37.5 gr

PROBLEM 2: Convert 10 grains to milligrams.

Known   Desired
gr:mg   ::gr :mg
1:60(65)::10:X

X = 600 mg or 650 mg

Note: *Because conversion gives approximate values, the answer could be 600 mg or 650 mg. If the problem uses 1 gr = 60 mg, the answer is 600 mg. However, the bottle may be labeled 10 gr = 650 mg. Both 600 mg and 650 mg are correct.*

PRACTICE PROBLEMS | Conversion by Weight

Answers can be found on page 40.

Grams and Grains

1. 10 g = _____ gr   **4.** 0.03 g = _____ gr

2. 0.5 g = _____ gr   **5.** 3 gr = _____ g

3. 0.1 g = _____ gr   **6.** 1½ gr = _____ g

Grains and Milligrams

1. 4 gr = _____ mg   **5.** 150 mg = _____ gr

2. 1½ gr = _____ mg   **6.** 30 mg = _____ gr

3. 7½ gr = _____ mg   **7.** 15 mg = _____ gr

4. ½ gr = _____ mg   **8.** 0.6 mg = _____ gr

Ratio and Proportion: Grams, Milligrams, and Grains

1. 2.5 g = _____ mg   **4.** 500 mg = _____ g

2. 0.5 g = _____ gr   **5.** 1 gr = _____ g

3. 100 mg = _____ g   **6.** ¼ gr = _____ mg

Conversion in Metric, Apothecary, and Household Systems by LIQUID VOLUME

LITERS AND OUNCES   1 L = 32 oz

a. To convert liters and quarts to ounces, *multiply* the number of liters by 32, the constant value.

b. To convert ounces to liters or quarts, *divide* the number of ounces by 32, the constant value.

EXAMPLES   PROBLEM 1: Change 3 liters to ounces.

3 L × 32 = 96 oz, or fl ℥ (ounces)

PROBLEM 2: Change 64 ounces to liters.

64 oz ÷ 32 = 2 L (liters)

OUNCES AND MILLILITERS   1 oz = 30 ml

a. To convert ounces to milliliters, *multiply* the number of ounces by 30, the constant value.

b. To convert milliliters to ounces, *divide* the number of milliliters by 30, the constant value.

EXAMPLES   PROBLEM 1: Change 5 ounces to milliliters.

5 oz × 30 = 150 ml (milliliters)

PROBLEM 2: Change 120 milliliters to ounces.

120 ml ÷ 30 = 4 oz or fl ℥ (ounces)

MILLILITERS AND DROPS 1 ml = 15 drops (gtt) (number of drops may vary according to the size of the dropper)

a. To convert milliliters to drops, *multiply* the number of milliliters by 15, the constant value.

b. To convert drops to milliliters, *divide* the number of minims or drops by 15, the constant value.

EXAMPLES   PROBLEM 1: Change 4 milliliters to drops.

4 ml × 15 = 60 minims or 60 drops

PROBLEM 2: Change 10 drops (gtt) to milliliters.

10 gtt ÷ 15 = ⅔ ml or 0.667 ml or 0.7 ml

RATIO AND PROPORTION

The ratio method is useful when converting smaller units within the three systems.

If it is difficult for you to recall these methods, then use the ratio and proportion method to convert from one system to the other.

you must MEMORIZE

> 30 ml = 1 oz = 8 dr = 2 T = 6t

These are equivalent values.

EXAMPLES

PROBLEM 1: Change 20 ml to teaspoons.

Known   Desired
ml:t :: ml:t
30:6 :: 20:X

30 X = 120
X = 4 t (teaspoons)

PROBLEM 2: Change 15 ml to tablespoons.

Known   Desired
ml:T :: ml:T
30:2 :: 15:X
30 X = 30
X = 1 T (tablespoon)

PROBLEM 3: Change 5 oz to tablespoons.

Known   Desired
oz:T :: oz:T
1:2 :: 5:X
X = 10 T (tablespoons)

PRACTICE PROBLEMS II **Conversion by Liquid Volume**

Answers can be found on page 40.

Liters and Ounces

1. 2.5 L = _____ oz (fl oz, fl ℥)   **3.** 40 oz (fl oz, fl ℥) = _____ L

2. 0.25 L = _____ oz   **4.** 24 oz = _____ L

Ounces and Milliliters

1. 4 oz (fl oz, fl ℥) = _____ ml   **4.** 45 ml = _____ oz

2. 6½ oz = _____ ml   **5.** 150 ml = _____ oz

3. ½ oz = _____ ml   **6.** 15 ml = _____ oz

Milliliters and Drops

1. 1.5 ml = _____ gtt   **3.** 20 gtt = _____ ml

2. 12 ml = _____ gtt   **4.** 8 gtt = _____ ml

ANSWERS

I   Conversion by Weight

Grams and Grains

1. $10 \times 15 = 150$ gr
2. $0.5 \times 15 = 7.5$ or $7\frac{1}{2}$ gr
3. $0.1 \times 15 = 1.5$ or $1\frac{1}{2}$ gr
4. $0.03 \times 15 = 0.45$ or 0.5 gr
5. $3 \div 15 = 0.2$ g
6. $1.5 \div 15 = 0.1$ g

Grains and Milligrams

1. $4 \times 60 = 240$ mg
2. $1.5 \times 60 = 90$ (100) mg
3. $7.5 \times 60 = 450$ mg
4. $0.5 \times 60 = 30$ mg
5. $150 \div 60 = 2.5$ or $2\frac{1}{2}$ gr
6. $30 \div 60 = 0.5$ or $\frac{1}{2}$ gr
7. $15 \div 60 = \frac{1}{4}$ gr
8. $0.6 \div 60 =$

$$60\overline{)0.60} = 0.01 \text{ or } \frac{1}{100} \text{ gr}$$

Ratio and Proportion: Grams, Milligrams, and Grains

1. g : mg :: g : mg
   1 : 1000 :: 2.5 : X
   $\quad$ X = 2500 mg
   or
   Move decimal point three spaces to the right (conversion within the metric system)
   2.5 g = 2.500 mg

2. g : gr :: g : gr
   1 : 15 :: 0.5 : X
   $\quad$ X = 7.5 or $7\frac{1}{2}$ gr

3. mg : g :: mg : g
   1000 : 1 :: 100 : X
   1000 X = 100
   $\quad$ X = 0.1 g

4. mg : g :: mg : g
   1000 : 1 :: 500 : X
   1000 X = 500
   $\quad$ X = 0.5 g

5. g : gr :: g : gr
   1 : 15 :: X : 1
   15 X = 1
   $\quad$ X = 0.06 g

6. gr : mg :: gr : mg
   1 : 60 :: 0.25 : X
   $\quad$ X = 60×0.25
   $\quad$ X = 15 mg

II   Conversion by Liquid Volume

Liters and Ounces

1. $2.5 \text{ L} \times 32 = 80$ oz
2. $0.25 \text{ L} \times 32 = 8$ oz
3. $40 \text{ oz} \div 32 = 1.25$ L
4. $24 \text{ oz} \div 32 = 0.75$ L

Ounces and Milliliters

1. $4 \text{ oz} \times 30 = 120$ ml
2. $6.5 \text{ oz} \times 30 = 195$ ml
3. $0.5 \text{ oz} \times 30 = 15$ ml
4. $45 \text{ ml} \div 30 = 1\frac{1}{2}$ oz
5. $150 \text{ ml} \div 30 = 5$ oz
6. $15 \text{ ml} \div 30 = \frac{1}{2}$ oz

Milliliters and Drops

1. $1.5 \text{ ml} \times 15 = 22.5$ or 23 gtt
2. $12 \, \text{℥} \times 1 = 12$ gtt (1 ℥ = 1 gtt)
3. $20 \text{ gtt} \div 15 = 1.3$ ml
4. $8 \text{ gtt} \div 15 = 0.5$ ml

SUMMARY PRACTICE PROBLEMS

Before dosage problems can be completed, one system of measurement must be selected. If a medication is ordered in one system and the drug label is in another system, then conversion to one of the systems is necessary. As previously stated, it may be easier to convert to the system used on the drug label.

There are three methods of conversion for the three systems: (1) memorization of a conversion table, (2) conversion methods, and (3) ratio method. You need to convert not only within three systems but also within the same system if units are not the same, e.g., grams and milligrams. Again, units of measurement *must* be the same to solve problems.

REMEMBER   *Multiply* when converting from larger to smaller units, and *divide* when converting from smaller to larger units.

Weight: Metric and Apothecary Conversion

Fill in the blanks with the correct terms and make the conversions.

1. To convert grams to grains, _____ the number of grams by

   _____; to convert grains to grams, _____ the

   number of grains by _____.

   a. 2 g = _____ gr   d. 0.02 g = _____ gr

   b. 7½ gr (gr viiss) = _____ g   e. 150 gr = _____ g

   c. 3 gr = _____ g   f. 0.06 g = _____ gr

2. To convert grains to milligrams, _____ the number of grains by

   _____; to convert milligrams to grains, _____ the

   number of milligrams by _____.

   a. 3 gr (gr iii) = _____ mg   d. 5 gr = _____ mg

   b. 10 mg = _____ gr   e. 7½ gr = _____ mg

   c. ¼ gr = _____ mg   f. 0.4 mg = _____ gr

3. Ratio and proportion.
   Remember: 1 g or 1000 mg = 15 gr; 60 (65) mg = 1 gr

   a. Change 5 g to gr

   _____

   b. Change 120 mg to gr

   _____

Volume: Metric, Apothecary, and Household Conversion

4. To convert liters and quarts to ounces, _____ the number
   of liters by _____; to convert ounces to liters and
   quarts, _____ the number of ounces by _____.

   a. 3 L = _____ oz (fl ℥)   **d.** ½ L = _____ oz

   b. 1½ qt = _____ oz   **e.** 8 oz = _____ L or qt

   c. 64 oz (fl ℥) = _____ qt   **f.** 24 oz = _____ qt

5. To convert ounces to milliliters, _____ the number of ounces by
   _____; to convert milliliters to ounces, _____ the
   number of milliliters by _____.

   a. 1½ oz = _____ ml   **d.** 75 ml = _____ oz (fl ℥)

   b. 15 ml = _____ oz (fl ℥)   **e.** 3 oz (fl ℥) = _____ ml

   c. 60 ml = _____ oz   **f.** 8 oz = _____ ml

6. To convert milliliters to drops, _____ the number of milliliters by
   _____; to convert drops to milliliters, _____ the
   number of drops by _____.

   a. 15 ml = _____ gtt   **d.** 4 ml = _____ gtt

   b. 10 gtt = _____ ml   **e.** 30 gtt = _____ ml

   c. 18 gtt = _____ ml   **f.** ½ ml = _____ gtt

7. Ratio and proportion.
   Remember: 30 ml = 1 oz = 8 dr = 2 T = 6 t

   a. Change 16 oz (fl ℥) to L or qt

   _____

   b. Change 1½ oz to T

   _____

   c. Change 1 T to t

   _____

   d. Change 20 ml to t

   _____

   e. Change 2½ oz to ml

   _____

   f. Change 4 oz to ml

   _____

8. Client intake for lunch included a carton of milk (8 oz), cup of coffee (6 oz), small glass of apple juice (4 oz), and jello (4 oz). How many milliliters (ml) did the client consume?

ANSWERS SUMMARY PRACTICE PROBLEMS

1. multiply, 15; divide, 15
   a. 2 g × 15 = 30 gr
   b. 7.5 gr ÷ 15 = ½ or 0.5 g
   c. 3 gr ÷ 15 = 0.2 g
   d. 0.02 g × 15 = 0.3 or ⅓ gr
   e. 150 gr ÷ 15 = 10 g
   f. 0.06 g × 15 = 0.9 or 1 gr (round off to 1)

2. multiply, 60; divide, 60
   a. 3 gr × 60 = 180 mg
   b. 10 mg ÷ 60 = $^{10}/_{60}$ = ⅙ gr
   c. 0.25 gr × 60 = 15 mg
   d. 5 gr × 60 = 300 mg
   e. 7.5 gr × 60 = 450 mg
   f. 0.4 mg ÷ 60 = $^{4}/_{600}$ = $^{1}/_{150}$ gr

3. Ratio and proportion
   Known   Desired
   a. g : gr ∷ g : gr
      1 : 15 ∷ 5 : X
           X = 75 gr
   b. gr : mg ∷ gr : mg
      1 : 60 ∷ X : 120
      60 X = 120
         X = 2 gr
   or
   mg : gr ∷ mg : gr
   60 : 1 ∷ 120 : X
   60 X = 120
      X = 2 gr

4. multiply, 32; divide, 32
   a. 3 L × 32 = 96 oz
   b. 1.5 qt × 32 = 48 oz
   c. 64 oz ÷ 32 = 2 qt
   d. 0.5 L × 32 = 16 oz
   e. 8 oz ÷ 32 = $^{8}/_{32}$ = ¼ L or ¼ qt
   f. 24 oz ÷ 32 = $^{24}/_{32}$ = ¾ qt

5. multiply, 30; divide, 30
   a. 1½ oz × 30 = 45 ml
   b. 15 ml ÷ 30 = $^{15}/_{30}$ = ½ oz
   c. 60 ml ÷ 30 = 2 oz
   d. 75 ml ÷ 30 = 2½ oz
   e. 3 oz × 30 = 90 ml
   f. 8 oz × 30 = 240 ml

6. multiply, 15; divide, 15
   a. 15 ml × 15 = 225 gtt
   b. 10 gtt ÷ 15 = $^{10}/_{15}$ = ⅔ ml
   c. 18 gtt ÷ 15 = 1⅕ ml
   d. 4 ml × 15 = 60 gtt
   e. 30 gtt ÷ 15 = 2 ml
   f. ½ ml × 15 = 7.5 gtt

7. Ratio and proportion

    Known Desired

  a. L:oz::L:oz

      1:32::X:16

      32 X = 16

         X = ½ L

  b. oz:T::oz:T

      1:2::1½:X

        X = 3 T

  c. T:t::T:t

      2:6::1:X

      2 X = 6

        X = 3 t

  d. ml:t::ml:t

      30:6::20:X

      30 X = 120

        X = 4 t

  e. oz:ml::oz:ml

      1:30::2½:X

        X = 75 ml

  f. oz:mL::oz:ml

      1:30::4:X

        X = 120 ml

8. (1 ounce = 30 ml)

          milk = 240 ml

       coffee = 180 ml

  apple juice = 120 ml

         jello = <u>120 ml</u>

               660 ml

The client's intake for lunch is 660 ml.

Interpretation of Drug Labels, Drug Orders, Bar Codes, Charting, "5 Rights," and Abbreviations

OBJECTIVES

- Identify brand names, generic names, drug forms, dosages, expiration dates, and lot numbers on drug labels.
- Give examples of drugs with "look-alike" drug names.
- Recognize the components of a drug order.
- Explain the computer-based medication administration system.
- Recognize the use of bar code for unit drug dose.
- Identify the drug information for charting.
- Name the "5 rights" in drug administration and give examples of each.
- Utilize the chart related to the "5 rights."
- Provide meanings of abbreviations: drug form, drug measurement, and routes and times of drug administration.

OUTLINE

INTERPRETING DRUG LABELS
    Military Time versus
        Traditional (Universal) Time
DRUG DIFFERENTIATION
    Drug Orders
    Computer-Based Medication
      Administration
    Bar Code
    Charting Medications
    Methods of Drug Distribution

THE "5 RIGHTS" IN DRUG
    ADMINISTRATION
ABBREVIATIONS
    Drug Form
    Drug Measurements
    Routes of Drug
      Administration
    Times of Drug Administration

INTERPRETING DRUG LABELS

Pharmaceutical companies label drugs with their brand name of the drug in large letters and the generic name in smaller letters. The form of the drug (tablet, capsule, liquid, or powder) and dosage are printed on the drug label.

Many of the calculation problems in this book use drug labels. By using drug labels, the student can practice solving drug problems that are applicable to clinical practice. The student should know what information is on a drug label and how this information is used in drug calculations. All drug labels provide seven basic items of data: (1) brand (trade) name, (2) generic name, (3) dosage, (4) form of the drug, (5) expiration date, (6) lot number, and (7) name of the manufacturer.

 Additional information on "How to Read a Drug Label" is available on the CD-ROM.

EXAMPLE   DRUG LABEL

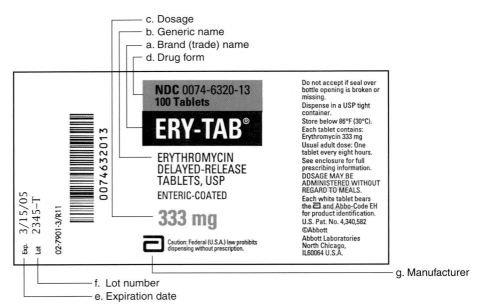

a. **The brand (trade) name** is the commercial name given by the pharmaceutical company (manufacturer of the drug). It is printed in large, bold letters.

b. **The generic name** is the chemical name given to the drug, regardless of the drug manufacturer. It is printed in smaller letters, usually under the brand name.

c. **The dosage strength** is the drug dose per drug form (tablet, capsule, liquid) as stated on the label.

d. **The form of the drug** (tablet, capsule, liquid) relates to the dosage strength.

e. **The expiration date** refers to the length of time the drug can be used before losing its potency. Drugs should not be administered after the expiration date. The nurse must check the expiration date of all drugs he or she administers to them.

f. The lot number identifies the drug batch in which the medication was produced. Occasionally, a drug is recalled according to the lot number.

g. The manufacturer is the pharmaceutical company that produces the brand name drug.

Examples of drug labels are given, and practice problems for reading drug labels follow the examples.

EXAMPLE 1   ORAL DRUG (SOLID FORM)

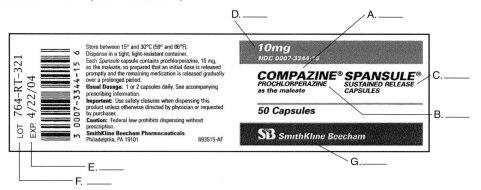

a. Brand (trade) name is Compazine
b. Generic name is prochlorperazine
c. Drug form is a sustained release capsule (SR capsule)
d. Dosage is 10 mg per capsule
e. Expiration date is 4/22/04 (after this date, the drug should be discarded)
f. Lot number is 764-RT-321
g. Manufacturer is SmithKline Beecham Pharmaceuticals

EXAMPLE 2   ORAL DRUG (LIQUID FORM)

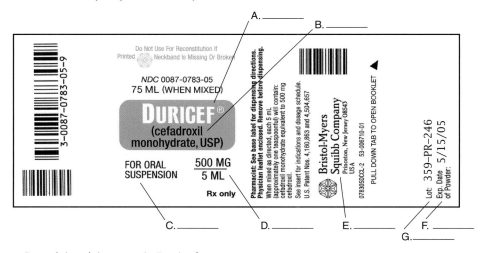

a. Brand (trade) name is Duricef
b. Generic name is cefadroxil monohydrate

c. Drug form is oral suspension
d. Dosage is 500 mg per 5 ml
e. Manufacturer is Bristol-Myers Squibb Company
f. Expiration date is 5/15/05
g. Lot number is 359-PR-246

EXAMPLE 3   INJECTABLE DRUG

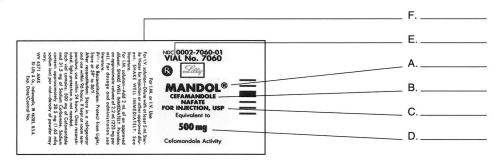

a. Brand name is Mandol
b. Generic name is cefamandole nafate
c. Drug form is drug powder that must be reconstituted in a liquid form for use
d. Dosage is 500 mg drug powder
e. Drug container is vial
f. IV: reconstitute by using at least 5 ml of sterile water for injection, which then must be diluted in 50 to 100 ml of IV fluids.
   IM: 2 ml of a diluent should be added. The total amount of the drug would then equal 2.2 ml. The powder increases the liquid form by 0.2 ml.

PRACTICE PROBLEMS I **Interpretation of Drug Labels**

Answers can be found on pages 64 and 65.

1.

Store below 86°F (30°C).	NDC 0049-5340-66		4238
Dispense in tight, light-resistant containers (USP).	100 Capsules		MADE IN USA
DOSAGE AND USE See accompanying prescribing information.	**Sinequan®** (doxepin HCl)		
*Each capsule contains doxepin hydrochloride equivalent to 10 mg doxepin.	**10 mg***		
CAUTION: Federal law prohibits dispensing without prescription.	Distributed by **Pfizer Roerig** Division of Pfizer Inc, NY, NY 10017		

a. Brand (trade) name _____   d. Dosage _____

b. Generic name _____   e. Manufacturer _____

c. Drug form _____

2.

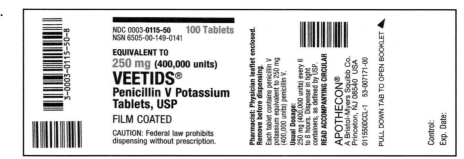

a. Brand (trade) name _____

b. Generic name _____

c. Drug form _____

d. Dosage _____ mg _____ units

e. Manufacturer _____

3.

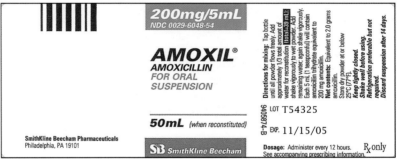

a. Brand (trade) name _____   e. Lot number _____

b. Generic name _____   f. Expiration date _____

c. Drug form _____   g. Manufacturer _____

d. Dosage _____

4.

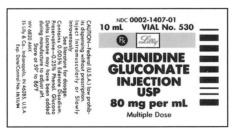

a. Brand (trade) name _____   d. Drug container _____

b. Generic name _____   e. Dosage _____

c. Drug form _____   f. Expiration date _____

5.

NDC 0006-7646-03
5 mL INJECTION
DECADRON® Phosphate
(DEXAMETHASONE SODIUM PHOSPHATE)
24 mg per mL
Dexamethasone Phosphate Equivalent

7222305

STERILE
USUAL ADULT DOSAGE:
See accompanying circular.
Sealed under nitrogen.
Protect from light.
Store container in carton until contents have been used. Protect from freezing.
CAUTION: Federal (USA) law prohibits dispensing without prescription.
FOR INTRAVENOUS USE ONLY
Dist by
MERCK & CO., INC.
West Point, PA 19486, USA

5 mL | No. 7646   Sensitive to heat—Do not autoclave

Lot   Exp.

a. Brand (trade) name _____   c. Drug form _____

b. Generic name _____   d. Dosage _____

6.

NDC 0015-7225-20
EQUIVALENT TO
1 gram NAFCILLIN
NAFCILLIN SODIUM FOR INJECTION, USP
Buffered-For IM or IV Use
CAUTION: Federal law prohibits dispensing without prescription.
APOTHECON®
A BRISTOL-MYERS SQUIBB COMPANY

When reconstituted with 3.4 mL diluent, (SEE INSERT:INTRAMUS-CULAR ROUTE), each vial contains 4 mL solution. Each mL of solution contains nafcillin sodium, as the monohydrate, equivalent to 250 mg nafcillin, buffered with 10 mg sodium citrate. Read accompanying circular for complete stability data.
Usual Dosage: Adults—500 mg every 4 to 6 hours. Read accompanying circular for directions for IM or IV use.

APOTHECON®
A Bristol-Myers Squibb Company
Princeton, NJ 08540 USA
7225200RL-2

Cont:
Exp. Date: 11/30/05

a. Brand name _____

b. Generic name_____

c. Drug form_____

d. Drug label suggests adding_____ diluent

e. Method of administration _____

f. Dosage 1 gram = _____ ml

g. Expiration date _____

h. Manufacturer_____

Military Time versus Traditional (Universal) Time

Many nursing settings currently are using military time, a 24-hour clock, when administering medications and treatments. For example, in military time, 3 AM is 0300 and 3 PM is 1500; 7:15 AM is 0715 and 7:30 PM is 1930. The AM hours are the same as on the traditional clock, and for hours after 12 noon, 12 is added to the PM hours; see Figure 3-1. The use of the 24-hour clock reduces drug administration errors.

DRUG DIFFERENTIATION

Some drugs with similar names, such as quinine and quinidine, have different chemical drug structures. Extreme care must be exercised when administering drugs that "look alike" or that have similar spellings.

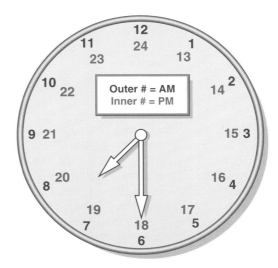

FIGURE 3-1 Military clock.

EXAMPLE 1   PERCOCET

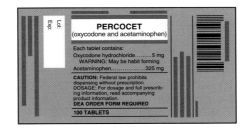

PERCODAN

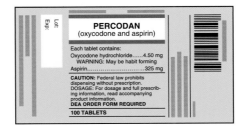

Percocet contains oxycodone and acetaminophen, whereas Percodan contains oxycodone and aspirin. A client may be allergic to aspirin or should not take aspirin; therefore it is important that the client be given Percocet. *Read the drug labels carefully.*

EXAMPLE 2   HYDROXYZINE AND HYDRALAZINE

Hydroxyzine is an antianxiety drug and hydralazine is an antihypertensive drug.

EXAMPLE 3   QUINIDINE AND QUININE

Quinidine sulfate is an antidysrhythmic drug, and quinine sulfate is an antimalarial drug.

Drug Orders

Medication orders may be prescribed and written by a physician (MD), an osteopathic physician (DO), a dentist (DDS), a podiatrist (DPM), or a licensed health care provider (HCP) who has been given authority by the state to write prescriptions. Drug prescriptions in private practice or in clinics are written on a small prescription pad and filled by a pharmacist at a drug store or hospital (see Fig. 3-2). For hospitalized patients, the drug orders may be written on a doctor's order sheet and signed by the physician or licensed health care provider (see Fig. 3-3), or a computerized drug order system may be used. If the order is given by telephone (TO), the order must be cosigned by the physician within 24 hours. Most health care institutions have policies concerning verbal or telephone drug orders. The nurse must know and follow the institution's policy.

The basic components of a drug order are (1) date and time the order was written, (2) drug name, (3) drug dosage, (4) route of administration, (5) frequency of administration, and (6) physician's or health care provider's signature. It is the nurse's responsibility to follow the physician's or health care provider's order, but if any one of these components is missing, the drug order is incomplete and cannot be carried out. If the order is illegible, is missing a component, or calls for an inappropriate drug or dosage, clarification must be obtained before the order is carried out.

Roger J. Smith, Jr., M.D.
678 Apple Street
Wilmington, Delaware 19810

(123) 456-7891

Name _____ Age _____

Address _____ Date _____

R~x~

Generic permitted _____
Label _____   _____ M.D.
Safety cap _____
Refill _____ times

FIGURE 3-2 Prescription pad medication order.

CITY HOSPITAL Dover, Delaware		PATIENT'S NAME Room #
Date	Time	Patient's Orders

FIGURE 3-3 Patient's orders.

Examples of drug orders and their interpretation are as follows:

6/3/05   9:10A   Digoxin 0.25 mg, po, qd
(give 0.25 mg of digoxin by mouth daily)

Ibuprofen 400 mg, po, q4h, PRN
(give 400 mg of ibuprofen by mouth every 4 hours as needed)

Cefadyl 500 mg, IM, q6h
(give 500 mg of Cefadyl intramuscularly every 6 hours)

Prednisone 5 mg, po, q8h × 5 days
(give 5 mg of prednisone by mouth every 8 hours for 5 days)

PRACTICE PROBLEMS II Interpretation of Drug Orders

Answers can be found on page 65.

Interpret these drug orders. For abbreviations that you do not know, see the section on abbreviations later in this chapter.

1. Tetracycline 250 mg, po, q6h

2. HydroDIURIL 50 mg, po, qd

_____

3. Meperidine 50 mg, IM, q3–4h, PRN

_____

4. Ancef 1 g, IV, q8h

_____

5. Prednisone 10 mg, tid × 5 days

_____

List what is missing in the following drug orders.

6. Codeine 30 mg, po, PRN for pain_____

7. Digoxin 0.25 mg, qd_____

8. Ceclor 125 mg, po_____

9. TheoDur 200 mg _____

10. Penicillin V K 200,000 U, for days _____

There are four types of drug orders: (1) standing order, (2) one-time (single) order, (3) PRN (whenever necessary) order, and (4) STAT (immediate) order (Table 3-1). Many of the drugs ordered for nonhospitalized patients are

---

Table 3-1

Types of Drug Orders

Types/Description	Examples
Standing orders: A standing order may be typed or written on the doctor's order sheet. It may be an order that is given for a number of days, or it may be a routine order for all patients who had the same type of procedure. Standing orders may include PRN orders.	Erythromycin 250 mg, po, q6h, 5 days Demerol 50 mg, IM, q3-4h, PRN, pain Colace 100 mg, po, hs, PRN
One-time (single) orders: One-time orders are given once, usually at a specified time.	Preoperative orders: Meperidine 75 mg, IM, 7:30 AM Atropine SO$_4$ 0.4 mg, IM, 7:30 AM
PRN orders: PRN orders are given at the patient's request and at the nurse's discretion concerning safety and need.	Pentobarbital 100 mg, hs, PRN Darvocet-N, tab 1, q4h, PRN
STAT orders: A STAT order is for a one-time dose of drug to be given immediately.	Regular insulin 10 U, SC, STAT

normally standing orders that can be renewed (refilled) for 6–12 months. Narcotic orders are *not* automatically refilled; if the narcotic use is extended, the physician writes another prescription or calls the pharmacy.

Computer-Based Medication Administration

Computer-based drug administration is a system developed to prevent medication errors. The Centers for Disease Control and Prevention (CDC) reported a rise in the number of medication-related deaths between 1983 and 1993. As a result, software systems have been designed to reduce medication inaccuracies to improve patient/client outcomes. The federal government, through the Department of Veterans Affairs Hospitals, has developed a software program that automates the medication administration process to improve accuracy and efficiency in documentation.

The process begins with the physician or health care provider order entry when medication is selected on screen from a scrolling list (Fig. 3-4). Once the medication is chosen, the next screen displays all the possible doses, routes, and schedules (Fig. 3-5). Once the physician selects those components of the order, he or she can view the screen and make changes.

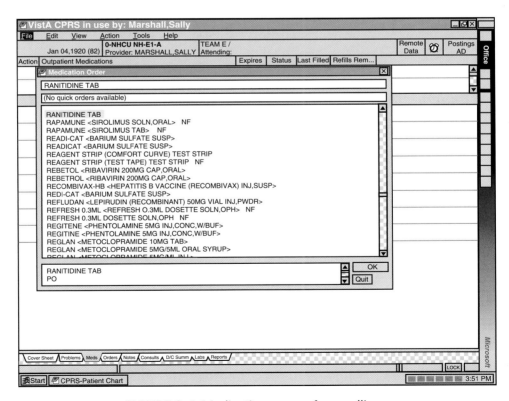

FIGURE 3-4 Medication screen for scrolling.

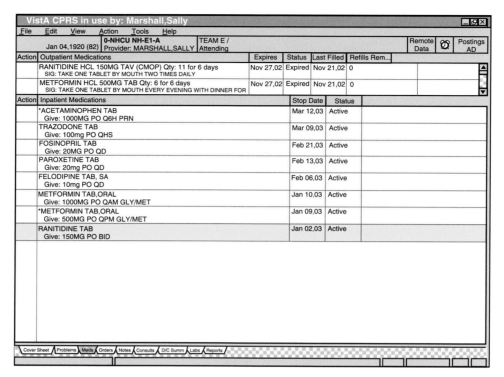

FIGURE 3-5 Medications chosen, doses, routes, and time.

If the screen information is correct, the physician signs the order with his or her distinctive electronic code, and the order is sent and processed in the pharmacy.

Bar Code

Today, most unit drug doses are prepared by the pharmacy with a **bar code** (Fig. 3-6). The pharmacy individually places the drug in a cellophane envelope or packet with a bar code number. The pharmacy delivers the bar-coded drugs to the hospital unit at specified times and the drugs are kept at the nurses' stations or cart. In some hospitals, the nurse "brings up" the medication administration record screen for the patient and uses a bar code reader to scan the patient's wrist band and bar code on the drug (Fig. 3-7). The software validates the correct patient, drug, and dosage with the right route and time. The software is intended to enhance patient safety by clarifying orders, improving communication, and augmenting clinical judgment.

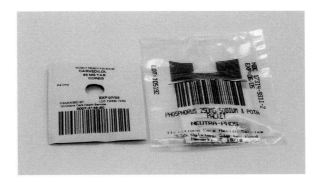

FIGURE 3-6 Bar code for unit drug dose.

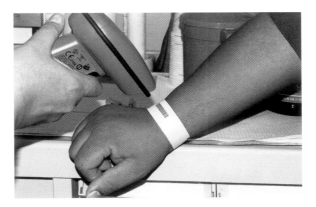

FIGURE 3-7 Bar code reader. It is used to scan the patient's wristband.

Charting Medications

Charting on medication records should be done immediately after the medications are given. Delay in charting could result in (1) forgetting to chart the drugs or (2) administration of the drugs by another nurse who thought the drugs were *not* given.

Medication records (charts) differ among health care facilities. Drug information that should be on the medication record includes (1) date drug was ordered, (2) drug name, (3) dosage, (4) route of aministration, (5) frequency of administration, (6) date and time drug was given, and (7) nurse's signature and initials. An example of a medication record is provided in Figure 3-8.

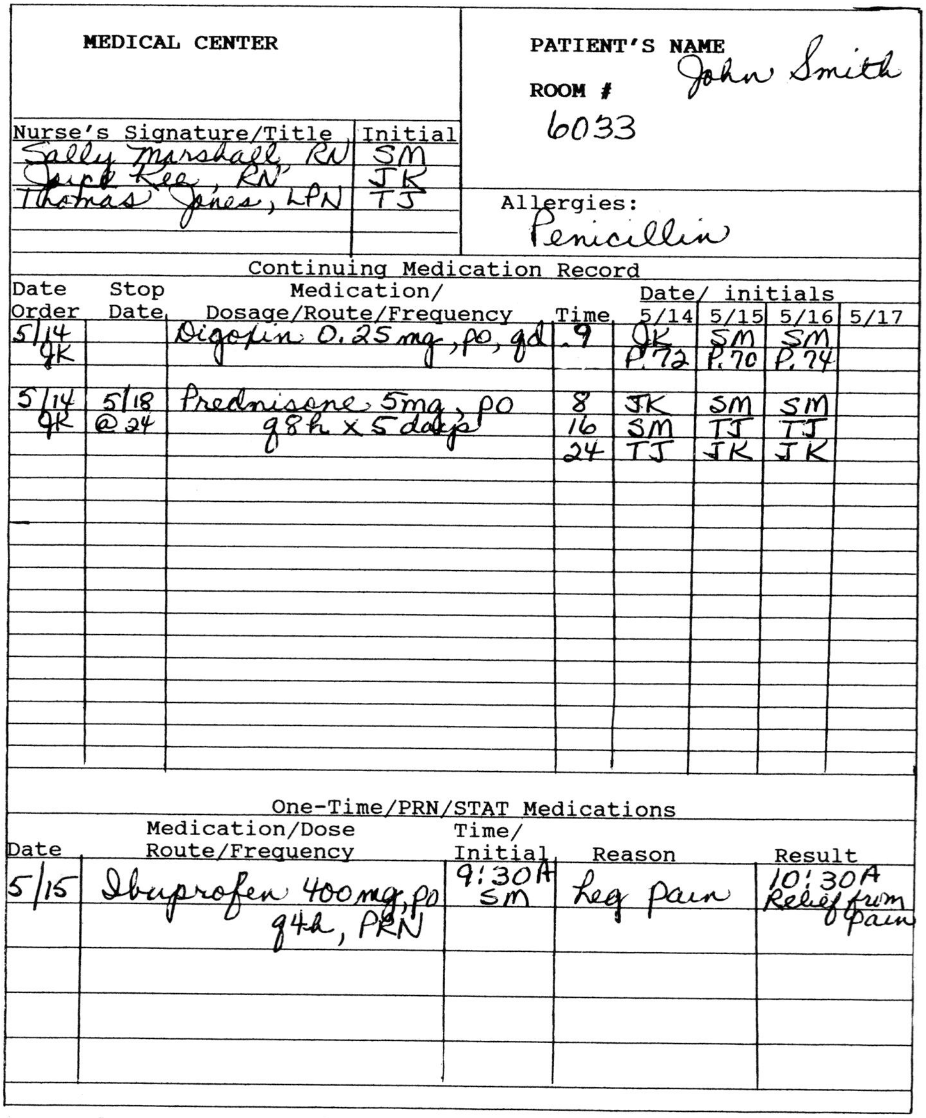

MEDICAL CENTER			PATIENT'S NAME John Smith				
			ROOM # 6033				
Nurse's Signature/Title		Initial					
Sally Marshall, RN		SM	Allergies: Penicillin				
Jack Kee, RN		JK					
Thomas Jones, LPN		TJ					

Continuing Medication Record

Date Order	Stop Date	Medication/ Dosage/Route/Frequency	Time	Date/ initials 5/14	5/15	5/16	5/17
5/14 JK		Digoxin 0.25 mg, po, qd	9	JK P.72	SM P.70	SM P.74	
5/14 JK	5/18 @ 24	Prednisone, 5mg, po q8h x 5 days	8	JK	SM	SM	
			16	SM	TJ	TJ	
			24	TJ	JK	JK	

One-Time/PRN/STAT Medications

Date	Medication/Dose Route/Frequency	Time/ Initial	Reason	Result
5/15	Ibuprofen 400mg, po q4h, PRN	9:30A SM	Leg Pain	10:30A Relief from pain

FIGURE 3-8 Medication record.

Methods of Drug Distribution

Two methods of drug distribution frequently used for administering medications are the stock drug method and the unit dose method. Unit dose method is described under bar code title. Table 3-2 describes these methods and lists the advantages and disadvantages of each.

Table 3-2

Methods of Drug Distribution

	Stock Drug Method	Unit Dose Method
Description	Drug is stored in a large container on the floor and is dispensed from the container for all patients.	Drug is packaged in single doses by the pharmacy for 24-hour dosing.
Advantages	Drug is always available, which eliminates time spent waiting for drug to arrive from the pharmacy. Cost efficiency is enhanced by having large quantities of the drug.	Fewer drug errors are made. Packaging saves the nurse time otherwise spent in preparing the drug dose. Correct dose is provided with *no* calculation needed. Drug is billed for specific number of doses.
Disadvantages	Drug error is more prevalent because the drug is "poured" by many persons. There are more drugs to choose from, which may cause error. Drug expiration date on the container may be missed.	There is time delay in receiving the drug from the pharmacy. If the doses are contaminated or damaged, they are not immediately replaceable.

THE "5 RIGHTS" IN DRUG ADMINISTRATION

To provide safe drug administration, the nurse should practice the "5 rights": the right client, the right drug, the right dose, the right time, and the right route (see "Checklist"). Three additional rights could be added: the right documentation, the right of the client to know the reason for administration of the drug, and the right of the client to refuse to take a medication.

Right Client

The client's identification band should always be checked before a medication is given. The nurse should do the following:
- Verify client by checking his or her identification bracelet.
- Ask the client his or her name. Do not call the client by name. Some individuals answer to any name.
- Check the name on the client's medication label.

Right Drug

To avoid error, the nurse should do the following:
- Check the drug label three times: (1) at first contact with the drug bottle, (2) before pouring the drug, and (3) after pouring the drug.
- Check that the drug order is complete and legible. If it is not, contact the physician or charge nurse.

Checklist for the "5 Rights" in Drug Administration

Right Client
- Check client's identification bracelet. ☐
- Ask the client for his or her name. ☐
- Check the name on the client's medication label. ☐

Right Drug
- Check that the drug order is complete and legible. ☐
- Check the drug label three times. ☐
- Check the expiration date. ☐
- Know the drug action. ☐

Right Dose
- Calculate the drug dose. ☐
- Know the recommended dosage range for the drug. ☐
- Recalculate the drug dose with another nurse if in doubt. ☐

Right Time
- Administer drug at the specified time(s). ☐
- Document any delay or omitted drug dose. ☐
- Administer drugs that irritate gastric mucosa with food. ☐
- Administer antibiotics at even intervals (q6h, q8h). ☐

Right Route
- Know the route for administration of the drug. ☐
- Use aseptic techniques when administering a drug. ☐
- Document the injection site on the patient's chart. ☐

- Know the drug action.
- Check the expiration date. Discard an outdated drug or return the drug to the pharmacy.
- If client questions the drug, recheck drug and drug dose. If in doubt, seek another health care provider's advice, e.g., pharmacist, physician, licensed health care provider. Some generic drugs differ in shape or color.

Right Dose

Stock drugs and unit doses are the two methods frequently used for drug distribution. Not all health care institutions use the unit dose method (drugs prepared by dose in the pharmacy or by the pharmaceutical company). If the institution uses the unit dose method, drugs in bottles should *not* be administered without the consent of the physician or pharmacist. The nurse should:
- Be able to calculate drug dose using the ratio and proportion, basic formula, or dimensional analysis method.

■ Know how to calculate drug dose by body weight (kg) or by body surface area (BSA; m²). Doses of potent drugs (e.g., anticancer agents) and doses for children are frequently determined by body weight or BSA.

■ Know the recommended dosage range for the drug. Check the *Physicians' Desk Reference,* the *American Hospital Formulary,* or another drug reference. If the nurse believes that the dose is incorrect or is not within the therapeutic range, he or she should notify the charge nurse, physician, or pharmacist and should document all communications.

■ Recalculate drug dose if in doubt, or have a colleague recheck the dose.

■ Question drug doses that appear to be incorrect.

■ Have a colleague check the drug dose of potent or specified drugs such as insulin, digoxin, narcotics, and anticancer agents. This procedure is required by some facilities.

Right Time

The drug dose should be given at a specified time to maintain a therapeutic drug serum level. Too-frequent dosing can cause drug toxicity, and missed doses can nullify the drug action and its effect. The nurse should:

■ Administer the drug at the specified time(s). Drugs can be given ½ hour before or after the time prescribed.

■ Omit or delay a drug dose according to specific circumstance, e.g., laboratory and diagnostic tests. Notify the appropriate personnel of the reason.

■ Administer drugs that are affected by foods, e.g., tetracycline, 1 hour before or 2 hours after meals.

■ Administer drugs that can irritate the gastric mucosa, e.g., potassium or aspirin, with food.

■ Know that drugs with a long half-life ($t_{1/2}$), e.g., 20 to 36 hours, are usually given once per day. Drugs with a short half-life, e.g., 1 to 6 hours, are given several times a day.

■ Administer antibiotics at even intervals (e.g., q8h [8-4-12] rather than tid [8-12-4]; q6h [6-12-6-12] rather than qid [8-12-4-8]) to maintain a therapeutic drug serum level.

Right Route

The right route is necessary for appropriate absorption of the medication. The more common routes of absorption are (1) oral (by mouth, po) tablet, capsule, pill, liquid, or suspension; (2) sublingual (under the tongue for venous absorption, *not* to be swallowed); (3) buccal (between gum and cheek); (4) topical (applied to the skin); (5) inhalation (aerosol sprays); (6) instillation (in nose, eye, ear, rectum, or vagina); (7) and four parenteral routes: intradermal, subcutaneous, intramuscular, and intravenous. The nurse should:

■ Know the drug route. If in doubt, check with the pharmacy. Ointment for the eye should have "ophthalmic" written on the tube. Drugs given sublingually (e.g., nitroglycerin tablet) should *not* be swallowed, because the effect of the drug would be lost.

- Administer injectables (subcutaneous and intramuscular) at appropriate sites (see Chapter 8).
- Use aseptic technique when administering drugs. Sterile technique is required with the parenteral routes.
- Document the injection site used on the client's chart or on another designated sheet.

ABBREVIATIONS

Selected abbreviations are given here in four categories: drug form, drug measurements, route of drug administration, and times of drug administration. These abbreviations are frequently used in drug therapy and in this text; therefore, nurses must know the meanings of these abbreviations.

Drug Form

Abbreviation	Meaning	Abbreviation	Meaning
aq	Water	SR	Sustained release
cap	Capsule	supp	Suppository
CD	Controlled dose	susp	Suspension
elix	Elixir	syr	Syrup
emuls	Emulsion	tab	Tablet
ext	Extract	tr, tinct	Tincture
mixt	Mixture	ung	Ointment
		XR	Extended release

Drug Measurements

Abbreviation	Meaning	Abbreviation	Meaning
cc	Cubic centimeter	ml	Milliliter
dl	Deciliter (one-tenth of a liter)	$\mathfrak{m}$, min	Minim
		ng	Nanogram
dr	Dram	oz	Ounce
fl dr	Fluid dram (fl ℥)	pt	Pint
fl oz	Fluid ounce (fl ℥)	qt	Quart
g, gm, G, Gm	Gram	$\overline{ss}$	One-half
gr	Grain	T.O.	Telephone order
gtt	Drops	T, tbsp	Tablespoon
kg	Kilogram	t, tsp	Teaspoon
l, L	Liter	U	Unit
m^2, M^2	Square meter	V.O.	Verbal order
mcg, μg	Microgram	$\times$	Times
mEq	Milliequivalent	$>$	Greater than
mg	Milligram	$<$	Less than

Routes of Drug Administration

Abbreviation	Meaning	Abbreviation	Meaning
A.D., ad	Right ear	NGT	Nasogastric tube
A.S., as	Left ear	O.D., od	Right eye
A.U., au	Both ears	O.S., os	Left eye
ID	Intradermal	O.U., ou	Both eyes
IM	Intramuscular	P.O., po, os	By mouth
IV	Intravenous	PR	Per rectum
IVPB	Intravenous piggyback	®	Right
		Rect	Rectal
KVO	Keep vein open	SC, subc, sc	Subcutaneous
Ⓛ	Left	Sl, sl, subl	Sublingual
		Vag	Vaginal

Times of Drug Administration

Abbreviation	Meaning	Abbreviation	Meaning
A.C., ac	Before meals	qd, od	Every day
ad lib	As desired	qh	Every hour
B.i.d., Bid, bid	Twice a day	q2h	Every 2 hours
BIW, b.i.w.	Two times a week	q4h	Every 4 hours
$\bar{c}$	With	q6h	Every 6 hours
h	Hour	q8h	Every 8 hours
hs	Hour of sleep	Q.i.d., Qid, qid	Four times a day
noct	At night	Qod, qod	Every other day
NPO	Nothing by mouth	$\bar{s}$	Without
P.C., pc	After meals	SOS	Once if necessary, if there is a need
per	By		
PRN	Whenever necessary, as needed	STAT	Give immediately
		T.i.d., Tid, tid	Three times a day
q	Every	TIW, t.i.w.	Three times a week
qAM	Every morning, every AM		

PRACTICE PROBLEMS III Abbreviations

Answers can be found on page 65.

If you have more than two incorrect answers, review the abbreviations and meanings. Then quiz yourself again.

1. cap _____

2. SR _____

3. fl oz _____

4. g, G _____

5. gr _____

6. L _____

7. ml _____

8. mcg, μg _____

9. mg _____

10. $\overline{ss}$ _____

11. T _____

12. t _____

13. > _____

14. A.U., au _____

15. IM _____

16. IV _____

17. KVO _____

18. O.S. _____

19. O.U. _____

20. SC _____

21. $\overline{c}$ _____

22. A.C., ac _____

23. hs _____

24. NPO _____

25. P.C., pc _____

26. q4h _____

27. Qid, qid, q.i.d. _____

28. Tid, tid, t.i.d. _____

29. Bid, bid, b.i.d. _____

30. STAT _____

ANSWERS

I Interpretation of Drug Labels

1. **a.** Sinequan
   b. doxepin
   c. capsule
   d. 10 mg per capsule
   e. Pfizer/Roerig

2. **a.** Veetids
   b. penicillin V potassium
   c. tablet
   d. 250 mg per tablet; 400,000 units per tablet
   e. Apothecon

3. **a.** Amoxil
   b. amoxicillin
   c. liquid for oral suspension when reconstituted
   d. 200 mg/5 ml
   e. Lot #T54325
   f. Expiration date: 11/15/05
   g. SmithKline Beecham

4. a. quinidine gluconate
   b. quinidine gluconate
      (same as brand name)
   c. liquid for injection
   d. vial (multiple dose vial),
      total amount is 10 ml
      per vial
   e. 80 mg per ml
   f. 10/11/04

5. a. Decadron phosphate
   b. dexamethasone sodium
      phosphate
   c. liquid for injection
   d. 24 mg per ml

6. a. nafcillin sodium
   b. nafcillin sodium (same as
      brand name)
   c. drug powder to be
      reconstituted
   d. 3.4 ml diluent
   e. IM or IV
   f. 1 gram = 4 ml
   g. 11/30/05
   h. Apothecon

II Interpretation of Drug Orders

1. Give 250 mg of tetracycline by mouth every 6 hours
2. Give 50 mg of HydroDIURIL by mouth every day
3. Give 50 mg of meperidine intramuscularly every 3 to 4 hours whenever necessary
4. Give 1 g of Ancef intravenously every 8 hours
5. Give 10 mg of prednisone three times a day for 5 days
6. frequency of administration
7. route of administration
8. frequency of administration
9. route and frequency of administration
10. route and frequency of administration and stop date

III Abbreviations

1. capsule
2. sustained release
3. fluid ounce
4. gram
5. grain
6. liter
7. milliliter
8. microgram
9. milligram
10. one-half
11. tablespoon
12. teaspoon
13. greater than
14. both ears
15. intramuscular
16. intravenous
17. keep vein open
18. left eye
19. both eyes
20. subcutaneous
21. with
22. before meals
23. hour of sleep
24. nothing by mouth
25. after meals
26. every 4 hours
27. four times a day
28. three times a day
29. two times a day
30. immediately

Alternative Methods for Drug Administration

OBJECTIVES

- Recognize the various methods for drug administration.
- Explain the steps (methods) in drug administration when the various methods are used.

OUTLINE

TRANSDERMAL PATCH

INHALATION

NASAL SPRAY AND DROPS

EYE DROPS AND OINTMENT

EAR DROPS

PHARYNGEAL SPRAY, MOUTHWASH, AND LOZENGE

TOPICAL PREPARATIONS: LOTION, CREAM, AND OINTMENT

RECTAL SUPPOSITORY

VAGINAL SUPPOSITORY, CREAM, AND OINTMENT

There are numerous methods for administering medications in addition to the oral (tablets, capsules, liquid) and parenteral (subcutaneous, intramuscular, intravenous) routes. Alternative methods for drug administration include transdermal patches; inhalation sprays; nasal sprays and drops; eye drops and ointments; ear drops; pharyngeal (throat) sprays, mouthwashes, and lozenges; topical lotions, creams, and ointments; rectal suppositories; and vaginal suppositories, creams, and ointments.

TRANSDERMAL PATCH

Purpose

The transdermal patch contains medication (Fig. 4-1); the patch is applied to the skin for slow, systemic absorption, usually over 24 hours. Use of the transdermal route avoids the gastrointestinal problems associated with some oral medications and provides a more consistent drug level in the client's blood.

METHOD Transdermal Patch

1. Cleanse the skin area where the patch will be applied. The area can be the chest, abdomen, arms, or thighs. Avoid areas that have hair.
2. Remove the transparent cover (inside) of the patch. Do not touch the inside of the patch.
3. Apply the patch to the chosen area with the dull, plastic side up.

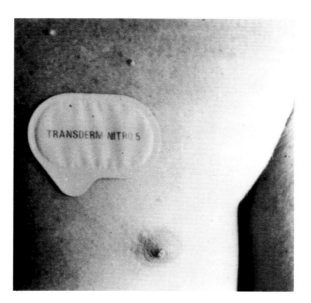

FIGURE 4-1 Transdermal nitrogycerin patch. (Courtesy of Summit Pharmaceutical.)

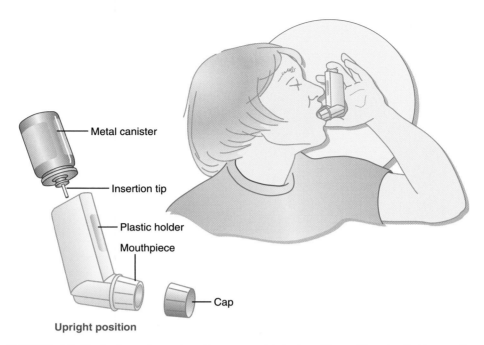

Metal canister

Insertion tip

Plastic holder

Mouthpiece

Cap

Upright position

FIGURE 4-2 Technique for using the aerosol inhaler. (From Kee, J., & Hayes, E. [2003]. *Pharmacology: A Nursing Process Approach* [4th ed.] Philadelphia: W. B. Saunders.)

INHALATION

Purpose

The drug inhaler delivers the prescribed dose to be absorbed by the mucosal lining of the respiratory tract (Fig. 4-2). The drug categories for respiratory inhalation are bronchodilators, which dilate bronchial tubes; glucocorticoids, which are anti-inflammatory agents; and mucolytics, which liquefy bronchial secretions.

Types

Two types of inhalers are the metered-dose inhaler (MDI) or nebulizer and the nasal inhaler.

The MDI can also be used with a spacer device, which enhances delivery of the medication. Figure 4-3 illustrates the advantage of a spacer device.

METHOD Metered-Dose Inhaler

1. Insert the medication canister into the plastic holder. If the inhaler has not been used recently or if it is being used for the first time, test spray before administering the metered dose.

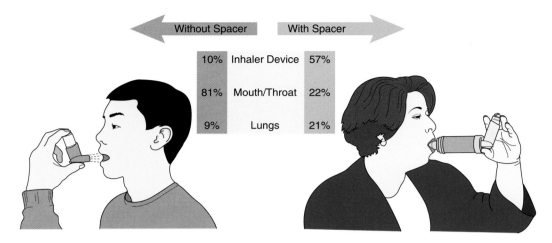

FIGURE 4-3 Distribution of medication with and without a spacer. (From American Lung Association. [1993]. *Understanding Lung Medications: How They Work—How to Use Them.* Wilmington, DE: American Lung Association, p. 5.)

2. Shake the inhaler well before using. Remove the cap from the mouthpiece.
3. Instruct the client to breathe out through the mouth, expelling air. Place the mouthpiece into the client's mouth, holding the inhaler upright (Fig. 4-2).
4. Instruct the client to keep his or her lips securely around the mouthpiece and inhale. While the client is inhaling, push the top of the medication canister once.
5. Instruct the client to hold his or her breath for a few seconds. Remove the mouthpiece and take your finger off the canister. Tell the client to exhale slowly.
6. If a second dose is required, wait 1 to 2 minutes and repeat steps 3 to 5.
7. Cleanse the mouthpiece.

METHOD Metered-Dose Inhaler with Spacer

1. Method is the same as the method used for the MDI just described (Fig. 4-3).

METHOD Nasal Inhaler

1. Instruct the client to blow his or her nose to clear the nostrils.
2. Insert the drug cartridge into the adapter (Fig. 4-4).
3. Shake the inhaler well before using. Remove the cap.
4. Place your finger on top of the cartridge.
5. Instruct the client to tilt his or her head back slightly. Place the tip of the adapter in one nostril; occlude the other nostril; and have client inhale while you press the adapter. Inform the client to exhale through his or her mouth.
6. Repeat the procedure with the other nostril if ordered.
7. Cleanse the tip of the adapter and dry thoroughly.

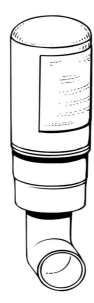

FIGURE 4-4 Nasal inhaler.

NASAL SPRAY AND DROPS

Purpose

Most drugs in nasal spray and drop containers are intended to relieve nasal congestion caused by upper respiratory tract infection and polyps by shrinking swollen nasal membranes. Types of drugs given by this method are vasoconstrictors and glucocorticoids.

METHOD Nasal Spray

1. Instruct the client to sit with his or her head tilted slightly back or slightly forward, according to the directions on the spray container (Fig. 4-5).
2. Insert the tip of the container in one nostril and occlude the other nostril.
3. Instruct the client to inhale as you squeeze the drug spray container. Repeat with the same nostril if ordered.
4. Repeat the procedure with the other nostril if ordered.
5. Encourage the client to keep his or her head tilted for several minutes until the drug action is effective. The nose should not be blown until the head is upright.

METHOD Nose Drops

1. Place the client in an upright position with his or her head tilted back.
2. Insert the dropper into the nostril without touching the nasal membranes.
3. Instill 2 drops of medications or the amount prescribed.
4. Instruct the client to keep his or her head back for 5 minutes and to breathe through the mouth.

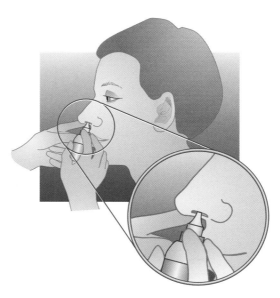

FIGURE 4-5 Administering nasal spray. (From Kee, J., & Hayes, E. [2003]. *Pharmacology: A Nursing Process Approach* [4th ed.]. Philadelphia: W. B. Saunders.)

5. Cleanse the dropper.
6. For the medication to reach the sinuses, the client should be in the supine position with head turned to one side and then the other so the medication can reach the frontal and maxillary sinuses. For the medication to reach the ethmoidal and sphenoidal sinuses, the client's head is lowered below his or her shoulders (Fig. 4-6).

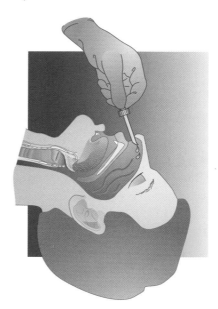

FIGURE 4-6 Administering nose drops. (From Kee, J., & Hayes, E. [2003]. *Pharmacology: A Nursing Process Approach* [4th ed.]. Philadelphia: W. B. Saunders.)

EYE DROPS AND OINTMENT

Purpose

Eye medications are prescribed for various eye disorders, such as glaucoma, infection, and allergies, and for eye examination and eye surgery.

METHOD Eye Drops

1. Instruct the client to lie or sit with his or her head tilted back.
2. Instruct the client to look up toward the ceiling and away from the dropper. Pull down the lower lid of the affected eye (Fig. 4-7). Place one drop of medication into the lower conjunctival sac. This prevents the drug from dropping onto the cornea.
3. Press gently on the medial nasolacrimal canthus (side closer to the nose) with a tissue to prevent systemic drug absorption.
4. If the other eye is affected, repeat the procedure in the other eye.
5. Inform the client to blink one or two times and then to keep the eyes closed for several minutes. Use a tissue to blot away excess drug fluid.

METHOD Eye Ointment

1. Instruct the client to lie or sit with his or her head tilted back.
2. Pull down the lower lid to expose the conjunctival sac of the affected eye (Fig. 4-8).

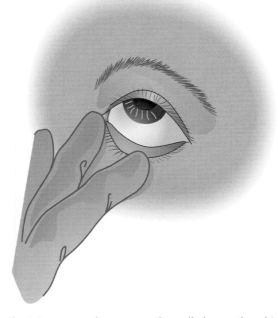

FIGURE 4-7 To administer eye drops, gently pull down the skin below the eye to expose the conjunctival sac. (From Kee, J., & Hayes, E. [2003]. *Pharmacology: A Nursing Process Approach* [4th ed.]. Philadelphia: W. B. Saunders.)

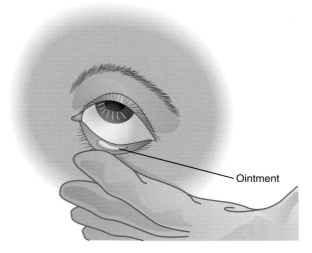

FIGURE 4-8 To administer eye ointment, squeeze a ¼-inch–wide strip of ointment onto the conjunctival sac. (From Kee, J., & Hayes, E. [2003]. *Pharmacology: A Nursing Process Approach* [4th ed.]. Philadelphia: W. B. Saunders.)

3. Squeeze a strip of ointment about ¼ inch long (unless otherwise indicated) onto the conjunctival sac. Medication placed directly onto the cornea can cause discomfort or damage.
4. If the other eye is affected, repeat the procedure.
5. Instruct the client to close his or her eyes for 2 to 3 minutes. The client's vision may be blurred for a short time.

EAR DROPS

Purpose

Ear medication is frequently prescribed to soften and loosen the cerumen (wax) in the ear canal, for anesthetic effect, to immobilize insects in the ear canal, and to treat infection such as fungal infection.

METHOD Ear Drops

1. Instruct the client to lie on the unaffected side or to sit upright with his or her head tilted toward the unaffected side.
2. Straighten the external ear canal (Fig. 4-9), as follows:
   Adult: Pull the auricle of the ear up and back.
   Child: Pull the auricle of the ear down and back.
3. Instill the prescribed number of drops. Avoid contaminating the dropper.
4. Instruct the client to remain in this position for 2 to 5 minutes to prevent the medication from leaking out of the ear.

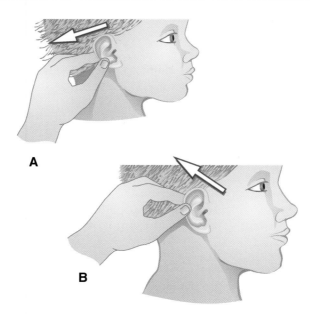

FIGURE 4-9 To administer ear drops, straighten the external ear canal by
(A) pulling down on the auricle in children and (B) pulling up and back on
the auricle in adults. (From Kee, J., & Hayes, E. [2003]. *Pharmacology: A Nursing
Process Approach* [4th ed.]. Philadelphia: W. B. Saunders.)

PHARYNGEAL SPRAY, MOUTHWASH, AND LOZENGE

Purpose

Sprays, mouthwashes, and lozenges can be prescribed to reduce throat irritation and for antiseptic and anesthetic effects. These methods are prescribed for a local effect on the throat and *not* for systemic use.

METHOD Pharyngeal Spray

1. Instruct the client to sit upright.
2. Place a tongue blade over the client's tongue to prevent the tongue from becoming numb if an anesthetic is being administered.
3. Hold the spray pump nozzle outside the client's mouth, and direct the spray to the back of the throat.

METHOD Pharyngeal Mouthwash

1. Instruct the client to sit upright.
2. Instruct the client to swish the solution around the mouth, but *not* to swallow the solution, and then to spit it into an emesis basin or sink.

METHOD Pharyngeal Lozenge

1. Instruct the client to sit upright.
2. Instruct the client to place the lozenge in his or her mouth and suck until it is fully dissolved. The lozenge should *not* be chewed or swallowed whole.

TOPICAL PREPARATIONS: LOTION, CREAM, AND OINTMENT

Purpose

Topical lotions, creams, and ointments are used to protect skin areas, prevent skin dryness, treat itching of skin areas, and relieve pain.

METHOD Topical Lotion

1. Cleanse skin area with soap and water or other designated solution.
2. Shake the lotion container. Use clean or sterile gloves to apply the medicated lotion. Rub the lotion thoroughly into the skin unless otherwise indicated.

METHOD A Topical Cream or Ointment

1. Cleanse the skin area.
2. Use clean or sterile glove(s) and a sterile tongue blade or gauze to apply the cream or ointment to the affected skin area. Use long, smooth strokes. A piece of sterile gauze can be placed over the medicated area after application to prevent soiling of clothing.

METHOD B Topical Cream or Ointment

1. Cleanse the skin area.
2. Squeeze a line of ointment from the tube onto your finger from the tip to the first skin crease; this is known as a fingertip unit (FTU) (Fig. 4-10). One FTU weighs about 0.5 g.
3. Use the guidelines shown in Figure 4-11 to determine the number of FTUs to apply to various body areas.
4. Apply the medication to the affected area.

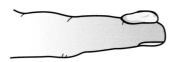

FIGURE 4-10 Fingertip unit: ointment squeezed from the tip of the finger to the first skin crease.

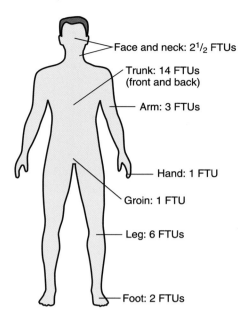

FIGURE 4-11 Number of fingertip units to various body areas.

RECTAL SUPPOSITORY

Purpose

Rectal medications are used to relieve vomiting when the client is unable to take oral medication, to relieve pain or anxiety, to promote defecation, and to administer drugs that could be destroyed by digestive enzymes.

METHOD Rectal Suppository

1. Place the client on his or her left side in the Sims' position (Fig. 4-12).
2. Use gloves or a finger cot on the index finger.

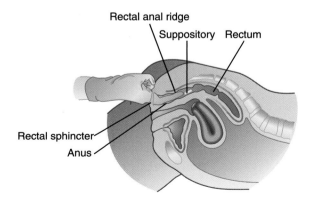

FIGURE 4-12 Inserting a rectal suppository. (From Kee, J., & Hayes, E. [2003]. *Pharmacology: A Nursing Process Approach* [4th ed.]. Philadelphia: W. B. Saunders.)

3. Expose the anus by lifting the upper portion of the buttock.
4. Lightly lubricate the suppository with water-soluble lubricant, and insert the narrow (pointed) end of the suppository through the anal sphincter muscle.
5. Instruct the client to remain in a supine position for 5 to 10 minutes.

VAGINAL SUPPOSITORY, CREAM, AND OINTMENT

Purpose

Vaginal medications are used to treat vaginal infection or inflammation.

METHOD Vaginal Suppository, Cream, and Ointment

1. Wear clean gloves.
2. Place the client in the lithotomy position (knees bent with feet on the table or bed).
3. Place the vaginal suppository at the tip of the applicator.

   or

   Connect the top of the vaginal cream or ointment tube with the tip of applicator. Squeeze the tube to fill the applicator.
4. Lubricate the applicator with water-soluble lubricant if necessary.
5. Insert applicator downward first and then upward and backward. (Fig. 4-13).
6. The client may use a light pad in the underwear to prevent soiling of clothing. Bedtime is the suggested time for vaginal drug administration.
7. Instruct the client to avoid using tampons after insertion of the vaginal medication.

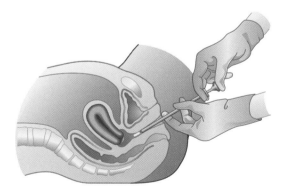

FIGURE 4-13 Inserting a vaginal suppository. (From Kee, J., & Hayes, E. [2003]. *Pharmacology: A Nursing Process Approach* [4th ed.]. Philadelphia: W. B. Saunders.)

Methods of Calculation

OBJECTIVES

- Determine the amount of drug needed for a specified time.
- Select a dosage formula, such as basic formula, ratio and proportion, fraction equation, or dimensional analysis, for solving drug dosage problems.
- Convert units of measurement to the same system and unit of measurement before calculating drug dosage.
- Calculate the dosage amount of tablets, capsules, and liquid volume (oral or parenteral) needed to administer the prescribed drug.

OUTLINE

DRUG CALCULATION
    Method 1: Basic Formula
    Method 2: Ratio and Proportion
    Method 3: Fractional Equation
    Method 4: Dimensional Analysis

Before drug dosage can be calculated, units of measurement must be converted to one system. If the drug is ordered in milligrams and comes in grains, then grains are converted to milligrams or milligrams are converted to grains.

Four methods for calculating drug dosages are: basic formula, ratio and proportion, fractional equation, and dimensional analysis. The ratio and proportion and fractional equation methods are similar. For drugs that require individualized dosing, body weight and body surface area are used. When body weight and body surface area calculations are used, one of the first four methods for calculation is necessary to determine the amount of drug needed from the container.

At some institutions, the nurse orders enough medication doses for a designated period. If the order requires 2 tablets, qid (4 times a day) for 5 days, then the number of tablets needed would be 2 tablets × 4 times a day × 5 days = 40 tablets.

 The CD-ROM presents three methods for calculating drug dosages: basic formula, ratio and proportion (in fractional equations), and dimensional analysis.

DRUG CALCULATION

The four methods as mentioned for drug calculations are (1) basic formula, (2) ratio and proportion, (3) fractional equation, and (4) dimensional analysis (factor labeling).

METHOD 1 Basic Formula

The following formula is often used to calculate drug dosages. The basic formula (BF) is the most commonly used method, and it is easy to remember.

$$\frac{D}{H} \times V = \text{Amount to give}$$

D or desired dose: Drug dose ordered by physician.
H or on-hand dose: Drug dose on label of container (bottle, vial, ampule).
V or vehicle: Form and amount in which the drug comes (tablet, capsule, liquid).

EXAMPLES   PROBLEM 1: Order: erythromycin (ERY-TAB) 0.5 g, po, q8h.
                Drug available:

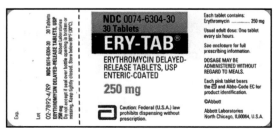

a. Both the dosage of the drug ordered and the dosage on the bottle are in the metric system; however, the units of measurement are different. Conversion is needed. To convert grams to milligrams, move the decimal point three spaces to the right (see Chapter 1, Metric System):

$$0.5 \text{ g} = 0.500 \text{ mg} = 500 \text{ mg}$$

b. BF: $\dfrac{D}{H} \times V = \dfrac{\overset{2}{\cancel{500}}}{\cancel{250}_{1}} \times 1 \text{ tab} = 2 \text{ tablets}$

Answer: erythromycin 0.5 g = 2 tablets

PROBLEM 2: Order: 0.5 g of ampicillin (Principen), po, bid.
Drug available:

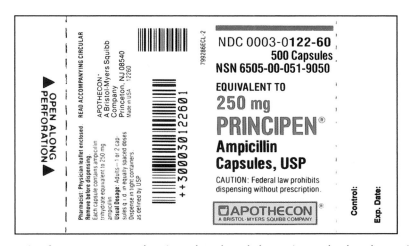

a. The unit of measurement that is ordered and the unit on the bottle are in the same system but in different units; therefore conversion of units within the same system must be done first. To convert grams to milligrams, move the decimal point three spaces to the right (see Chapter 1, Metric System):

$$0.5 \text{ g} = 0.500 \text{ mg} = 500 \text{ mg}$$

b. BF: $\dfrac{D}{H} \times V = \dfrac{500}{250} \times 1 \text{ capsule} = \dfrac{\overset{2}{\cancel{500}}}{\cancel{250}_{1}} = 2 \text{ capsules}$

Answer: ampicillin (Principen) 0.5 g = 2 capsules

PROBLEM 3: Order: phenobarbital gr ii, STAT.
Drug available: phenobarbital 30 mg per tablet.
a. Before calculating drug dosage, convert to one unit of measurement. To convert grains to milligrams, *multiply* the number of grains by 60 (see Chapter 2, Grains and Milligrams):

$$2 \text{ gr} \times 60 = 120 \text{ mg}$$

b. BF: $\dfrac{D}{H} \times V = \dfrac{120}{30} \times 1 = \dfrac{120}{30} = 4 \text{ tablets}$

Answer: phenobarbital gr ii = 4 tablets

PROBLEM 4: Order: meperidine (Demerol) 35 mg, IM, STAT.
Drug available:

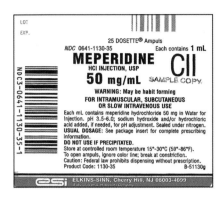

a. Conversion is not needed, because both are of the same unit of measurement.

b. BF: $\dfrac{D}{H} \times V = \dfrac{35}{50} \times 1 \text{ ml} = \dfrac{35}{50} = 0.7 \text{ ml}$

Answer: meperidine (Demerol) 35 mg = 0.7 ml

METHOD 2 Ratio and Proportion

Ratio and proportion (RP) is the oldest method used for calculating dosage problems:

$$
\begin{array}{ccccc}
\textit{Known} & & & \textit{Desired} & \\
H & : & V & :: & D & : & X \\
\text{on hand} & \text{vehicle} & \text{desired dose} & \text{amount to give}
\end{array}
$$

means
extremes

H and **V**: On the left side of the equation are the known quantities, which are dose on hand and vehicle.
D and **X**: On the right side of the equation are the desired dose and the unknown amount to give.
Multiply the means and the extremes. Solve for **X**.

EXAMPLES   PROBLEM 1: Order: erythromycin (ERY-TAB) 0.5 g, po, q8h.
Drug available:

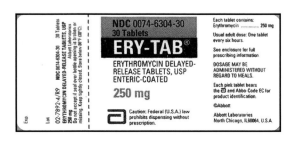

a. To convert grams to milligrams, move the decimal point three spaces to the right (see Chapter 1, Metric System):

$$0.5 \text{ g} = 0.500 \text{ mg} = 500 \text{ mg}$$

b. RP: H : V ::   D : X

250 mg:1 tab::500 mg:X tab

250 X = 500

X = 2 tablets

Answer: erythromycin 0.5 g = 2 tablets

Note: With ratio and proportion, the ratio on the left (milligrams to tablets) has the same relation as the ratio on the right (milligrams to tablets); the only difference is values.

PROBLEM 2: Order: aspirin (ASA) gr x, PRN.
         Drug available: aspirin 325 mg per tablet.

a. To convert to one system and unit of measurement. To convert grains to milligrams, *multiply* the number of grains by 60 (65) (see Chapter 2, Grains and Milligrams).

$$10 \text{ gr} \times 60 \ (65) = 600 \text{ or } 650 \text{ mg}$$

or

gr: mg :: gr : mg
1 : 60 (65) :: 10 : X
X = 600 or 650 mg

b. RP: H : V ::   D   : X

325 mg:1 tablet:: 600 (650) mg:X tablet

325 X = 600 (650)

X = 1.8 tablets or 2 tablets

(round off or use 650 instead of 600)

Answer: aspirin gr x = 2 tablets

PROBLEM 3: Order: amoxicillin 75 mg, po, qid.
         Drug available:

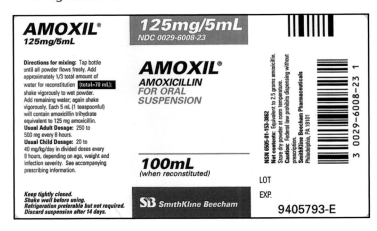

a. Conversion is not needed because both use the same unit of measurement.
b. RP: H   : V ::   D   : X
        125 mg:5 ml:: 75 mg:X ml
               125 X = 375
                   X = 3 ml

Answer: amoxicillin 75 mg = 3 ml

PROBLEM 4: Order: meperidine (Demerol) 60 mg, IM, STAT.
                Drug available:

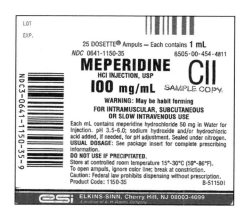

a. Conversion is not needed: the same unit of measurement is used.
b. RP: H   : V ::   D   : X
        100 mg:1 ml:: 60 mg:X ml
               100 X = 60
                   X = 0.6 ml

Answer: meperidine (Demerol) 60 mg = 0.6 ml

METHOD 3 Fractional Equation

The fractional equation (FE) method *is similar* to ratio and proportion, except it is written as a fraction.

$$\frac{H}{V} = \frac{D}{X}$$

H: The dosage on hand or in the container.
V: The vehicle or the form in which the drug comes (tablet, capsule, liquid).
D: The desired dosage.
X: The unknown amount to give.

Cross-multiply and solve for X.

EXAMPLES

PROBLEM 1: Order: kanamycin sulfate (Kantrex) 1 g, po, q6h × 3d.
Drug available:

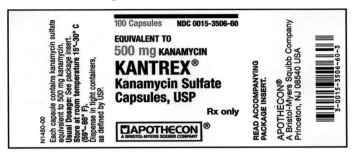

a. Convert grams to milligrams. Move the decimal point three spaces to the right.

$$1.0 \text{ g} = 1.\underset{\frown}{000} \text{ mg} = 1000 \text{ mg}$$

b. FE: $\dfrac{H}{V} = \dfrac{D}{X}$ $\dfrac{500 \text{ mg}}{1 \text{ capsule}} = \dfrac{1000}{X}$

$$500 \text{ X} = 1000$$
$$\text{X} = 2$$

Answer: kanamycin 1 g = 2 capsules

PROBLEM 2: Order: valproic acid (Depakene) 100 mg, po, tid.
Drug available: valproic acid (Depakene) 250 mg/5 ml suspension.

a. No unit conversion is needed.

b. FE: $\dfrac{H}{V} = \dfrac{D}{X}$ $\dfrac{250}{5} = \dfrac{100}{X}$

$$250 \text{ X} = 500$$
$$\text{X} = 2 \text{ ml}$$

Answer: valproic acid (Depakene) 100 mg = 2 ml

PROBLEM 3: Order: atropine gr ¹⁄₁₀₀, IM, STAT.
Drug available:

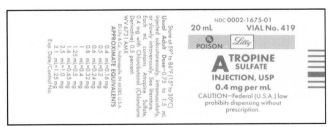

a. Two systems are involved: apothecary (grains) and metric (milligrams). Because the drug preparation is in milligrams, convert grains to milligrams (see Table 2-1 or Table 5-1; 0.6 mg = gr ¹⁄₁₀₀).

Table 5-1

Metric and Apothecary Conversions*

Metric		Apothecary
Grams (g)	Milligrams (mg)	Grains (gr)
1	1000	15
0.5	500	7½
0.3	300 (325)	5
0.1	100	1½
0.06	60 (64)	1
0.03	30 (32)	½
0.015	15 (16)	¼
0.010	10	$\frac{1}{6}$
0.0006	0.6	$\frac{1}{100}$
0.0004	0.4	$\frac{1}{150}$
0.0003	0.3	$\frac{1}{200}$

Liquid (Approximate)

30 ml (cc) = 1 oz (fl ʒ) = 2 tbsp (T) = 6 tsp (t)
15 ml (cc) = ½ oz = 1 T = 3 t
1000 ml (cc) = 1 quart (qt) = 1 liter (L)
500 ml (cc) = 1 pint (pt)
5 ml (cc) = 1 tsp (t)
4 ml (cc) = 1 fl dr (fl ʒ)
1 ml (cc) = 15 minims = 15 drops (gtt)

*Metric and apothecary equivalents frequently used in drug dosage conversions.

Also, you could use the RP method:

$$gr:mg :: gr : mg$$
$$1:60 :: \frac{1}{100} : X$$
$$X = \frac{60}{100}$$
$$X = 0.6 \text{ mg}$$

b. FE: $\dfrac{H}{V} = \dfrac{D}{X}$ $\dfrac{0.4}{1} = \dfrac{0.6}{X}$

$$0.4 X = 0.6$$
$$X = 1.5 \text{ ml}$$

Answer: atropine gr $\frac{1}{100}$ = 1.5 ml

METHOD 4 Dimensional Analysis

The dimensional analysis (DA) method (also called *factor labeling* or *the label factor method*) calculates dosages with three factors as follows:
1. Drug label factor: The form of the drug dose (V) with its equivalence in units (H), e.g., 1 capsule = 500 mg.

2. **Conversion factor (C):** It will help if you memorize the following common factor conversions:

Metric Equivalent:
1 g = 1000 mg
1 mg = 1000 mcg (μg)

Metric-Apothecary Equivalent:
1 g = 15 gr
1000 mg = 15 gr
1 gr = 60 mg

3. **Drug order factor:** The dosage desired (D).

These three factors are set up in an equation that allows you to cancel the units, giving you the correct answer in the correct units for delivery.

$$V = \frac{V \text{ (vehicle)} \times C \text{ (H)} \times D \text{ (desired)}}{H \text{ (on hand)} \times C \text{ (D)} \times 1}$$
(drug label) (conversion factor) (drug order)

As with other methods for calculation, the three components, **D, H,** and **V,** are necessary to solve the drug problem. With dimensional analysis, the conversion factor is built into the equation and is included when the units of measurements of the drug order and drug container differ. If the two are of the same units of measurement, the conversion factor is eliminated from the equation.

EXAMPLES

PROBLEM 1: Order: kanamycin (Kantrex) 1 g, po, q6h × 3 days.
Drug available:

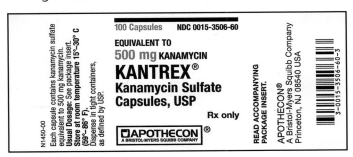

Factors: 500 mg = 1 capsule (from drug label)
1 g/1 (from drug order)
Conversion factor: 1 g = 1000 mg

$$\text{DA: cap} = \frac{1 \text{ cap} \times \overset{2}{\cancel{1000}} \text{ mg} \times 1 \cancel{g}}{\underset{1}{\cancel{500}} \text{ mg} \times 1 \cancel{g} \times 1}$$

(drug label) × (conversion factor) × (drug order)
(cancel units and numbers from numerator and denominator)

1 cap × 2 = 2 caps

Answer: kanamycin 1 g = 2 capsules

PROBLEM 2: Order: acetaminophen (Tylenol) gr XV, po, PRN.
Drug available:

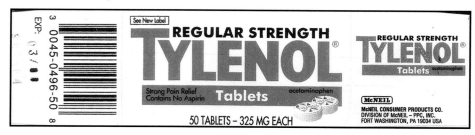

Factors: 325 mg = 1 tablet (from drug label)
15 gr/1 (from drug order)
Conversion factor: 1000 mg = 15 gr
How many tablet(s) would you give?

$$DA: tab = \frac{1 \text{ tab} \times 1000 \text{ mg} \times 15 \text{ gr}}{325 \text{ mg} \times 15 \text{ gr} \times 1} = \frac{1000}{325} = 3.07 \text{ tab or 3 tab}$$

Answer: acetaminophen gr XV = 3 tablets

Tylenol is also available in 500-mg tablets (extra-strength tablets).

PROBLEM 3: Order: Cipro (ciprofloxacin) 500 mg, po, q12h.
Drug available:

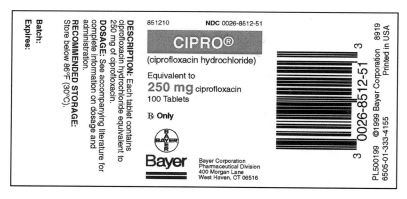

No conversion factor is needed because both are stated in milligrams (mg)

$$DA: tab = \frac{1 \text{ tab} \times \overset{2}{500} \text{ mg}}{\underset{1}{250} \text{ mg} \times 1} = 2 \text{ tablets}$$

Answer: Cipro 500 mg = 2 tablets

SUMMARY PRACTICE PROBLEMS

Solve the following calculation problems using Method 1, 2, 3, or 4. To convert units within the metric system (grams to milligrams), refer to Chapter 1. To convert apothecary to metric units and vice versa, refer to Chapter 2 or Table 5-1. For reading drug labels, refer to Chapter 3. Several of the calculation problems have drug labels. Drug dosage and drug form are printed on the drug label.

Extra practice problems are available in the chapters on oral drugs, injectable drugs, and pediatric drug administration.

1. Order: doxycycline hyclate (Vibra-Tab), po, initially 200 mg; then 50 mg, po, bid. Drug available:

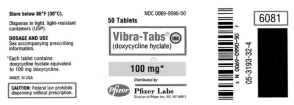

    a. How many tablet(s) would you give as the initial dose? _____

    b. How many tablets would you give for *each* dose after the initial

       dose? _____

2. Order: sulfisoxazole (Gantrisin) 1 g.
   Drug available: sulfisoxazole (Gantrisin) 250 mg per tablet.
   How many tablet(s) would you give? _____

3. The physician ordered erythromycin 500 mg, po, q8h, for 7 days. Drug available:

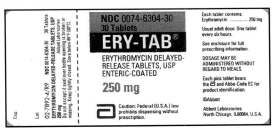

    a. How many tablets would you order for 7 days? _____

    b. How many tablets would you give every 8 hours? _____

4. Order: clarithromycin (Biaxin) 100 mg, po, q6h.
   Drug available:

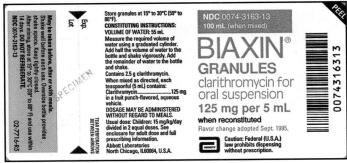

How many milliliters should the client receive per dose? _____

5. Order: phenytoin (Dilantin) 50 mg, po, bid.
Drug available:

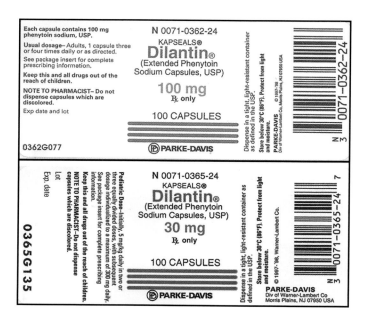

    a. Which Dilantin container would you select? _____

    b. How many Dilantin capsules would you give per dose? _____

6. Order: methyldopa (Aldomet) 150 mg, po, tid.
Drug available:

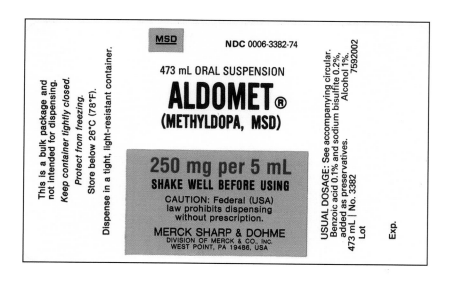

How many milliliters would you give per dose? _____

7. Order: dexamethasone (Decadron) 0.5 mg, po, qid.
Drug available:

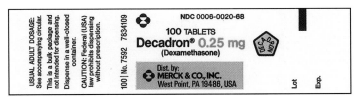

a. How many tablets would you give per dose? _____

b. How many milligrams would the client receive per day? _____

8. Order: diltiazem (Cardizem) SR 120 mg, po, bid for hypertension.
Drugs available:

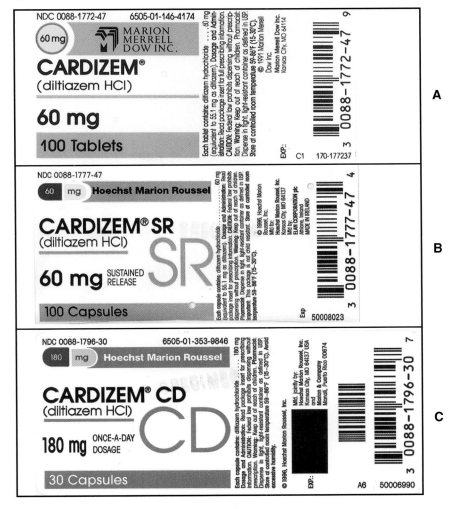

a. Which drug bottle should be selected? _____

b. How many tablet(s) should the client receive per dose? _____

9. Order: cimetidine (Tagamet) 0.2 g, po, qid.
Drug available:

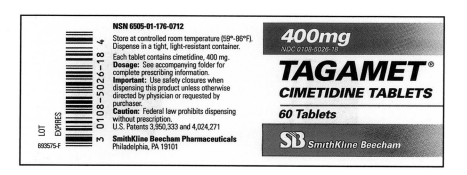

How many tablet(s) would you give per dose? _____

10. Order: codeine gr 1, po, STAT.
Drug available:

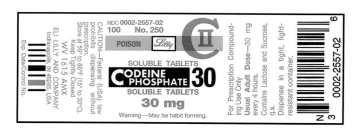

How many tablet(s) should the client receive? _____

11. Order: methylprednisolone (Medrol) 75 mg, IM.
Drug available: Medrol 125 mg per 2 ml per ampule.

How many milliliters would you give? _____

Additional Dimensional Analysis (Factor Labeling)

12. Order: aminocaproic acid 1.5 g, po, STAT.
Drug available: aminocaproic acid 500 mg tablet.
Factors: 500 mg = tablet (drug label)
Conversion factor: 1 g = 1000 mg

How many tablet(s) would you give? _____

13. Order: ampicillin (Principen) 50 mg/kg/day, po, in 4 divided
doses (q6h).
Client weighs 88 pounds, or 40 kg (88 ÷ 2.2 = 40 kg).

Drug available:

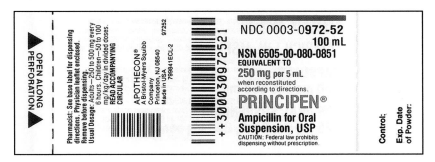

Factors: 250 mg = 5 ml (drug label)
Conversion factor: none (both are in milligrams)

   a. How many milligrams per day should the client receive? _____

   b. How many milligrams per dose should the client receive? _____

   c. How many milliliters should the client receive per dose (q6h)? _____

14. Order: cimetidine (Tagamet) 0.8 g, po, hs.
Drug available:

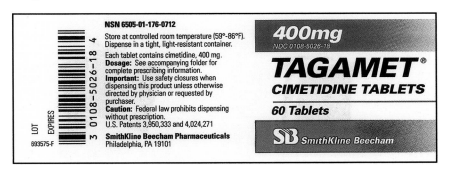

Factors: 400 mg = 1 tablet (drug label)
       0.8 g/1 (drug order)
Conversion factor: 1 g = 1000 mg (units of measurements are not the same; conversion factor is needed)

How many tablet(s) would you give? _____

15. Order: codeine gr i (1), po, STAT.
Drug available:

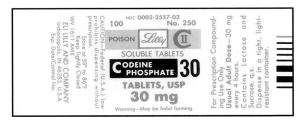

Factors: 30 mg = 1 tablet (drug label)
gr 1/1 (drug order)
Conversion factor: 1 gr = 60 mg

How many tablet(s) would you give? _____

16. Order: amikacin (Amikin) 250 mg, IM, q6h.
Drug available:

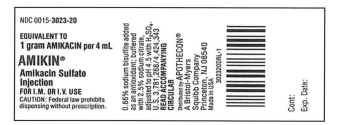

Factors: 1 g = 4 ml (drug label)
250 mg/1 (drug order)
Conversion factor: 1 g = 1000 mg

How many milliliters would you give? _____

ANSWERS SUMMARY PRACTICE PROBLEMS

1. a. Initially: BF: $\dfrac{D}{H} \times V = \dfrac{\overset{2}{\cancel{200}}}{\underset{1}{\cancel{100}}} \times 1 =$
2 tablets

or RP: H : V :: D : X
100 mg : 1 tab :: 200 mg : X
100 X = 200
X = 2 tablets

FE (cross-multiply):

$\dfrac{100}{1} \times \dfrac{200}{X} = 2$ tablets
100 X = 200
X = 2

or DA: No conversion factor

Tablet(s) $= \dfrac{1 \times \overset{2}{\cancel{200}}}{\underset{1}{\cancel{100}} \times 1} = 2$ tablets

b. Daily: RP: H : V :: D : X
100 mg : 1 tab :: 50 mg : X
100 X = 50
X = ½ tablet

or DA: No conversion factor

Tablet(s) $= \dfrac{1\ \text{tab} \times \overset{1}{\cancel{50\ \text{mg}}}}{\underset{2}{\cancel{100\ \text{mg}}} \times 1} = \text{½ tablet}$

2. 4 tablets
3. a. 2 tablets × 3 doses per day × 7 days = 42 tablets
   b. 2 tablets every 8 hours

4. BF: $\dfrac{D}{H} \times V = \dfrac{100}{\underset{25}{\cancel{125}}} \times \overset{1}{\cancel{5}} = \dfrac{100}{25} = 4$ ml

or RP: H : V :: D : X
125 : 5 :: 100 : X
125 X = 500
X $= \dfrac{500}{125} = 4$ ml

$$\text{DA: ml} = \frac{5 \text{ ml} \times \overset{4}{\cancel{100}} \text{ mg}}{\underset{5}{\cancel{125}} \text{ mg} \times 1} = \frac{20}{5} = 4 \text{ ml}$$

5. a. The nurse could *not* use either of the Dilantins.

   b. A capsule *cannot* be cut in half. The physician should be notified. Dilantin dose should be changed.

6. BF: $\dfrac{D}{H} \times V = \dfrac{150}{\underset{50}{\cancel{250}}} \times \overset{1}{\cancel{5}}$

              $\dfrac{150}{50} = 3 \text{ ml}$

or RP: H :V :: D :X
          250:5 :: 150:X
          250 X = 750
             X = 3 ml

7. a. BF: $\dfrac{D}{H} \times V = \dfrac{0.5}{0.25}$

      $0.25\overline{)0.50} = 2 \text{ tablets}$

or RP: H : V :: D : X
   0.25:1 tablet :: 0.5:X tablets
        0.25 X = 0.5
          X = 2 tablets

   b. 2 mg

8. a. Cardizem SR 60 mg

   b. 2 SR capsules per dose

9. Change grams to milligrams by moving the decimal three spaces to the right (see Chapter 1, Metric System).

$$0.2 \text{ g} = 0.\underset{\smile}{200} \text{ mg (200 mg)}$$

BF: $\dfrac{D}{H} \times V = \dfrac{200}{400} \times 1 \text{ tablet}$

           $= \dfrac{200}{400} = \frac{1}{2} \text{ tablet}$

or RP: H : V :: D : X
  400 mg:1 tablet :: 200 mg:X tablet
         400 X = 200
         X = $\dfrac{200}{400} = 0.5$ or $\frac{1}{2}$ tablet

or DA: With conversion factor

$$\text{Tablets} = \frac{1 \text{ tab} \times \overset{10}{\cancel{1000}} \text{ mg} \times 0.2 \cancel{g}}{\underset{4}{\cancel{400}} \text{ mg} \times 1 \cancel{g} \times 1} = \frac{2.0}{4} = \frac{1}{2} \text{ tablet}$$

10. Change grains to milligrams (see Chapter 2 or Table 5-1): 1 gr = 60 mg.

BF: $\dfrac{D}{H} \times V = \dfrac{60}{30} \times 1$

          $= \dfrac{60}{30} = 2 \text{ tablets}$

or RP: H : V :: D : X
  30 mg:1 tablet :: 60 mg:X tablet
         30 X = 60
           X = 2 tablets

11. BF: $\dfrac{D}{H} \times V = \dfrac{75}{125} \times 2$

           $= \dfrac{150}{125} = 1.2 \text{ ml}$

or RP: H :V :: D :X
     125:2 :: 75:X
     125 X = 150
       X = 1.2 ml

  or FE: $\dfrac{125}{2} = \dfrac{75}{X}$

      125 X = 150
        X = 1.2 ml

or DA: No conversion factor needed

$$\text{ml} = \frac{2 \text{ ml} \times \overset{3}{\cancel{75}} \text{ mg}}{\underset{5}{\cancel{125}} \text{ mg} \times 1} = \frac{6}{5} = 1.2 \text{ ml solution}$$

Additional Dimensional Analysis (Factor Labeling)

12. $\text{Tablets} = \dfrac{1 \text{ tablet} \times \overset{2}{\cancel{1000}} \cancel{mg} \times 1.5 \cancel{g}}{\underset{1}{\cancel{500}} \cancel{mg} \times 1 \cancel{g} \times 1} = \dfrac{3.0}{1} = 3 \text{ tablets}$

13. a. 50 mg/kg/day

$50 \times 40 = 2000$ mg

   b. 2000 mg ÷ 4 = 500 mg per dose.

   c. $\text{ml} = \dfrac{5 \text{ ml} \times \overset{2}{\cancel{500}} \cancel{mg}}{\underset{1}{\cancel{250}} \cancel{mg} \times 1} = \dfrac{10}{1} = 10 \text{ ml}$

14. $\text{Tablets} = \dfrac{1 \text{ tablet} \times \overset{10}{\cancel{1000}} \cancel{mg} \times 0.8 \cancel{g}}{\underset{4}{\cancel{400}} \cancel{mg} \times 1 \cancel{g} \times 1} = \dfrac{10 \times 0.8}{4} = \dfrac{8}{4} = 2 \text{ tablets}$

15. $\text{Tablets} = \dfrac{1 \text{ tablet} \times \overset{2}{\cancel{60}} \cancel{mg} \times 1 \cancel{gr}}{\underset{1}{\cancel{30}} \cancel{mg} \times 1 \cancel{gr} \times 1} = 2 \text{ tablets}$

16. $\text{Milliliters} = \dfrac{4 \text{ ml} \times 1 \cancel{g} \times \overset{1}{\cancel{250}} \cancel{mg}}{1 \cancel{g} \times \underset{4}{\cancel{1000}} \cancel{mg} \times 1} = \dfrac{4}{4} = 1 \text{ ml}$

Methods of Calculation for Individualized Drug Dosing

OBJECTIVES

- Calculate the drug dosage needed according to body weight and body surface area (BSA) for clients who are children, clients receiving chemotherapy, and persons with extremity losses.
- Calculate the BSA using the square root.
- Recognize that individuals with extremity losses may need individualized drug dosing.

OUTLINE

CALCULATION FOR INDIVIDUALIZED DRUG DOSING
    Body Weight (BW)
    Body Surface Area (BSA)

CALCULATION FOR INDIVIDUALIZED DRUG DOSING

The two methods for individualizing drug dosing are body weight (BW) and body surface area (BSA).

Body Weight (BW)

Drug dosing by actual body weight is the primary way medication is individualized for adults and children. Manufacturers supply dosing information in the package insert. The insert data provide the dosage based on the patient's weight in kilograms (kg). The first step is to convert pounds to kilograms (if necessary). The second step is to determine the drug dose per body weight by multiplying drug dose × body weight (BW) × frequency (day or per day in divided doses). The third step is to choose one of the four methods of drug calculation for the amount of drug to be given.

EXAMPLES

PROBLEM 1: Order: fluorouracil (5-FU), 12 mg/kg/day IV, not to exceed 800 mg/day. The adult weighs 140 pounds.

a. Convert pounds to kilograms. Divide number of pounds by 2.2.
   Remember: 1 kg = 2.2 lb

$$140 \div 2.2 = 64 \text{ kg}$$

b. Dosage/BW: mg × kg × 1 day =
   12 × 64 × 1 = 768 mg IV per day

Answer: fluorouracil (5-FU), 12 mg/kg/day = 768 mg or 750 to 800 mg

PROBLEM 2: Give cefaclor (Ceclor), 20 mg/kg/day in three divided doses. The child weighs 20 pounds.
Drug available:

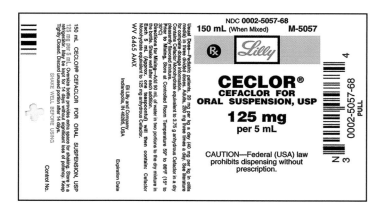

a. Convert pounds to kilograms

$$20 \div 2.2 = 9 \text{ kg}$$

b. Dosage/BW: 20 mg × 9 kg × 1 day = 180 mg per day.

180 mg ÷ 3 divided doses = 60 mg

BF: $\dfrac{D}{H} \times V = \dfrac{60}{125} \times 5$ or RP: H : V :: D : X   or FE: $\dfrac{125}{5} = \dfrac{60}{X}$

$= \dfrac{300}{125} = 2.4$ ml

125 : 5 :: 60 : X

125 X = 300

X = 2.4 ml

125 X = 300

X = 2.4 ml

or DA: ml $= \dfrac{\overset{1}{\cancel{5}} \text{ ml} \times \overset{12}{\cancel{60}} \text{ mg}}{\underset{\underset{5}{25}}{\cancel{125}} \text{ mg} \times 1} = \dfrac{12}{5} = 2.4$ ml

Answer: cefacelor (Ceclor) 20 mg/kg/day = 2.4 ml per dose three times per day

Drug dosing by ideal body weight (IBW) or lean body mass (LBM) is used for medication that is poorly absorbed and distributed throughout the body fat.
IBW Formula
Male: 50 kg + 2.5 kg for each inch over 5 feet
Female: 45.5 kg + 2.3 kg for each inch over 5 feet

EXAMPLE

Female is 5'2"

IBW is 45.5 kg + 2(2.3 kg) = 45.5 kg + 4.6 kg = 50.1 kg

Adjusted body weight is used for dosing some medication for obese individuals or pregnant women.

Adjusted Body Weight Formula
IBW + 0.3 (Actual Body Weight − IBW) = Adjusted Body Weight (Male)
IBW + 0.2 (Actual Body Weight − IBW) = Adjusted Body Weight (Female)

EXAMPLE

Female is 5'2" and weighs 100.5 kg

50.1 kg + 0.2(100.5 kg × 50.1 kg) =
50.1 + 0.2(100.5 − 50.1) =
50.1 + 0.2(50.4) =
50.1 kg + 10.08 kg = 60.09 kg

Body Surface Area

Body surface area is an estimated mathematical function of height and weight. BSA is considered to be the most accurate way to calculate drug dosages since the correct dosage is more proportional to the surface area. BSA is commonly used in chemotherapy and some drug dosages for infants and children.

The BSA inches and pounds formula is:

$$\text{BSA} = \sqrt{\dfrac{\text{ht(in)} \times \text{wt(lb)}}{3131}}$$

BSA with the Square Root

BSA can be calculated by using the square root and a fractional formula of height and weight divided by a constant, one for the metric system and another for inches and pounds. Now that calculators are readily available, research has shown that this method results in fewer errors than drawing intersecting lines on a nomogram. Conversion of weight and height to the same system of measure is necessary first.

The BSA metric formula is:

$$BSA = \sqrt{\frac{ht(cm) \times wt(kg)}{3600}}$$

EXAMPLES

PROBLEM 1: Order: cisplatin (Platinol) 50 mg/m²/cycle IV. Client weighs 84.5 kg and is 168 cm tall. Use the BSA metric formula.

a. $BSA = \sqrt{\dfrac{168 \text{ cm} \times 84.5 \text{ kg}}{3600}}$

$BSA = \sqrt{\dfrac{14196}{3600}}$

$BSA = \sqrt{3.94}$
$BSA = 1.98 \text{ m}^2$

b. 50 mg × 1.98 m² = 99 mg/m², or 100 mg/m²

PROBLEM 2: Order: melphalon (Alkeran) 16 mg/m² q 2 weeks. Client is 68 inches tall and weighs 172 pounds. Use the BSA inches and pounds formula.

a. $BSA = \sqrt{\dfrac{68 \text{ in} \times 172 \text{ lb}}{3131}}$

$BSA = \sqrt{\dfrac{11696}{3131}}$

$BSA = \sqrt{3.73}$
$BSA = 1.9 \text{ m}^2$

b. 16 mg × 1.9 m² = 30.4 mg/m² or 30 mg/m²

BSA with a Nomogram

The BSA in square meters (m²) is determined by the person's height and weight and where these points intersect on the nomogram scale (Figs. 6-1 and 6-2). The nomogram charts were developed from the square root formulas and correlated with heights and weights to simplify drug dosing before calculators were readily available. When a nomogram is used, points on the scale must be carefully plotted. An error in plotting points or drawing intersecting lines can lead to reading the incorrect BSA, resulting in dosing errors.

To calculate the dosage by BSA, multiply the drug dose × m², e.g., 100 mg × 1.6 m² = 160 mg/m². The advantage of using the nomogram is that no conversions from pounds to kilograms or inches to centimeters are needed.

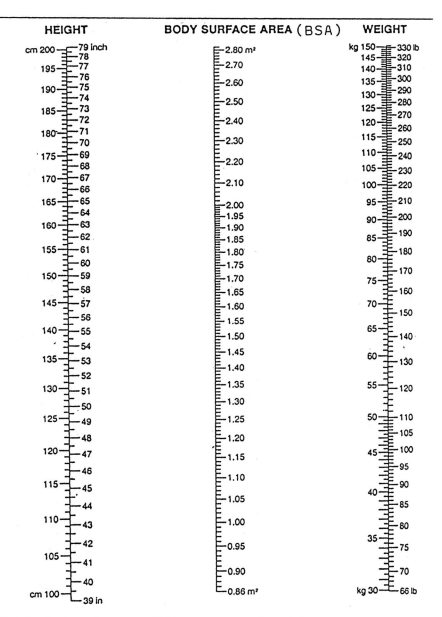

FIGURE 6-1 Body surface area (BSA) nomogram for adults. *Directions:* (1) find height; (2) find weight; (3) draw a straight line connecting the height and weight. Where the line intersects on the BSA column is the body surface area (m²). (From Deglin, J. H., Vallerand, A. H., Russin, M. M. [1991]. *Davis's Drug Guide for Nurses,* 2nd ed. Philadelphia: F. A. Davis, p. 1218. Used with permission from Lentner C. [ed.]. [1991]. *Geigy Scientific Tables,* 8th ed., Vol. 1. Basel, Switzerland: Ciba-Geigy, pp. 226-227.)

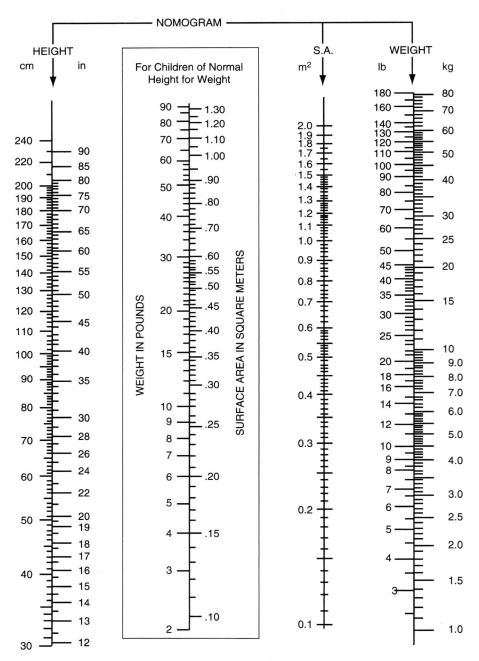

FIGURE 6-2 West nomogram for infants and children. *Directions:* (1) find height; (2) find weight; (3) draw a straight line connecting the height and weight. Where the line intersects on the SA column is the body surface area (m²). (Modified from data of E. Boyd and C. D. West, in Behrman, R. E., Kliegman, R. M., and Jenson H.B. [2000]. *Nelson Textbook of Pediatrics,* 16th ed. Philadelphia: W. B. Saunders.)

EXAMPLES   PROBLEM 1: Order: cyclophosphamide (Cytoxan) 100 mg/m²/day, po. Client weighs 150 pounds and is 5'8" (68 inches) tall.
a. 68 inches and 150 pounds intersect the nomogram scale at 1.88 m² (BSA).
b. BSA: 100 mg × 1.9 m² = 190 mg/m²/day of Cytoxan.

$$1.88 \text{ m}^2 = 188 \text{ mg/m}^2/\text{day or } 190 \text{ mg/m}^2/\text{day}$$

PROBLEM 2: Order: cytarabine (cytosine arabinoside) 200 mg/m²/day IV × 5 days for a client with myelocytic leukemia. The client is 64 inches tall and weighs 130 pounds.
a. 64 inches and 130 pounds intersect the nomogram scale at 1.69 m² (BSA), or 1.7 m² (BSA) rounded off to the nearest tenth.
b. BSA: 200 mg × 1.69 m² = 340 mg/m² IV daily for 5 days.

$$1.69 \text{ m}^2 = 338 \text{ mg/m}^2 \text{ or } 340 \text{ mg/m}^2$$

SUMMARY PRACTICE PROBLEMS

1. Order: sulfisoxazole (Gantrisin) 50 mg/kg daily in 4 divided doses (q6h). Client weighs 44 pounds.

   How many milligrams should the client receive per dose? _____

2. Order: azithromycin (Zithromax), po. First day: 10 mg/kg/d; next 4 days: 5 mg/kg/d. Client weighs 44 pounds.
   Drug available:

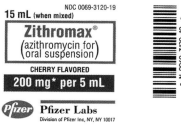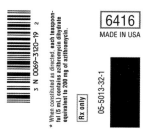

   a. How much does the child weigh in kilograms? _____

   b. How many milliliters should the child receive for the first

      day? _____

   c. How many milliliters should the child receive each day for the next

      4 days (second to fifth days)? _____

3. Order: ticarcillin disodium (Ticar), 200 mg/kg/d in 4 divided doses, IV. Client weighs 176 pounds.
   Max dose: 40 q/d.

Drug available:

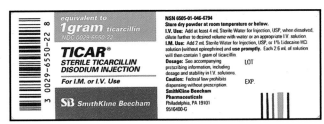

a. How many kilograms does the client weigh? _____

b. How many milligrams per day _____ mg/d; and how many milligrams per dose? _____ mg, q6h; or how many grams per dose? _____ g, q6h.

4. Order: kanamycin (Kantrex) 15 mg/kg/day in 3 divided doses (q8h), IV. Drug is to be diluted in 100 mg of D₅W. The client weighs 180 pounds. Drug available:

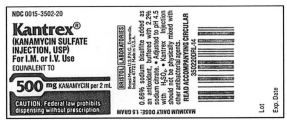

a. How many milligrams should the client receive per day? _____

b. How many milligrams should the client receive per dose? _____

c. How many milliliters should the client receive per dose? _____

5. Order: sulfisoxazole (Gantrisin) 2 g/m² daily in 4 divided doses (q6h). The client weighs 110 pounds and is 60 inches tall.

How many milligrams should the client receive per dose? _____

6. Order: doxorubicin (Adriamycin) 60 mg/m² IV per month. Client weighs 120 pounds and is 5'2" (62 inches) tall.

How many milligrams should the client receive? _____

7. Order: etoposide (VePesid) 100 mg/m²/d × 5 days. Client weighs 180 pounds and is 70 inches tall.
Drug available:

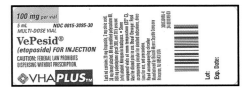

    a. What is the BSA? _____

    b. How many milligrams should the client receive? _____

    c. How many milliliters are needed? _____

BSA by Square Root

8. Order: vinblastine sulfate (Velban) 7.4 mg/m² IV × 1. Client's height is 115 cm and weight is 52 kg. Use the BSA metric formula to determine dosage. Drug available:

How many milligrams should the client receive? _____

9. Order: etoposide (VePesid) 50 mg/m² day IV. Client's height is 72 inches and weight is 190 pounds.

How many milligrams should the client receive? _____

10. Patient with advanced colorectal cancer
Order: Fluorouracil 250 mg/m²/day × 7 days
Patient's height and weight: 6'2", 218 lb

    a. What is patient's BSA m²? _____ (use square root)

    b. What is the daily dose? _____

    c. What is the total dosage for 7 days? _____

11. Order: Docetaxel 60 mg/m²/dose in 200 ml of normal saline solution over 60 minutes. Patient's height and weight: 5'8", 136 lb

    a. What is patient's BSA m²? _____

    b. What is the total dosage of docetaxel? _____

    c. What is the concentration per milliliter? _____

12. Order: Gemcitabine 800 mg/m²/dose in 100 ml of normal saline solution over 30 minutes. Patient's height and weight: 6'6", 150 lb
Drug available: 1 gm/25 ml

    a. What is patient's BSA in square meters? _____

    b. What is the total dose of gemcitabine? _____

    c. How many milliliters should you prepare? _____

13. Order: Liposome doxorubicin 20 mg/m² in 250 ml D₅W IV over 30 minutes. Patient's height and weight: 6', 129 lb
Drug available: Doxorubicin 20 mg/10 ml

    a. What is patient's BSA in square meters? _____

    b. What is the total dose of doxorubicin? _____

    c. How many milliliters should you prepare? _____

14. Order: Irinotecan 60 mg/m² in 500 ml D5 ½ NS IV over 90 minutes. Patient's height and weight: 6', 202 lb
Drug available: Irinotecan 20 mg/ml

    a. What is patient's BSA in square meters? _____

    b. What is the total dose of irinotecan? _____

    c. How many milliliters should you prepare? _____

15. Order: Cisplatin 80 mg/m² in 500 ml normal saline solution over 90 minutes. Patient's height and weight: 6', 200 lb
Drug available: Cisplatin 1 mg/ml

    a. What is patient's BSA in square meters? _____

    b. What is the total dose of cisplatin? _____

16. Order: Adriamycin 50 mg/m² in 3 individual doses mixed with 1000 ml normal saline solution per dose continuous infusion over 24 hr. Patient's height and weight: 5'8", 139 lb
Drug available: Adriamycin 10 mg/5 ml

    a. What is patient's BSA in square meters? _____

    b. What is the total dosage? _____

    c. What is the divided dose? _____

ANSWERS SUMMARY PRACTICE PROBLEMS

1. Change 44 pounds to kilograms: 44 ÷ 2.2 = 20 kg
   50 mg × 20 kg × 1 day = 1000 mg of Gantrisin per day
   1000 mg ÷ 4 times per day (q6h) = 250 mg q6h
2. a. 20 kg
   b. First day: 10 mg × 20 kg = 200 mg

$$BF: \frac{D}{H} \times V = \frac{\overset{1}{\cancel{200}} \text{ mg}}{\underset{1}{\cancel{200}} \text{ mg}} \times 5 \text{ ml} = 5 \text{ ml} \quad \textbf{or} \quad RP:$$

   H : V :: D : X
   200 mg : 5 ml :: 200 mg : X
   200 X = 1000
   X = 5 ml

or DA: ml = $\dfrac{5\ ml \times \overset{1}{\cancel{200}}\ mg}{\underset{1}{\cancel{200}}\ mg \times 1}$ = 5 ml

First day give 5 ml

  c. Second to fifth days (next 4 days): 5 mg × 20 kg = 100 mg
  Give 2.5 ml/d. Same answer worked out by BF, RP, and DA

3. **a.** Client weighs 80 kg
   b. 200 mg × 80 = 16,000 mg per day; 4000 mg per dose or 4 g per dose (q6h)

4. Change 180 pounds to kilograms: 180 ÷ 2.2 = 81.8 kg
   a. 15 mg × 82 kg = 1230 mg per day
   b. 1230 ÷ 3 times a day (q8h) = 410 mg (400 mg, q8h)

   c. BF: $\dfrac{D}{H} \times V = \dfrac{400}{500} \times 2$ **or** RP: H : V :: D : X

   $= \dfrac{800}{500} = 1.6$ ml   500 mg : 2 ml :: 400 mg : X ml
   500 X = 800
   X = 1.6 ml

   Give kanamycin 1.6 ml

5. 60 inches and 110 pounds intersect the nomogram scale at 1.5 m².
   BSA: 2 g × 1.5 m² = 3 g or 3000 mg per day
   3000 mg ÷ 4 times per day = 750 mg

6. 62 inches and 120 pounds intersect the nomogram scale at 1.6 m².
   BSA: 60 mg × 1.6 m² = 96 mg of Adriamycin

7. **a.** With the use of the nomogram, the BSA is 2.06
   b. 100 mg × 2.06 = 206 mg or 200 mg.
   c. The amount of VePesid administered should be 10 ml

   BF: $\dfrac{D}{H} \times V = \dfrac{200}{100} \times 5 = 10$ ml   **or**   RP: 100 mg : 5 ml :: 200 mg : X

   100 X = 1000
   X = 10 ml

   or DA: ml = $\dfrac{5\ ml \times \overset{2}{\cancel{200}}\ mg}{\underset{1}{\cancel{100}}\ mg \times 1}$ = 10 ml

BSA by Square Root

8. **a.** BSA = $\sqrt{\dfrac{115\ cm \times 52\ kg}{3600}}$

   BSA = $\sqrt{\dfrac{5980}{3600}}$

   BSA = $\sqrt{1.66}$

   BSA = 1.28 m²

   b. 7.4 mg × 1.28 m² = 9.4 mg/m²

9. a. $\text{BSA} = \sqrt{\dfrac{72 \text{ in} \times 190 \text{ lb}}{3131}}$

$\text{BSA} = \sqrt{\dfrac{13680}{3131}}$

$\text{BSA} = \sqrt{4.36}$

$\text{BSA} = 2.0 \text{ m}^2$

b. $50 \text{ mg} \times 2.0 \text{ m}^2 = 100 \text{ mg/m}^2$

10. a. $\sqrt{\dfrac{74 \times 218}{3131}} = 2.26 \text{ m}^2$

b. $250 \text{ mg} \times 2.26 \text{ m}^2 = 565 \text{ mg/m}^2$

c. $565 \text{ mg} \times 7 = 3955 \text{ mg}$

11. a. $\sqrt{\dfrac{68 \times 136}{3131}} = 1.7 \text{ m}^2$

b. $60 \text{ mg} \times 1.7 \text{ m}^2 = 102 \text{ mg/m}^2$

12. a. $\sqrt{\dfrac{78 \times 150}{3131}} = 1.9 \text{ m}^2$

b. $800 \text{ mg} \times 1.9 \text{ m}^2 = 1520 \text{ mg/m}^2$

c. BF: $\dfrac{D}{H} \times V = \dfrac{1520 \text{ mg}}{1000 \text{ mg}} \times \dfrac{25 \text{ ml}}{1} = \dfrac{38000}{1000} = 38 \text{ ml}$

RP: $1000 \text{ mg} : 25 \text{ ml} :: 1520 \text{ mg} : X$

$1000 X = 38000$

$X = 38 \text{ ml}$

DA: $\text{ml} = \dfrac{25 \text{ ml} \times 1520 \text{ m\!\!/g}}{1000 \text{ m\!\!/g} \times 1} = 38 \text{ ml}$

13. a. $\sqrt{\dfrac{71 \times 129}{3131}} = 1.72 \text{ m}^2$

b. $20 \text{ mg} \times 1.72 \text{ m}^2 = 34 \text{ mg}$

c. BF: $\dfrac{D}{H} \times V = \dfrac{34 \text{ mg}}{20 \text{ mg}} \times 10 \text{ ml} = \dfrac{340}{20} = 17 \text{ ml}$

RP: $20 \text{ mg} : 10 \text{ ml} :: 34 \text{ mg} : X$

$20 X = 340$

$X = 17 \text{ ml}$

DA: $\text{ml} = \dfrac{10 \text{ ml} \times 34 \text{ m\!\!/g}}{20 \text{ m\!\!/g} \times 1} = 17 \text{ ml}$

14. **a.** $\sqrt{\dfrac{72 \times 202}{3131}} = 2.15$ m²

   b. 60 mg $\times$ 2.15 m² = 129 mg or 130 mg/m²

   c. BF: $\dfrac{D}{H} \times V = \dfrac{130 \text{ mg}}{20 \text{ mg}} \times 1$ ml $= \dfrac{130}{20} = 6.5$ ml

   RP: 20 mg:1 ml :: 130 mg:X
   $\qquad\qquad$ 20 X = 130
   $\qquad\qquad\quad$ X = 6.5 ml

   DA: ml $= \dfrac{1 \text{ ml} \times 130 \text{ mg}}{20 \text{ mg} \times 1} = 6.5$ ml

15. **a.** $\sqrt{\dfrac{72 \times 200}{3131}} = 2.14$ m²

   b. 80 mg $\times$ 2.14 m² = 171 mg or 170 mg/m²

16. **a.** $\sqrt{\dfrac{68 \times 193}{3131}} = 1.73$ m²

   b. 50 mg $\times$ 1.73 m² = 86.5 mg/m²
   c. 86.5 mg/3 doses = 28.8 mg

PART III

CALCULATIONS FOR ORAL, INJECTABLE, AND INTRAVENOUS DRUGS

Oral and Enteral Preparations with Clinical Applications

OBJECTIVES

- State the advantages and disadvantages of administering oral medications.
- Calculate oral dosages from tablets, capsules, and liquids using given formulas.
- Give the rationale for diluting and not diluting oral liquid medications.
- Explain the method for administering sublingual medication.
- Calculate the amount of drug to be given per day in divided doses.
- Determine the amount of tube feeding solution needed for dilution according to the percent ordered.
- Determine the amount of water needed to dilute liquid medication.

OUTLINE

TABLETS AND CAPSULES
  Calculation of Tablets and Capsules
LIQUIDS
  Calculation of Liquid Medications
SUBLINGUAL TABLETS
  Calculation of Sublingual Medications
ENTERAL NUTRITION AND DRUG ADMINISTRATION
  Enteral Feedings
  Enteral Medications

Oral administration of drugs is considered a convenient and economical method of giving medications. Oral drugs are available as tablets, capsules, powders, and liquids. Oral medications are referred to as po (per os, or by mouth) drugs and are absorbed by the gastrointestinal tract, mainly from the small intestine.

There are some disadvantages in administering oral medications, such as (1) variation in absorption rate caused by gastric and intestinal pH and food consumption within the gastrointestinal tract; (2) irritation of the gastric mucosa causing nausea, vomiting, or ulceration (e.g., with oral potassium chloride); (3) retention or inactivation of the drug in the body because of reduced liver function; (4) destruction of drugs by digestive enzymes; (5) aspiration of drugs into the lungs by seriously ill or confused patients; and (6) discoloration of tooth enamel, e.g., with a saturated solution of potassium iodide (SSKI). Oral administration is an effective way to give medications in many instances, and at times it is the route of choice.

Body weight and body surface area are discussed in Chapter 6. When solving drug problems that require body weight or body surface area, refer to Chapter 6.

Enteral nutrition and enteral medication are discussed toward the end of the chapter. Calculations of percent for enteral feeding solutions and enteral medication are also discussed.

TABLETS AND CAPSULES

Most tablets are scored and can be broken in halves and sometimes in quarters (Fig. 7-1). Half of a tablet may be indicated when the drug does not come in a lesser strength. Half-tablets may not be broken equally; therefore, the patient may receive less than or more than the required dose. Also, crushing a drug tablet does not ensure that the patient will receive the entire drug dose. Some of the crushed tablet could be lost. Instead of halving or crushing a drug tablet, use the liquid form of the drug, if available, to ensure proper drug dosage.

Capsules are gelatin shells containing powder or time pellets. Caplets (solid-looking capsules) are hard-shell capsules. Time-release capsules should re-

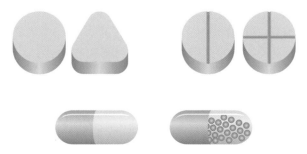

FIGURE 7-1   Shapes of tablets. (From Kee, J., & Hayes, E. [2003]. *Pharmacology: A Nursing Process Approach* [4th ed.]. Philadelphia: W. B. Saunders.)

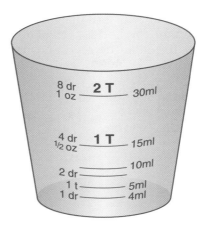

FIGURE 7-2 Medicine cup for liquid measurement. (From Kee, J., & Hayes, E. [2003]. *Pharmacology: A Nursing Process Approach* [4th ed.]. Philadelphia: W. B. Saunders.)

main intact and not be divided in any way. Many drugs that come in capsules also come in liquid form. When a smaller dose is indicated and is not available in tablet or capsule form, the liquid form of the drug is used (Fig. 7-2).

- A tablet that is NOT scored should not be broken. At times when this is necessary, a pill cutter may be used.
- Instead of breaking or crushing a tablet, use the liquid form if available.
- Time-release capsules should not be crushed and diluted, because the entire medication could be absorbed rapidly.
- Enteric-coated tablets must NOT be crushed, because the medication could irritate the stomach. Enteric-coated tablets are absorbed by the small intestine.
- Tablets or capsules that are irritating to the gastric mucosa should be taken with 6 to 8 ounces of fluid, with meals, or immediately after meals.

Calculation of Tablets and Capsules

The following steps should be taken to determine the drug dose:
1. Check the drug order.
2. Determine the drug available (generic name, brand name, and dosage per drug form).
3. Set up the method for drug calculation (basic formula, ratio and proportion, fraction equation, or dimensional analysis).
4. Convert to like units of measurement within the same system before solving the problem. Use the unit of measure on the drug container to calculate the drug dose.
5. Solve for the unknown **(X).**

Decide which of the methods of calculation you wish to use and then use that same method for calculating all dosages. In the following examples, the basic formula, the ratio and proportion, and dimensional analysis methods are used.

Basic Formula (BF)

$$\frac{D \text{ (desired dose)}}{H \text{ (on-hand dose)}} \times V = \text{(vehicle)}$$

Ratio and proportion (RP)

$$H \quad : \quad V \quad :: \quad D \quad : X$$

on hand   vehicle   desired dose   X

Dimensional Analysis (DA)

$$V = \frac{V \times C\ (H) \times D}{H \times C\ (D) \times 1}$$

NOTE: C = conversion factor if needed.

EXAMPLES

PROBLEM 1: Order: pravastatin sodium (Pravachol) 20 mg, qd
Drug available:

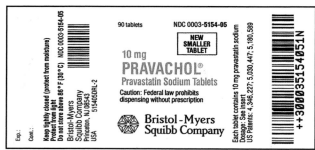

Methods: BF: $\dfrac{D}{H} \times V$

$$\frac{20}{10} \times 1 = 2 \text{ tablets}$$

RP: H : V :: D : X
10 mg : 1 tab :: 20 mg : X tab

$$10\,X = 20$$
$$X = 2 \text{ tablets}$$

DA: no conversion factor

$$\text{tab} = \frac{1 \text{ tab} \times \overset{2}{\cancel{20}} \text{ mg}}{\underset{1}{\cancel{10}} \text{ mg} \times \quad 1} = 2 \text{ tablets}$$

Answer: Pravachol 20 mg = 2 tablets, daily.

PROBLEM 2: Order: erythromycin (ERY-TAB) 0.5 g, qid.
Drug available:

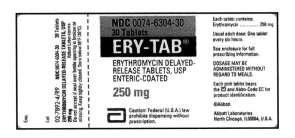

Note: Grams (g) and milligrams (mg) are both units in the metric system. *Remember:* when changing grams (larger unit) to milligrams (smaller unit), move the decimal point three spaces to the right. Refer to Chapter 1, Table 2-1, or Table 5-1. Because the drug dose on the drug label is in milligrams, conversion should be from grams to milligrams.

Methods: 0.5 g = 0.500 mg (Method A)

$$BF: \frac{D}{H} \times V = \frac{500}{250} \times 1 = \frac{500}{250} = 2 \text{ tablets}$$

or

RP: H : V ::   D : X
250 mg:1 tab :: 500 mg:X tab
250 X = 500
X = 2 tablets

or

$$DA: \text{tablet} = \frac{1 \text{ tab} \times \overset{4}{\cancel{1000}} \text{ mg} \times 0.5 \cancel{g}}{\underset{1}{\cancel{250}} \text{ mg} \times 1 \cancel{g} \times 1}$$

$$4 \times 0.5 = 2 \text{ tablets}$$

Answer: ERY-TAB 0.5 g = 2 tablets

PROBLEM 3: Order: aspirin gr x, po, STAT.
Drug available: aspirin 325 mg per tablet.

Note: The dose is ordered in the apothecary system, gr x, and the label on the drug bottle is in the metric system (325 mg). Use Table 2-1 or Table 5-1 to convert units.

Methods: 325 mg = gr v (5) and 650 mg = gr x (10)

$$BF: \frac{D}{H} \times V = \frac{10 \text{ gr}}{5 \text{ gr}} \times 1 = \frac{10}{5} = 2 \text{ tablets}$$

or

RP: H : V :: D : X
5 gr : 1 tab :: 10 gr : X tab

5 X = 10
X = 2 tablets

or

$$\frac{D}{H} \times V = \frac{650 \text{ mg}}{325 \text{ mg}} \times 1 = \frac{650}{325} = 2 \text{ tablets}$$

or

$$\text{DA: tablet} = \frac{1 \text{ tab} \times \overset{3}{\cancel{1000}} \text{ mg} \times \overset{2}{\cancel{10}} \text{ gr}}{\underset{1}{\cancel{325}} \text{ mg} \times \underset{3}{\cancel{15}} \text{ gr} \times 1} = \frac{6}{3} = 2 \text{ tablets}$$

Answer: Aspirin gr x = 2 tablets.

LIQUIDS

Liquid medications come as tinctures, elixirs, suspensions, and syrups. Some liquid medications are irritating to the gastric mucosa and must be well diluted before being given, e.g., potassium chloride (KCl). Usually, liquid cough medicines are not diluted. Medications in tincture form are always diluted.

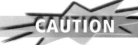

- Concentrated liquid medication that can irritate the gastric mucosa should be diluted in *at least* 6 ounces of fluid.
- Liquid medication that can discolor the teeth *should be well diluted* and taken through a drinking straw.

Calculation of Liquid Medications

EXAMPLES

PROBLEM 1: Order: potassium chloride (KCl) 20 mEq, bid.
Drug available: liquid potassium chloride 10 mEq per 5 ml.

Methods: BF: $\dfrac{D}{H} \times V = \dfrac{20}{10} \times 5 = \dfrac{100}{10} = 10 \text{ ml}$

or

RP: H : V :: D : X
10 mEq : 5 ml :: 20 mEq : X ml
10 X = 100
X = 10 ml

or

DA: no conversion factor

$$ml = \frac{5\ ml \quad \times\ \overset{2}{\cancel{20}}\ mEq}{\underset{1}{\cancel{10}}\ mEq \times \quad 1} = 10\ ml$$

Answer: Potassium chloride 20 mEq = 10 ml

PROBLEM 2: Order: amoxicillin (Amoxil) 0.25 g, po, tid.
Drug available:

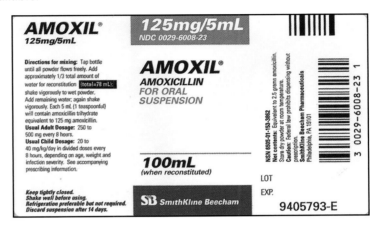

Change grams to milligrams: 0.25 g = 0.250 mg.

Methods: BF: $\dfrac{D}{H} \times V = \dfrac{250}{125} \times 5 = \dfrac{1250}{125} = 10\ ml$

or

RP: H   : V   ::   D   : X
      125 mg : 5 ml :: 250 mg : X ml

125 X = 1250
X = 10 ml

or

DA: $ml = \dfrac{5\ ml \quad \times\ \overset{8}{\cancel{1000}}\ mg \times \overset{1}{\cancel{0.25}}\ g}{\underset{1}{\cancel{125}}\ mg \times \quad \underset{4}{\cancel{1}}\ g \quad \times\ 1} = \dfrac{40}{4} = 10\ ml$

Answer: Amoxil 0.25 g = 10 ml

PROBLEM 3: Give SSKI 300 mg, q6h, diluted in water.
Drug available: saturated solution of potassium iodide, 50 mg per drop (gt), drops (gtt).

Methods: BF: $\dfrac{D}{H} \times V = \dfrac{300}{50} \times 1 = \dfrac{300}{50} = 6\ gtt$

or

RP: H : V ::   D : X
50 mg : 1 gt :: 300 mg : X gtt
50 X = 300
X = 6 gtt

or

$$\text{DA: gtt} = \frac{1 \text{ gt} \times \overset{6}{\cancel{300}} \text{ mg}}{\underset{1}{\cancel{50}} \text{ mg} \times 1} = 6 \text{ gtt}$$

Answer: SSKI 300 mg = 6 gtt (drops)

SUBLINGUAL TABLETS

Few drugs are administered sublingually (tablet placed under the tongue). Sublingual tablets are small and soluble and are quickly absorbed by the numerous capillaries on the underside of the tongue.

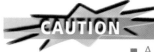

■ A sublingual tablet, e.g., nitroglycerin (NTG), should not be swallowed. If the drug is swallowed, the desired immediate action of the drug is decreased or lost.
■ Fluids *should not* be taken until the drug has dissolved.

Calculation of Sublingual Medications

EXAMPLES   PROBLEM 1: Order: nitroglycerin (Nitrostat) 0.6 mg, sublingually (SL). Drug available:

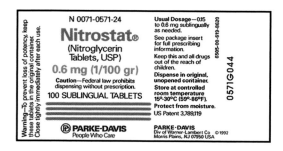

Note: The systems and weights must be the same. See Table 2-1 or Table 5-1. The label has both systems of measurement.

$$0.6 \text{ mg} = \text{gr } \frac{1}{100}$$

Methods: $\text{BF: } \dfrac{D}{H} \times V = \dfrac{0.6}{0.6} \times 1 = \dfrac{0.6}{0.6} = 1 \text{ SL tablet}$

or

RP: H : V ::   D : X

$$\frac{1}{100} \text{ gr} : 1 \text{ tab} :: \frac{1}{100} \text{ gr} : X \text{ tab}$$

$$\frac{1}{100} X = \frac{1}{100}$$

$$X = \frac{1}{100} \times \frac{100}{1} = 1 \text{ SL tablet}$$

or

DA: no conversion factor

$$\text{SL tab} = \frac{1 \text{ tab} \times \overset{1}{\cancel{0.6 \text{ mg}}}}{\underset{1}{\cancel{0.6 \text{ mg}}} \times 1} = 1 \text{ SL tablet}$$

Answer: nitroglycerin (Nitrostat) 0.6 mg = 1 SL tablet

PROBLEM 2: Order: isosorbide dinitrate (Isordil) 5 mg sublingually.
Drug available: Isordil 2.5 mg per tablet.

Methods: BF: $\dfrac{D}{H} \times V = \dfrac{5}{2.5} \times 1 = 2$ SL tablets

or

RP: H : V :: D : X
    2.5 mg : 1 tab :: 5 mg : X tab
          2.5 X = 5
               X = 2 SL tablets

or

DA: no conversion factor

$$\text{SL tablet} = \frac{1 \text{ SL tab} \times \overset{2}{\cancel{5 \text{ mg}}}}{\underset{1}{\cancel{2.5 \text{ mg}}} \times 1} = 2 \text{ SL tablets}$$

Answer: Isordil 5 mg = 2 SL tablets

PRACTICE PROBLEMS I **Oral Medications**

Answers can be found on page 139.

For each question, calculate the correct dosage that should be administered.

1. Order: doxycycline hyclate (Vibra-Tabs) 50 mg, po, q12h
   Drug available:

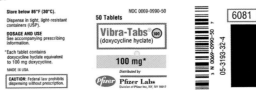

a. How many tablets(s) would you give for each dose? _____

2. Order: sulfisoxazole (Gantrisin) 0.5 g.
Drug available: Gantrisin 250 mg per tablet.

3. Order: digoxin (Lanoxin) 0.5 mg.
Drug available:

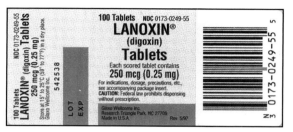

4. Order: codeine gr 1, prn, q4h.
Drug available:

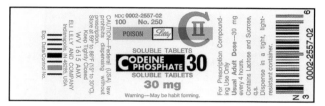

5. Order: potassium chloride 40 mEq, po.
Drug available: potassium chloride 20 mEq/15 ml.

6. Order: Cefaclor (Ceclor) 250 mg, q8h.
Drug available:

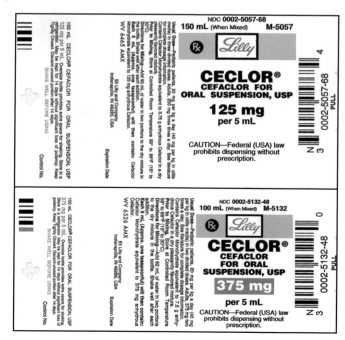

a. Which Ceclor bottle would you select? Why? _____

b. How many milliliters per dose should the patient receive? _____

7. Order: ProSom (estazolam) 2 mg, po, hs.
Drug available: 1 mg tablet

a. How many tablet(s) should be given?_____

b. What time of day would you administer ProSom? _____

8. Order: cefuroxime axetil (Ceftin) 400 mg, q12h.
Drug available:

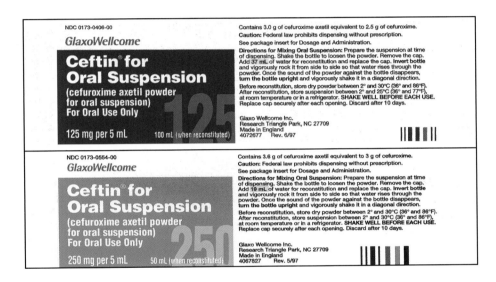

a. How many milliliters should the client receive?_____

b. Which drug bottle would you use? _____

Why? _____

9. Order: Dicloxacillin (Dynapen) 100 mg, q6h.
Drug available:

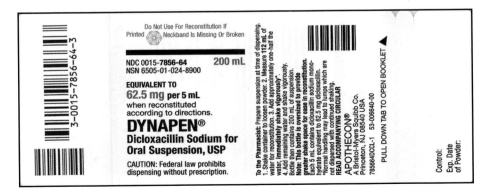

How many milliliters should the client receive? _____

10. Order: HydroDiuril 50 mg, po, qd.
Drug available:

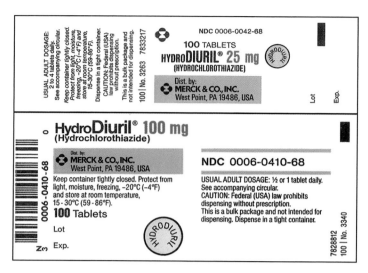

   a. Which drug bottle would you use? _____

   b. How many tablet(s) would you give, if the tablet(s) are not

       scored? _____

       Explain. _____

11. Order: simvastatin (Zocor) 30 mg, qd.
Drug available:

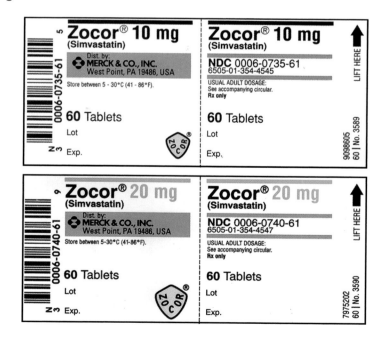

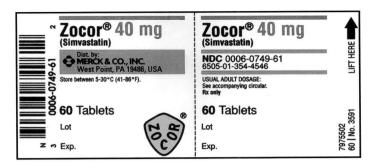

a. Which bottle(s) of Zocor would you select? Why?

_____

b. How many tablet(s) should the client receive? _____

12. Order: cefadroxil (Duricef) 0.4 g, po, q6h.
    Drug available:

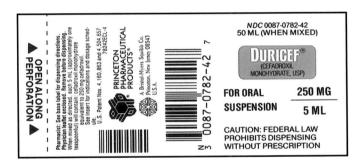

How many milliliters should the client receive per dose? _____

13. Order: phenobarbital gr ss.
    Drug available: phenobarbital 15 mg per tablet.

    How many tablet(s) should the client receive? _____

14. Order: cefprozil (Cefzil) 100 mg, po, q12h.
    Drug available:

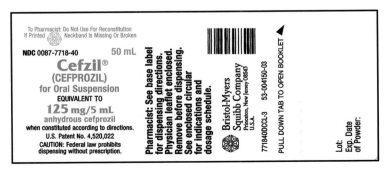

How many milliliters should the client receive per dose? _____

15. Order: rofecoxib (Vioxx) 25 mg, po, qd, prn, for pain.
Drug available:

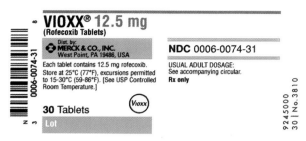

How many tablet(s) of Vioxx would you give? _____

16. Order: nitroglycerin gr $\frac{1}{150}$, SL, STAT.
Drug available:

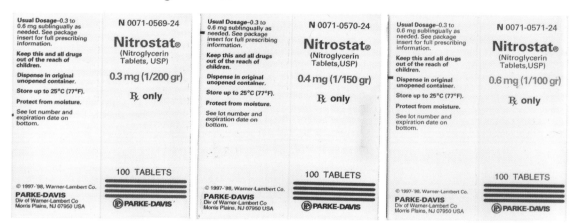

Which Nitrostat SL tablet would you give? (Refer to Table 2-1 or Table 5-1 if

necessary.) _____

17. Order: Mycostatin 250,000 U oral swish and swallow, qid.
Drug available:

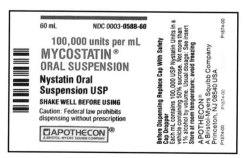

Calculate the correct dosage. _____

18. Order: diazepam (Valium) 2½ mg.
Drug available: Valium 5 mg scored tablet.
Calculate the correct dosage. _____

19. Order: ondansetron HCl (Zofran) 6 mg, 30 min before chemotherapy, then q8h × 2 more doses.
Drug available:

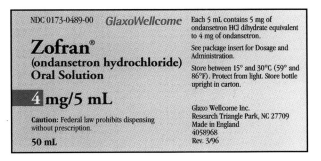

How many milliliters would you give per dose?

_____

20. Order: allopurinol 450 mg, po, qd.
Drug available: allopurinol 300 mg scored tablet.
Calculate the correct dosage.

21. Order: cefadroxil (Duricef) 1 g, po, as a loading dose; then cefadroxil 0.5 g, po, q12h.
Drug available:

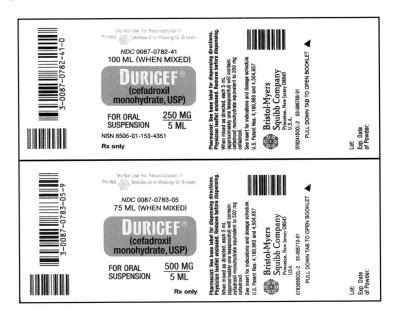

a. Which drug bottle would you select? _____

b. How many milliliters would you give as the loading dose?

_____

c. How many milliliters per 0.5 g? _____

22. Order: amoxicillin/clavulanate potassium (Augmentin) 0.5 g, po, q8h.
Drug available:

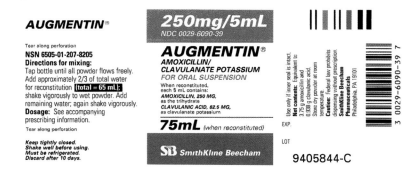

How many milliliters should the client receive per dose? _____

Questions 23-27 relate to additional dimensional analysis (factor labeling). Refer to Chapter 5 as necessary.

23. Order: methyldopa (Aldomet) 0.5 g, po, qd.
Drug available: drug label: _____ mg = _____ tablet.

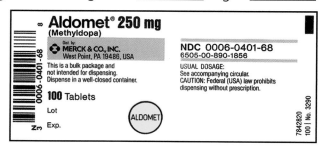

Factors: 250 mg = 1 tablet (drug label)
           0.5 g/1 (drug order)
Conversion factors: 1 g = 1000 mg

How many tablet(s) of methyldopa 250 mg would you give? _____

24. Order: Vasotec 5 mg, po, bid.
Drug available:

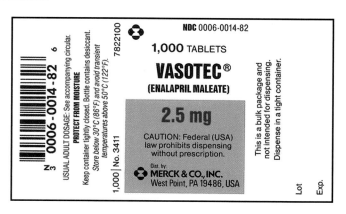

Factors: 2.5 mg = 1 tablet (drug label); 5 mg/1 (drug order)
Conversion factor: none

How many tablet(s) should the client receive? _____

25. Order: amoxicillin (Amoxil) 0.4 g, po, q6h.
    Drug available:

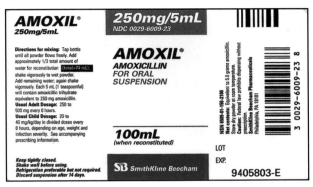

Factors: 250 mg/5 mL (drug label); 0.4 g/1 (drug order)
Conversion factor: 1 g = 1000 mg

How many milliliters would you give? _____

26. Order: acetaminophen (Tylenol) gr x, po.
    Drug available:

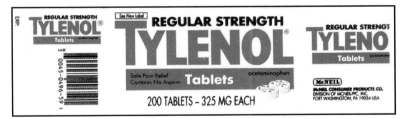

Factors: _____

Conversion factor: _____

How many acetaminophen tablets would you give? _____

27. Order: oxacillin sodium 125 mg, po, q6h.
    Drug available:

How many milliliters would you give? _____

Questions 28-32 relate to body weight and body surface area. Refer to Chapter 6 as necessary.

28. Order: valproic acid (Depakene) 10 mg/kg/day in three divided doses (tid), po. Client weighs 165 pounds. How much Depakene should be administered

tid? _____

29. Order: cyclophosphamide (Cytoxan) 4 mg/kg/day, po. Client weighs 154 pounds. How much Cytoxan would you give per day?

_____

30. Order: mercaptopurine 2.5 mg/kg/day po or 100 mg/m² body surface area po. The client weighs 132 pounds and is 64 inches tall. The estimated body surface area according to the nomogram is 1.7 m². The amount of drug the

client should receive according to body weight is _____ and according

to body surface area is _____.

31. Order: ethosuximide (Zarontin) 20 mg/kg/day in 2 divided doses (q12h). Client weighs 110 pounds (110 ÷ 2.2 = 50 kg). Drug available:

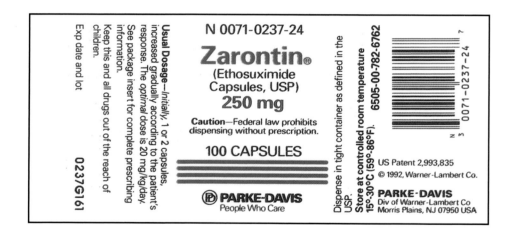

a. How many milligrams should the client receive per day? _____

b. How many tablet(s) should the client receive per dose? _____

32. Order: minocycline HCl (Minocin) 4 mg/kg/day in 2 divided doses (q12h). Client weighs 132 pounds (132 ÷ 2.2 = 60 kg). Drug available: Minocin 50 mg/5 ml.

a. How many milligrams should the client receive per day?_____

b. How many milliliters should the client receive per dose? _____

Additional practice problems for "Oral Dosage" are available on the CD-ROM in the "Calculating Doses" section.

ENTERAL NUTRITION AND DRUG ADMINISTRATION

When the client is unable to take nourishment by mouth, enteral feeding (tube feeding) is usually preferred over intravenous therapy. Candidates for enteral feedings are clients with neurological deficits who have difficulty swallowing; debilitated clients; clients with burns and malnutrition disorders; clients with upper gastric obstructions; and clients who have undergone radical head and neck surgery. The cost of enteral feedings is much less than that of intravenous therapy and there is less risk of infection.

Drugs that can be administered orally can be given via enteral tube. The drug must be in liquid form or dissolved into a liquid. Medications in time-release, enteric-coated, or sublingual form and bulk-forming laxatives can not be administered enterally.

Enteral Feedings

Enteral feeding can be administered through a tube inserted into the nose (nasogastric), mouth (orogastric), stomach (gastrostomy), or jejunum (jejunostomy) (Fig. 7-3). The nasogastric and orogastric routes are primarily for short-term use and cause nasal and pharyngeal irritation if use is prolonged. The gastrostomy and jejunostomy routes are for long-term feeding and require a surgical procedure for insertion of the tube.

Enteral feedings may be given as a bolus (intermittent) or as a continuous drip feeding over a specified period. With bolus feedings, the amount of solution administered is approximately 200 ml or less, and feeding times per day are more frequent. Continuous feedings can be given by gravity flow from a bag or by infusion pump (Fig. 7-4).

There are many types of enteral feeding solutions designed to meet the nutritional needs of clients. Names of common feeding solutions are listed in Table 7-1

Although enteral feeding solutions are formulated to be given full strength, this strength may not be tolerated. Solutions that are highly concentrated (hyperosmolar or hypertonic) when given in full strength can cause vomiting, cramping, or excessive diarrhea. When gastrointestinal symptoms occur, the enteral solution can be diluted with water. In many situations, clients have better gastrointestinal tolerance when the strength of the solution is gradually increased. However, in adults, the tube feeding may be

Table 7-1		
Common Enteral Formulations		
Ensure	Isocal	Nepho
Ensure Plus	Sustacal	Ultracal
Ensure HN	Sustacal HC	Jevity
Osmolite	Vital	Criticare
Osmolite HN	Pulmocare	Promote

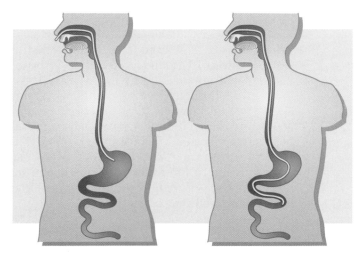

Nasogastric   Nasoduodenal/nasojejunal

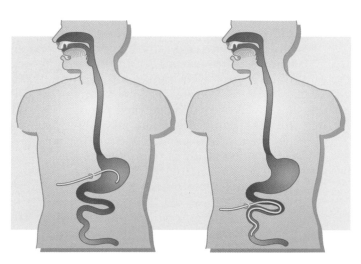

Gastrostomy   Jejunostomy

FIGURE 7-3 Types of gastrointestinal tubes for enteral feedings. A *nasogastric* tube is passed from the nose into the stomach. A *weighted nasoduodenal/nasojejunal* tube is passed through the nose into duodenum/jejunum. A *gastrostomy* tube is introduced through a temporary or permanent opening on the abdominal wall (stoma) into the stomach. A *jejunostomy* tube is passed through a stoma directly into the jejunum. (From Kee, J., & Hayes, E. [2003]. *Pharmacology: A Nursing Process Approach* [4th ed.]. Philadelphia: W. B. Saunders.)

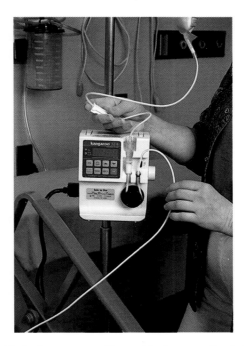

FIGURE 7-4 Enteral infusion pump. (From Lindeman, C., & McAthie, M. [1999]. *Fundamentals of Contemporary Nursing Practice.* Philadelphia: W. B. Saunders.)

started at a rate of 10 to 30 ml/hr if not diluted, depending on the health status of the individual. It may take 3 to 5 days for gastrointestinal tolerance to appear.

If diarrhea continues, changing to a fiber-containing formula may decrease or eliminate it. The liquid medication should be checked to make sure that it does not contain sorbitol, which has a laxative effect after several doses. Switching from liquid to tablets may be necessary. In some clients, hypoalbuminemia could be a cause of diarrhea, which can lead to malabsorption within the intestines. The prealbumin level is a better indicator of hypoalbuminemia than the serum albumin test. Other causes of diarrhea may be fecal impaction, *Clostridium difficile,* pseudomembranous colitis, and gut atrophy. A stool specimen should be analyzed for *C. difficile* toxin. If *C. difficile* toxin is detected, antidiarrheal drugs should not be prescribed because diarrhea helps to eliminate the toxin. The cause of diarrhea should be determined.

Blood sugar levels should be monitored during enteral therapy. This is important for patients who are acutely ill, those with septic conditions, those recovering from acute trauma, and those receiving steroids. If hyperglycemia occurs, decreasing the tube feeding rate or concentration may help.

When enteral feedings are less than full strength, they are ordered in percent (%). The nurse must calculate the amount of feeding solution and the amount of water that should be given.

Calculation of Percent for Enteral Feeding Solutions

Percent (%) of a solution indicates its strength. Percent is a portion of 100, e.g., 20% is 20 of 100 parts (20/100). The basic formula, ratio and proportion, or a percentage problem can be used to determine percent.

D: desired percent
H: on-hand volume (100)
V: desired total volume
X: unknown amount of solution

METHODS A & B Basic Formula *and* Ratio and Proportion

$$\frac{D}{H}\left(\frac{\text{desired \%}}{\text{on-hand volume}}\right) \times V \text{ (desired total volume)}$$

or

$$\begin{array}{ccccccc} H & : & V & :: & D & : & X \\ \text{on-hand} & : & \text{desired} & :: & \text{desired} & : & \text{unknown} \\ \text{volume} & & \text{total volume} & & \% & & \text{amount of} \\ & & & & & & \text{solution} \end{array}$$

or

METHOD C Percentage Problem

Desired total volume × desired % (in hundredths) = amount of tube feeding (TF) solution

After the tube feeding, 30 ml (cc) of water should be given to clear the tubing. The tube is clamped after a bolus feeding.

EXAMPLES

PROBLEM 1: A client has been receiving intravenous fluids for 5 days. A nasogastric tube was inserted, and 250 ml (cc) of 50% Ensure solution was ordered q4h for 1 day. Calculate how much Ensure and water are needed to make 250 ml (50% solution).

Methods: 50% solution is 50 in 100 parts.

$$\frac{D}{H}\left(\frac{\text{desired \%}}{\text{on-hand volume}}\right) \times V \text{ (desired total volume)}$$

$$\frac{50}{100} \times 250 = \frac{12,500}{100} = 125 \text{ ml of Ensure}$$

or

$$\begin{array}{ccccc} H & : & V & :: D : & X \\ 100 & : & 250 \text{ ml} & :: 50 : & X \text{ ml} \end{array}$$
$$100\, X = 12,500$$
$$X = 125 \text{ ml of Ensure}$$

or

$$250 \text{ ml} \times 0.50 \text{ (50\%)} = 125 \text{ ml of TF solution}$$

How much water should be added?

$$\text{Total amount} - \text{Amount of TF} = \text{Amount of water}$$
$$250 \text{ ml} \quad - \quad 125 \text{ ml} \quad = \quad 125 \text{ ml}$$

Answer: 125 ml of Ensure + 125 ml of water

PROBLEM 2: Three days later, the client's tube feeding order is changed. The client is to receive 250 ml (cc) of 70% Osmolite solution q6h.

How much Osmolite solution and water should be mixed to equal 250 ml?

Methods: 70% solution is 70 in 100 parts.

$$\frac{D}{H} \times V = \frac{70}{100} \times 250 = \frac{17,500}{100} = 175 \text{ ml of Osmolite}$$

or

$$H : V \quad :: D : X$$
$$100 : 250 \text{ ml} :: 70 : X \text{ ml}$$
$$100 X = 17,500$$
$$X = 175 \text{ ml of Osmolite}$$

or

$$250 \text{ ml} \times 0.70 \text{ (70\%)} = 175 \text{ ml of TF solution}$$

How much water should be added?

$$\text{Total amount} - \text{Amount of TF} = \text{Amount of water}$$
$$250 \text{ ml} \quad - \quad 175 \text{ ml} \quad = \quad 75 \text{ ml}$$

Answer: 175 ml of Osmolite + 75 ml of water

PROBLEM 3: One week later, the client's tube feeding order is changed to 250 ml (cc) of 40% Ensure Plus. How much Ensure Plus and water should be mixed to equal 250 ml?

Methods: 40% solution is 40 in 100 parts.

$$\frac{D}{H} \times V = \frac{40}{100} \times 250 = \frac{10,000}{100} = 100 \text{ ml of Ensure Plus}$$

or

$$H : V \quad :: D : X$$
$$100 : 250 \text{ ml} :: 40 : X \text{ ml}$$
$$100 X = 10,000$$
$$X = 100 \text{ ml of Ensure Plus}$$

or

$$250 \text{ ml} \times 0.40 \text{ (40\%)} = 100 \text{ ml of TF solution}$$

How much water should be added?

$$\text{Total amount} - \text{Amount of TF} = \text{Amount of water}$$
$$250 \text{ ml} \quad - \quad 100 \text{ ml} \quad = \quad 150 \text{ ml}$$

Answer: 100 ml of Ensure Plus + 150 ml of water

Percent of Enteral Solutions

Answers can be found on page 144.

1. Order: 200 ml of 25% Sustacal solution q4h through a nasogastric tube. How much Sustacal solution and water should be mixed to equal

   200 ml?_____

2. Order: 300 ml of 75% Pulmocare solution q6h through a nasogastric tube. How much Pulmocare solution and water should be mixed to equal

   300 ml?_____

3. Order 500 ml of 60% Ensure Plus solution q8h through a nasogastric tube. How much Ensure Plus solution and water should be mixed to equal

   500 ml?_____

4. Order: 400 ml of 30% Osmolite solution q6h through a nasogastric tube. How much Osmolite solution and water should be mixed to equal

   400 ml?_____

Enteral Medications

Oral medications in liquid, tablet, or capsule form can be administered when properly diluted through the feeding tube as a bolus and then flushed from the enteral tube with water.

All liquid medication is hyperosmolar (>1000 mOsm/kg) when compared with the osmolality of the secretions of the gastrointestinal tract (130 to 350 mOsm/kg). Although the hyperosmolality of liquid medication was once thought to be well tolerated by the gastrointestinal tract, research indicates that cramping, distention, vomiting, and diarrhea can be caused by the administration of undiluted hypertonic liquid medications and electrolyte solutions. Liquid medication should be diluted with water to reduce osmolality to 500 mOsm/kg to decrease gastrointestinal intolerance.

Table 7-2 lists the osmolalities of various commercial drug solutions and suspensions.

Most tablets can be crushed and dissolved in water. Clogged feeding tubes can result if the medication is not adequately diluted or if the tube is not frequently flushed. New feeding pumps are designed to include a flush bag to periodically clear the feeding tube and prevent clogging.

Calculation of Dilution for Enteral Medications

To determine the amount of water needed to dilute a liquid medication, the following information must be obtained:
1. The volume of the drug from the drug order
2. The osmolality of the drug (check drug literature or ask pharmacist)
3. 500 mOsm may be used as a constant for the desired osmolality

Table 7-2

Osmolalities of Various Commercial Drug Solutions and Suspensions

Product	Manufacturer	Average Osmolality (m/Osm/kg)
Acetaminophen elixir, 65 mg/ml	Roxane	5400
Acetaminophen with codeine elixir	Wyeth-Ayerst	4700
Amoxicillin suspension, 50 mg/ml	Squibb	2250
Ampicillin suspension, 50 mg/ml	Squibb	2250
Cascara aromatic fluid extract	Roxane	1000
Cephalexin suspension, 50 mg/ml	Dista	1950
Cimetidine solution, 60 mg/ml	SmithKline Beecham	5500
Co-trimoxazole suspension	GlaxoWellcome	2200
Dexamethasone solution, 1 mg/ml	Roxane	3100
Dextromethorphan HBr syrup, 2 mg/ml	Parke-Davis	5950
Digoxin elixir, 50 μg/ml	GlaxoWellcome	1350
Diphenhydramine HCl elixir, 2.5 mg/ml	Roxane	850
Diphenoxylate/atropine suspension	Roxane	8800
Docusate sodium syrup, 3.3 mg/ml	Roxane	3900
Erythromycin E.S. suspension, 40 mg/ml	Abbott	1750
Ferrous sulfate liquid, 60 mg/ml	Roxane	4700
Furosemide solution, 10 mg/ml	Hoechst Marion Roussel	2050
Haloperidol concentrate, 2 mg/ml	McNeil	500
Hydroxyzine HCl syrup, 2 mg/ml	Roerig	4450
Kaolin-pectin suspension	Roxane	900
Lactulose syrup, 0.67 g/ml	Roerig	3600
Lithium citrate syrup, 1.6 mEq/ml	Roxane	6850
Magnesium citrate solution	Medalist	1000
Metoclopramide HCl syrup, 1 mg/ml	A. H. Robins	8350
Milk of magnesia suspension	Pharmac. Assoc.	1250
Multivitamin liquid	Upjohn	5700
Nystatin suspension, 100,000 U/ml	Squibb	3300
Paregoric tincture	Roxane	1350
Phenytoin sodium susp., 25 mg/ml	Parke-Davis	1500
Potassium chloride liquid, 10%	Roxane	3550
Potassium iodide sat sol (SSKI), 1 g/ml	Upsher-Smith	10950
Prochlorperazine syrup, 1 mg/ml	SmithKline Beecham	3250
Promethazine HCl syrup, 1.25 mg/ml	Wyeth-Ayerst	3500
Sodium phosphate liquid, 0.5 g/ml	C. B. Fleet	7250
Theophylline solution, 5.33 mg/ml	Berlex	800
Thioridazine suspension, 20 mg/ml	Sandoz	2050

From: Estoup, M. (1994). Approaches and limitations of medication delivery in patients with enteral feeding tubes. *Critical Care Nurse*, Vol 14(1), Table 2, p. 70. Reprinted with permission of *Critical Care Nurse*, February, 1994.

METHOD

Step 1 Calculate the volume of drug:

$$BF: \frac{D}{H} \times V \quad \textbf{or} \quad RP: H:V::D:X \quad \textbf{or} \quad DA: V = \frac{V \times C\,(H) \times D}{H \times C\,(D) \times 1}$$

Step 2 Find osmolality of drug:

$$\frac{Known\ mOsm}{Desired\ mOsm} \times Volume\ of\ drug = Total\ volume\ of\ liquid$$

Step 3 Water for dilution:

$$Total\ volume\ of\ liquid - Volume\ of\ drug = Volume\ of\ water\ for\ dilution$$

EXAMPLES

PROBLEM 1: Order: acetaminophen 650 mg, q6h, PRN for pain.
Drug available: acetaminophen elixir 65 mg/ml.
Average mOsm/kg = 5400.

Step 1: Calculate the volume of drug:

$$BF: \frac{D}{H} \times V = \frac{650}{65} \times 1 = 10\ ml$$

or

$$RP: \quad H \quad : \quad V \quad :: \quad D \quad : \quad X$$
$$65\ mg:1\ ml::650\ mg:X\ ml$$
$$65\ X = 650$$
$$X = 10\ ml$$

or

DA: no conversion factor

$$ml = \frac{1\ ml \times \overset{10}{\cancel{650}}\ \cancel{mg}}{\underset{1}{\cancel{65}}\ \cancel{mg} \times 1} = 10\ ml$$

Step 2: Find osmolality of drug:

$$\frac{Known\ mOsm\ (5400)}{Desired\ mOsm\ (500)} \times Volume\ of\ drug\ (10) = \frac{5400}{500} \times 10 = 108\ ml$$

Step 3: Water for dilution:

$$Total\ volume\ of\ drug\ (108\ ml) - Volume\ of\ drug\ (10\ ml)$$
$$= 98\ ml\ volume\ of\ water\ for\ dilution$$

PROBLEM 2: Order: Colace 50 mg bid.
Drug available: docusate sodium 3.3 mg/ml.
Average mOsm/kg = 3900.

Step 1: Calculate the volume of drug:

$$BF: \frac{D}{H} \times V = \frac{50}{3.3} \times 1 = 15.1\ ml$$

or

RP: H : V ::   D : X
3.3 mg : 1 ml :: 50 mg : X
3.3 X = 50
X = 15.1 or 15 ml

or

DA: no conversion factor

$$ml = \frac{1\ ml \times 50\ mg}{3.3\ mg \times 1} = \frac{50}{3.3} = 15\ ml$$

Step 2: Find osmolality of drug:

$$\frac{Known\ mOsm\ (3900)}{Desired\ mOsm\ (500)} \times Volume\ of\ drug\ (15\ ml)$$

$$= \frac{3900}{500} \times 15 = 117\ ml$$

Step 3: Water for dilution:

Total volume of drug (117 ml) − Volume of drug (15 ml)
= 102 ml volume of water for dilution

PRACTICE PROBLEMS III Enteral Medications

Answers can be found on page 144.

Calculate the amount of water needed to reduce the osmolality to 500 mOsm for the following medications:

1. Order: amoxicillin suspension 250 mg by tube, qid.
   Drug available: amoxicillin suspension 50 mg/ml.

2. Order: metoclopramide HCl syrup 10 mg, q ac and hs per tube.
   Drug available: metoclopramide 1 mg/ml.

3. Order: KCl oral solution 40 mEq, qd by tube.
   Drug available: KCl 10% oral solution, 20 mEq/15 ml.

4. Order: thioridazine suspension 50 mg, tid by tube.
   Drug available: thioridazine suspension 20 mg/ml.

ANSWERS

I Oral Medications

1. **a.** BF: $\frac{D}{H} \times V = \frac{50}{100} \times 1$

$$= 100\overline{)50.0}^{.5} = 0.5 = \text{½ tablets}$$

or

RP: H : V :: D : X
100 mg : 1 tab :: 50 mg : X tab

$$100 \, X = 50$$
$$X = 0.5 \text{ or } \frac{1}{2} \text{ tablets}$$

or

DA: no conversion factor

$$\text{tab} = \frac{1 \text{ tab} \times \overset{1}{\cancel{50}} \text{ mg}}{\underset{2}{\cancel{100}} \text{ mg} \times 1} = \frac{1}{2} \text{ tablet}$$

2. 0.5 g = 500 mg (Method A) or see Table 2-1 or Table 5-1.

BF: $\dfrac{D}{H} \times V = \dfrac{500}{250} \times 1 = \dfrac{500}{250} = 2$ tablets

or

RP: H : V ::   D   :   X
250 mg : 1 tab :: 500 mg : X tab

$$250 \, X = 500$$
$$X = 2 \text{ tablets}$$

or

DA: tab = $\dfrac{1 \text{ tab} \times \overset{4}{\cancel{1000}} \text{ mg} \times 0.5 \text{ g}}{\underset{1}{\cancel{250}} \text{ mg} \times 1 \cancel{g} \times 1} = 4 \times 0.5 = 2$ tablets

3. 2 tablets

4. Change grains to milligrams (milligram value is on the drug label). Refer to Table 2-1 or Table 5-1: 1 gr = 60 mg.

BF: $\dfrac{D}{H} \times V = \dfrac{60}{30} \times 1 = 2$ tablets

or

RP: H : V :: D : X
30 mg : 1 tab :: 60 mg : X tab

$$30 \, X = 60$$
$$X = 2 \text{ tablets}$$

5. 30 ml

6. a. Select the 125 mg/5 ml bottle. It is a fractional dosage with the 375 mg/5 ml bottle (3.3 ml).

b. BF: $\dfrac{D}{H} \times V = \dfrac{250}{125} \times 5 \text{ ml} = \dfrac{1250}{125} = 10$ ml of Ceclor

or

RP: H : V :: D : X
125 : 5 :: 250 : X

$$125 \, X = 1250$$
$$X = 10 \text{ ml of Ceclor}$$

or

DA: ml = $\dfrac{5 \text{ ml} \times \overset{2}{\cancel{250}} \text{ mg}}{\underset{1}{\cancel{125}} \text{ mg} \times 1} = 10$ ml

7. **a.** 2 tablets of ProSom
   b. hs: hour of sleep or at bedtime

8. **a.** BF: $\dfrac{D}{H} \times V = \dfrac{400}{125} \times 5 = \dfrac{2000}{125} = 16$ ml of Ceftin

   or

   BF: $\dfrac{D}{H} \times V = \dfrac{400}{250} \times 5 = \dfrac{2000}{250} = 8$ ml of Ceftin

   b. Either Ceftin bottle could be used. For fewer milliliters, select the 250 mg/5 ml bottle.

9. BF: $\dfrac{D}{H} \times V = \dfrac{100}{62.5} \times 5$ ml $= \dfrac{500}{62.5} = 8$ ml of Dynapen

   or

   RP: H : V :: D : X
   62.5 : 5 :: 100 : X
   62.5 X = 500
   X = 8 ml

10. **a.** The HydroDiuril 25 mg tablet bottle is preferred. A half-tablet from the HydroDiuril 100 mg tablet bottle can be used; however, breaking or cutting the 100 mg tablet can result in an inaccurate dose.
    b. From the HydroDiuril 25 mg bottle, give 2 tablets. From the HydroDiuril 100 mg bottle, give ½ tablet (if the tablet is scored).

11. **a.** Select a 10 mg and 20 mg Zocor bottle.
    b. Give 1 tablet from each bottle.

12. Change grams to milligrams by moving the decimal point three spaces to the right:
    0.400 g = 400 mg. Also see Table 2-1 or Table 5-1.

    BF: $\dfrac{D}{H} \times V = \dfrac{400}{250} \times 5$ ml $= \dfrac{2000}{250} = 8$ ml

    or

    RP: H : V :: D : X
    250 mg : 5 ml :: 400 mg : X ml
    250 X = 2000
    X = 8 ml

    or

    DA: ml $= \dfrac{5 \text{ ml} \times \overset{4}{\cancel{1000}} \text{ mg} \times 0.4 \text{ g}}{\underset{1}{\cancel{250}} \text{ mg} \times 1 \text{ g} \times 1} = 20 \times 0.4 = 8$ ml

13. Use the metric system. According to Table 2-1 or Table 5-1, gr $\overline{ss}$ = 30 mg. Give 2 tablets.

14. BF: $\dfrac{D}{H} \times V = \dfrac{100}{125} \times 5$ ml $= \dfrac{500}{125} = 4$ ml

    or

    RP: H : V :: D : X
    125 mg : 5 ml :: 100 mg : X
    125 X = 500
    X = 4 ml

    or

DA: no conversion factor

$$ml = \frac{5\ ml\ \times\ \overset{4}{\cancel{100}}\ \cancel{mg}}{\underset{5}{\cancel{125}}\ \cancel{mg}\ \times\ 1} = \frac{20}{5} = 4\ ml$$

15. Give 2 tablets of Vioxx

16. Nitrostat 0.4 mg

17. 2½ ml

18. ½ tablet

19. BF: $\dfrac{D}{H} \times V = \dfrac{6}{4} \times 5 = \dfrac{30}{4} = 7.5\ ml$ of Zofran

20. 1½ tablets

21. **a.** For loading dose and maintenance doses, the 500 mg/5 ml is preferred, but either bottle could be used.

    b. Loading dose: change grams to milligrams:

       1.000 g = 1000 mg

       Using the 250 mg/5 ml bottle:

       BF: $\dfrac{D}{H} \times V = \dfrac{1000}{\underset{50}{\cancel{250}}} \times \overset{1}{\cancel{5}}\ ml = \dfrac{1000}{50} = 20\ ml$

       or

       RP: H   : V ::   D   : X

          250 mg:5 ml :: 1000 mg:X ml

                250 X = 5000

                    X = 20 ml

       or

       DA: $ml = \dfrac{5\ ml\ \times\ \overset{2}{\cancel{1000}}\ mg\ \times\ \cancel{1}\ \cancel{g}}{\underset{1}{\cancel{500}}\ \cancel{mg}\ \times\ \cancel{1}\ \cancel{g}\ \times\ 1} = 10\ ml$ (using 500 mg/5 ml)

       Using the 500 mg/5 ml bottle: give 10 ml per dose of Duricef.

    c. Maintenance doses per dose, change grams to milligrams

       0.500 g = 500 mg

       Using the 250 mg/5 ml bottle:

       BF: $\dfrac{D}{H} \times V = \dfrac{500}{250} \times 5\ ml = 10\ ml$

       or

       RP: H   : V ::   D   :X

          250 mg:5 ml :: 500 mg:X

                250 X = 2500

                    X = 10 ml

       or

       DA: $ml = \dfrac{5\ ml\ \times\ \overset{4}{\cancel{1000}}\ mg\ \times\ 0.5\ \cancel{g}}{\underset{1}{\cancel{250}}\ \cancel{mg}\ \times\ 1\ \cancel{g}\ \times\ 1} = 20 \times 0.5 = 10\ ml$ (using 250 mg/5 ml)

       Using the 500 mg/5 ml: give 5 ml per dose of Duricef.

22. 10 ml

Additional Dimensional Analysis

23. Drug label: 250 mg = 1 tablet

$$\text{tablets} = \frac{1 \text{ tab} \times \overset{4}{\cancel{1000}} \text{ \cancel{mg}} \times 0.5 \text{ \cancel{g}}}{\underset{1}{\cancel{250}} \text{ \cancel{mg}} \times 1 \text{ \cancel{g}} \times 1} = 0.5 \times 4 = 2 \text{ tablets}$$

24. $$\text{tablets} = \frac{1 \times \overset{2}{\cancel{5.0}} \text{ \cancel{mg}}}{\underset{1}{\cancel{2.5}} \text{ \cancel{mg}} \times 1} = 2 \text{ tablets of Vasotec}$$

25. $$\text{ml} = \frac{5 \text{ ml} \times \overset{4}{\cancel{1000}} \text{ \cancel{mg}} \times 0.4 \text{ \cancel{g}}}{\underset{1}{\cancel{250}} \text{ \cancel{mg}} \times 1 \text{ \cancel{g}} \times 1} = 8 \text{ ml}$$

Give 8 ml per dose of amoxicillin.

26. Factors: 325 mg = 1 tablet; gr $\times$ (10)/1
Conversion factor: 1 gr = 60 mg

$$\text{tablets} = \frac{1 \text{ tab} \times \overset{12}{\cancel{60}} \text{ \cancel{mg}} \times \overset{2}{\cancel{10}} \text{ \cancel{gr}}}{\underset{\underset{13}{65}}{\cancel{325}} \text{ \cancel{mg}} \times 1 \text{ \cancel{gr}} \times 1} = \frac{24}{13} = 1.84 \text{ or } 2 \text{ tablets}$$

60 (64) mg = 1 gr (approximate weights). Round off to the nearest whole number.

27. Factors: 250 mg = 5 ml; 125 mg/1
Conversion factor: *none*

$$\text{ml} = \frac{5 \text{ ml} \times \overset{1}{\cancel{125}} \text{ \cancel{mg}}}{\underset{2}{\cancel{250}} \text{ \cancel{mg}} \times 1} = \frac{5}{2} = 2\frac{1}{2} \text{ or } 2.5 \text{ ml}$$

28. 165 lb = 75 kg (change pounds to kilograms by dividing by 2.2 into 165 pounds, or 165 ÷ 2.2)
10 mg $\times$ 75 = 750 mg
750 ÷ 3 = 250 mg, tid

29. 154 lb = 70 kg
4 mg $\times$ 70 = 280 mg/day

30. 132 lb = 60 kg
2.5 mg $\times$ 60 = 150 mg **or** 100 $\times$ 1.7 = 170 mg

31. **a.** 20 mg/50 kg/day = 20 $\times$ 50 = 1000 mg per day
b. 2 tablets of Zarontin per dose (500 mg per dose)

32. **a.** 4 mg/60 kg/day = 4 $\times$ 60 = 240 mg per day **or** 120 mg, q12h

b. BF: $\dfrac{D}{H} \times V = \dfrac{120}{\underset{10}{\cancel{50}}} \times \overset{1}{\cancel{5}} \text{ ml} = \dfrac{120}{10} = 12 \text{ ml}$

or
RP: H : V :: D : X
50 : 5 :: 120 : X

50 X = 600

$X = \dfrac{600}{50} = 12 \text{ ml}$

or

$$DA: ml = \frac{5\ ml\ \times\ \overset{12}{\cancel{120}}\ mg}{\underset{5}{\cancel{50}}\ mg\ \times\ 1} = \frac{60}{5} = 12\ ml$$

Give 12 ml per dose of minocycline.

II Percent of Enteral Solutions

1. BF: $\dfrac{D}{H} \times V = \dfrac{25}{100} \times 200 = \dfrac{200}{4} = 50$ ml of Sustacal

   or

   RP: 100 : 200 :: 25 : X

   100 X = 5000

   X = 50 ml of Sustacal

   or

   $$DA: ml = \frac{\overset{2}{\cancel{200}}\ ml\ \times\ 25\ mg}{\underset{1}{\cancel{100}}\ mg\ \times\ 1} = 50\ ml$$

   or

   200 ml × 0.25 (25%) = 50 ml of Sustacal

   Total amount − Amount of TF = Amount of water

      200 ml   −   50 ml   =   150 ml

   50 ml of Sustacal + 150 ml of water

2. 225 ml of Pulmocare + 75 ml of water

3. BF: $\dfrac{D}{H} \times V = \dfrac{60}{100} \times 500 = \dfrac{30,000}{100} = 300$ ml of Ensure Plus

   or

   RP: 100 : 500 :: 60 : X

   100 X = 30,000

   X = 300 ml of Ensure Plus

   or

   500 ml × 0.60 (60%) = 300 ml of Ensure Plus

   Total amount − Amount of TF = Amount of water

      500 ml   −   300 ml   =   200 ml

   300 ml of Ensure Plus + 200 ml of water

4. 120 ml of Osmolite + 280 ml of water

III Enteral Medications

1. *Step 1* BF: $\dfrac{D}{H} \times V = \dfrac{\overset{5}{\cancel{250}}}{\underset{1}{\cancel{50}}} \times 1 = 5$ ml

   or

   RP: H : V :: D : X

      50 : 1 :: 250 : X

      50 X = 250

        X = 5 ml

   or

DA: no conversion factor

$$ml = \frac{1\ ml \times \overset{5}{\cancel{250}}\ \cancel{mg}}{\underset{1}{\cancel{50}}\ \cancel{mg} \times 1} = 5\ ml$$

Step 2 $\dfrac{\text{Known mOsm (2250)}}{\text{Desired mOsm (500)}} \times$ Volume of drug (5)

$$= BF:\ \frac{2250}{500} \times 5\ ml = 22.5\ ml$$

Step 3 Total volume of liquid (22.5) − Volume of drug (5) = 17.5 ml liquid (water)

Total: 22.5 ml to be administered (17.5 ml liquid + 5 ml drug = 22.5 ml)

2. *Step 1* BF: $\dfrac{D}{H} \times V = \dfrac{10}{1} \times 1 = 10\ ml$

or

RP: H : V :: D : X

1 mg : 1 ml :: 10 mg : X

X = 10 ml

or

DA: $ml = \dfrac{1\ ml \times 10\ \cancel{mg}}{1\ \cancel{mg} \times 1} = 10\ ml$

Step 2 $\dfrac{\text{Known mOsm (8350)}}{\text{Desired mOsm (500)}} \times$ Volume of drug (10)

$$= \frac{8350}{500} \times 10 = 167\ ml\ \text{(liquid and drug)}$$

Step 3 Total volume of liquid (167 ml) − Volume of drug (10 ml) = 157 ml liquid (water)

3. *Step 1* BF: $\dfrac{D}{H} \times V = \dfrac{\overset{2}{\cancel{40}}}{\underset{1}{\cancel{20}}} \times 15 = 30\ ml$

or

RP: H : V :: D : X

20 mEq : 15 ml :: 40 mEq : X

20 X = 600

X = 30 ml

or

DA: $ml = \dfrac{15\ ml \times \overset{2}{\cancel{40}}\ mEq}{\underset{1}{\cancel{20}}\ mEq \times 1} = 30\ ml$

Step 2 $\dfrac{\text{Known mOsm (3550)}}{\text{Desired mOsm (500)}} \times$ Volume of drug (30)

$$= \frac{3550}{500} \times 30 = 213\ ml\ \text{(liquid and drug)}$$

Step 3 Total volume of liquid (213) − Volume of drug (30) = 183 ml liquid (water)

4. *Step 1* BF: $\dfrac{D}{H} \times V = \dfrac{\cancel{50}}{\underset{2}{\cancel{20}}} \times 1 = 2.5$ ml

or

RP: H : V ::   D   : X

   20 mg : 1 ml :: 50 mg : X

              20 X = 50

                  X = 2.5 ml

or

DA: ml $= \dfrac{1 \text{ ml } \times 50 \cancel{\text{ mg}}}{20 \cancel{\text{ mg}} \times \quad 1} = \dfrac{50}{20} = 2.5$ ml

Step 2 $\dfrac{\text{Known mOsm (2050)}}{\text{Desired mOsm (500)}} \times$ Volume of drug (2.5) = 10.25 ml (liquid and drug)

Step 3 Total volume of liquid (10.25 ml) − Volume of drug (2.5 ml) = 7.75 ml liquid (water)

Injectable Preparations with Clinical Applications

OBJECTIVES

- Select the correct syringe and needle for a prescribed injectable drug.
- Calculate dosage of drugs for subcutaneous and intramuscular routes from solutions in vials and ampules.
- Explain the procedure for preparing and calculating medications in powder form for injectable use.
- Determine prescribed insulin dosage in units using an insulin syringe.
- Explain the methods for mixing two insulin solutions in one insulin syringe and for mixing two injectable drugs in one syringe.
- Explain the various methods of insulin administration.
- State the various sites for intramuscular injections.
- Explain how to administer intradermal, subcutaneous, and intramuscular injections.

OUTLINE

INJECTABLE PREPARATIONS
    Vials and Ampules
    Syringes
    Needles
INTRADERMAL INJECTIONS
SUBCUTANEOUS INJECTIONS
    Calculations for Subcutaneous
      Injections
INSULIN INJECTIONS
TYPES OF INSULIN

MIXING INSULINS
    Insulin Pen Injectors
    Intranasal Insulin
    Insulin Jet Injectors
    Insulin Pumps
INTRAMUSCULAR INJECTIONS
    Drug Solutions for Injection
    Reconstitution of Powdered
      Drugs
MIXING OF INJECTABLE DRUGS

Medications administered by injection can be given intradermally (under the skin), subcutaneously (SC, into fatty tissue), intramuscularly (IM, into the muscle), and intravenously (IV, into the vein). Intravenous injectables are discussed in Chapter 9. Injectable drugs are ordered in grams, milligrams, micrograms, grains, or units. The preparations of injectable drugs may be packaged in a solvent (diluent or solution) or in a powdered form.

This chapter is divided into five sections: (1) injectable preparations, such as vials, ampules, syringes, needles, and pre-filled cartridges; (2) intradermal injections; (3) subcutaneous injections, including heparin; (4) insulin injections; and (5) intramuscular injections from prepared liquid and reconstituted powder in vials and ampules, and the mixing of drugs in a syringe. Examples and practice problems follow each section, and the answers to the practice problems are located at the end of the chapter.

INJECTABLE PREPARATIONS

Vials and Ampules

Drugs are packaged in vials (sealed rubber-top containers) for single and multiple doses and in ampules (sealed glass containers) for a single dose. Multiple-dose vials can be used more than once because of their self-sealing rubber top; however, ampules are used only once after the glass-necked container is opened. The drug is in either liquid or powder form in vials and ampules. When drugs in solution deteriorate rapidly, they are packaged in dry form and solvent (diluent) is added before administration. If the drug is in powdered form, mixing instructions and dose equivalents such as milligrams (mg) per milliliter (ml) are usually given; if not, check the drug information insert. After the dry form of the drug is reconstituted with sterile water, bacteriostatic water, or saline solution, the drug must be used immediately or refrigerated. Usually, the reconstituted drug in the vial is used within 48 hours to 1 week; check the drug information insert. A vial and an ampule are shown in Figure 8-1.

The route by which the injectable drug can be given, such as SC, IM, or IV, is printed on the drug label.

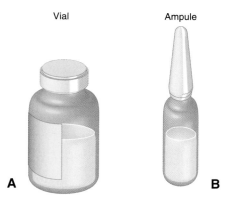

Vial   Ampule

A   B

FIGURE 8-1 **A,** Vial. **B,** Ampule. (From Kee, J., & Hayes, E. [2003]. *Pharmacology: A Nursing Process Approach* [4th ed.]. Philadelphia: W. B. Saunders.)

Syringes

Types of syringes used for injections include 3-ml and 5-ml calibrated syringes, metal and plastic syringes for pre-filled cartridges, tuberculin syringes, and insulin syringes. There are 10-ml, 20-ml, and 50-ml syringes that are used mostly for drug preparations. A syringe is composed of a barrel (outer shell), plunger (inner part), and the tip, where the needle joins the syringe (Fig. 8-2).

Three-Milliliter Syringe

The 3-ml syringe is calibrated in tenths (0.1 ml). The amount of fluid in the syringe is determined by the rubber end of the plunger that is closer to the tip of the syringe (Fig. 8-3). Remember, milliliter (ml) and cubic centimeter (cc) are used interchangeably. An advance in safety needle technology is the SafetyGlide shielding hypodermic needle (Fig. 8-4). The purpose of this type of needle is to reduce needlestick injuries.

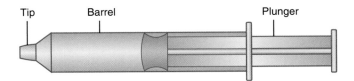

FIGURE 8-2 Parts of a syringe.

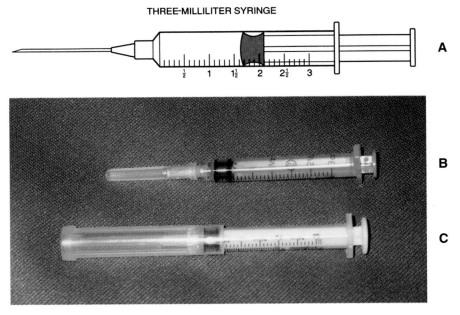

FIGURE 8-3 Three-milliliter syringes: **A,** 3-ml syringe with 0.1-ml markings; **B,** 3-ml syringe with a needle cover; **C,** 3-ml syringe with a protective cover over the needle after injection. (From Kee, J., & Hayes, E. [2003]. *Pharmacology: A Nursing Process Approach* [4th ed.]. Philadelphia: W. B. Saunders.)

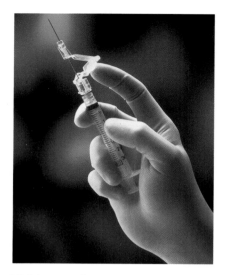

FIGURE 8-4 BD SafetyGlide™ needle. (From Becton, Dickinson and Company copyright 2003 BD.)

Five-Milliliter Syringe

The 5-ml syringe is calibrated in 0.2 ml. A 5-ml syringe is usually used when the fluid needed is more than 2½ ml. This syringe is frequently used to reconstitute a dry drug form with sterile water, bacteriostatic water, or saline solution. Figure 8-5 shows the 5-ml syringe and its markings and the 5-ml needleless syringe.

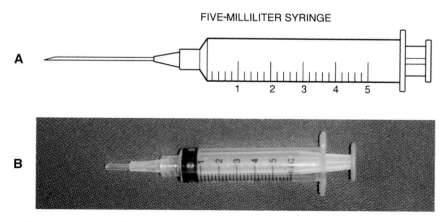

FIGURE 8-5 Five-milliliter syringes: **A,** 5-ml syringe with 0.2-ml markings; **B,** needleless 5-ml BD Syringe that can penetrate a rubber-top vial. (From Kee, J., & Hayes, E. [2003]. *Pharmacology: A Nursing Process Approach* [4th ed.]. Philadelphia: W. B. Saunders.)

Tuberculin Syringe

The tuberculin syringe is a 1-ml slender syringe that is calibrated in tenths (0.1 ml), hundredths (0.01 ml), and minims (Fig. 8-6). This syringe is used when the amount of drug solution to be administered is less than 1 ml and for pediatric and heparin dosages. The tuberculin syringe is also available in a one-half milliliter (ml) syringe. Figure 8-7 shows the ½-ml and the 1-ml tuberculin syringes.

Insulin Syringe

The insulin syringe has a capacity of 1 ml. Insulin is measured in units, and insulin dosage *must NOT* be calculated in milliliters. Insulin syringes are calibrated as 2 units per mark, and 100 units equal 1 ml (Fig. 8-8). *Insulin syringes, NOT tuberculin syringes, must be used for administering insulin.* Insulin syringes are available in lo-dose, ½-ml, and 1-ml sizes. The 1-ml insulin syringe may be purchased with a permanently attached needle or detachable needle (Fig. 8-9).

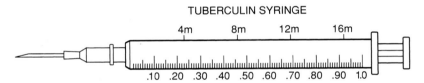

TUBERCULIN SYRINGE

FIGURE 8-6 Tuberculin syringe.

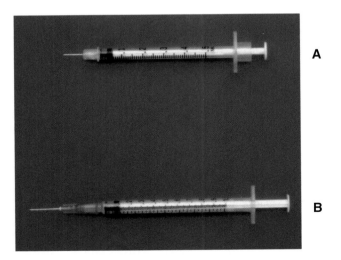

FIGURE 8-7 Two types of BD Tuberculin Syringes: **A,** ½-ml tuberculin syringe with a permanently attached needle; **B,** 1-ml tuberculin syringe with a detachable needle. (From Becton, Dickinson and Company copyright 2003 BD.)

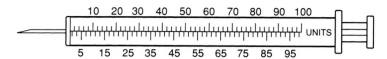

INSULIN SYRINGE

FIGURE 8-8 Insulin syringe. (From Kee, J., & Hayes, E. [2003]. *Pharmacology: A Nursing Process Approach* [4th ed.]. Philadelphia: W. B. Saunders.)

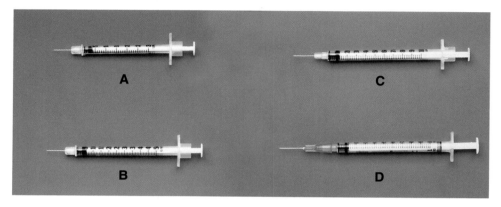

FIGURE 8-9 Four types of BD Insulin Syringes: **A,** $^{3}/_{10}$-ml insulin syringe with permanently attached needle; **B,** $^{1}/_{2}$-ml insulin syringe with a permanently attached needle; **C,** 1-ml insulin syringe with a permanently attached needle; **D,** 1-ml insulin syringe with a detachable needle. (From Becton, Dickinson and Company copyright 2003 BD.)

Pre-Filled Drug Cartridge and Syringe

Many injectable drugs are packaged in pre-filled disposable cartridges. The disposable cartridge is placed into a reusable metal or plastic holder. A pre-filled cartridge usually contains 0.1 to 0.2 ml of excess drug solution. On the basis of the amount of drug to be administered, the excess solution must be expelled before administration. Figure 8-10*A* shows a Carpuject syringe. Injectables are also supplied by pharmaceutical companies in ready-to-use pre-filled syringes that do not require a holder. Figure 8-10*B* shows a Tubex syringe.

Needles

A needle consists of (1) a hub (large metal or plastic part attached to the tip of the syringe), (2) a shaft (thin needle length), and (3) a bevel (end of the needle). Figure 8-11 shows the parts of a needle.

Needle size is determined by gauge (diameter of the lumen) and by length. The larger the gauge number, the smaller the diameter of the lumen. The smaller the gauge number, the larger the diameter of the lumen. The usual range of needle gauges is from 18 to 26. Needle length varies from $^{3}/_{8}$

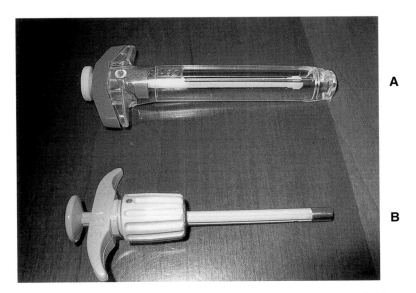

FIGURE 8-10 **A,** Carpuject syringe. **B,** Tubex syringe. (From Kee, J., & Hayes, E. [2003]. *Pharmacology: A Nursing Process Approach* [4th ed.]. Philadelphia: W. B. Saunders.)

PARTS OF A NEEDLE

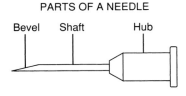

FIGURE 8-11 Parts of a needle. (From Kee, J., & Hayes, E. [2003]. *Pharmacology: A Nursing Process Approach* [4th ed.]. Philadelphia: W. B. Saunders.)

inch to 2 inches. Table 8-1 lists the needle sizes and lengths for use in intradermal, subcutaneous, and intramuscular injections.

When choosing the needle length for an intramuscular injection, the nurse must consider the size of the client and the amount of fatty tissue. A client with minimal fatty tissue may need a needle length of 1 inch. For an obese client, the length of the needle for an intramuscular injection may be $1\frac{1}{2}$ to 2 inches.

Table 8-1

Needle Size and Length

Type of Injection	Needle Gauge	Needle Lengths (inch)
Intradermal	25, 26	$\frac{3}{8}$, $\frac{1}{2}$, $\frac{5}{8}$
Subcutaneous	23, 25, 26	$\frac{3}{8}$, $\frac{1}{2}$, $\frac{5}{8}$
Intramuscular	19, 20, 21, 22	1, $1\frac{1}{2}$, 2

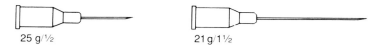

FIGURE 8-12 Two combinations of needle gauge and length.

Insulin syringes and pre-filled cartridges have permanently attached needles. With other syringes, needle sizes can be changed. Needle gauge and length are indicated on the syringe package or on the top cover of the syringe. These values appear as gauge/length, such as 21g/1½ inch. Figure 8-12 shows two types of needle gauge and length.

Research has shown that after an injection, medication remains in the hub of the syringe, where the needle joins the syringe. This volume can be as much as 0.2 ml. There is controversy as to whether air should be added to the syringe before administration to ensure that the total volume is given. The best practice is to follow the institution's policy.

Angles for Injection

For injections, the needle enters the skin at different angles. Intradermal injections are given at a 10- to 15-degree angle; subcutaneous injections, at a 45- to 90-degree angle; and intramuscular injections, at a 90-degree angle. Figure 8-13 shows the angles for intradermal, subcutaneous, and intramuscular injections.

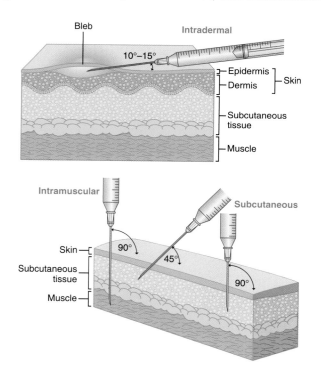

FIGURE 8-13 Angles for injection. (From Kee, J., & Hayes, E. [2003]. *Pharmacology: A Nursing Process Approach* [4th ed.]. Philadelphia: W. B. Saunders.)

I **Needles**

Answers can be found on page 183.

1. Which would have the larger needle lumen: a 21-gauge needle or a 25-gauge needle? _____

2. Which would have the smaller needle lumen: an 18-gauge needle or a 26-gauge needle? _____

3. Which needle would have a length of $1\frac{1}{2}$ inches: a 20-gauge needle or a 25-gauge needle? _____

4. Which needle would have a length of $\frac{5}{8}$ inch: a 21-gauge needle or a 25-gauge needle? _____

5. Which needle would be used for an intramuscular injection: a 21-gauge needle with a $1\frac{1}{2}$-inch length or a 25-gauge needle with a $\frac{5}{8}$-inch length? _____

INTRADERMAL INJECTIONS

Usually, an intradermal injection is used for skin testing for diagnostic purposes. Primary uses are for tuberculin and allergy testing. The tuberculin syringe (25 g/$\frac{1}{2}$ inch) holds 1 ml (16 minims) and is calibrated in 0.1 to 0.01 ml.

The inner aspect of the forearm is often used for diagnostic testing because there is less hair in the area and the test results are easily seen. The upper back can also be used as a testing site. The needle is inserted with the bevel upward at a 10- to 15-degree angle. Do not aspirate. Test results are read 48 to 72 hours after the intradermal injection. A reddened or raised area indicates a positive reaction.

SUBCUTANEOUS INJECTIONS

Drugs injected into the subcutaneous (fatty) tissue are absorbed slowly because there are fewer blood vessels in the fatty tissue. The amount of drug solution administered subcutaneously is generally 0.5 to 1 ml at a 45-, 60-, or 90-degree angle. Irritating drug solutions are given intramuscularly because they could cause sloughing of the subcutaneous tissue.

The two types of syringes used for subcutaneous injections are the tuberculin syringe (1 ml), which is calibrated in 0.1 and 0.01 ml, and the 3-ml syringe, which is calibrated in 0.1 ml (Fig. 8-14). The needle gauge commonly used is 25- or 26-gauge, and the length is usually $\frac{3}{8}$ to $\frac{5}{8}$ inch. Insulin is also administered subcutaneously and is discussed later in this chapter.

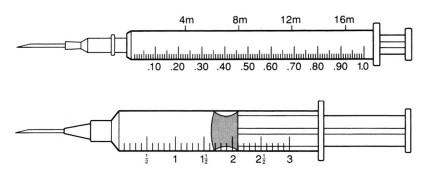

FIGURE 8-14 Syringes used for subcutaneous injections.

Calculations for Subcutaneous Injections

Formulas for solving problems of subcutaneous injections are the basic formula, ratio and proportion, fractional equation, and dimensional analysis (see Chapter 5). The following problems are examples of injections that can be given subcutaneously.

"Heparin Calculations" are available on the CD-ROM in the "Calculating Dosages" section.

EXAMPLES

PROBLEM 1: Order: heparin 5000 U, SC.
Drug available:

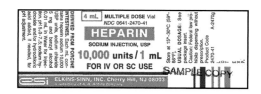

Methods:

Basic formula (BF)

$$\frac{D}{H} \times V = \frac{5000}{10,000} \times 1 = \frac{5}{10} = 0.5 \text{ ml}$$

or

Ratio and proportion (RP)

$$H \quad : \quad V \quad :: \quad D \quad : \quad X$$
$$10,000 \text{ U} : 1 \text{ ml} :: 5000 \text{ U} : X \text{ ml}$$

$$10,000 \text{ X} = 5000$$

$$X = \frac{5000}{10,000} = \frac{5}{10} = 0.5 \text{ ml}$$

or

Dimensional analysis (DA)

$$V = \frac{V \times C(H) \times D}{H \times C(D) \times 1}$$

$$ml = \frac{1\ ml \times 5{,}000\ \cancel{U}^{1}}{10{,}000\ \cancel{U}_{2} \times 1} = \frac{1}{2} \text{ or } 0.5\ ml$$

Answer: Heparin 5000 U = 0.5 ml

PROBLEM 2: Order: morphine 10 mg, SC.
Drug available:

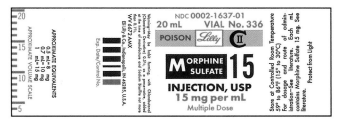

See label with approximate equivalents.

Methods: BF: $\dfrac{D}{H} \times V = \dfrac{10}{15} \times 1 = \dfrac{2}{3} = 0.67\ ml$ or $0.7\ ml$

or

H : V :: D : X
15 mg : 1 ml :: 10 mg : X ml

$$15\,X = 10$$

$$X = \frac{\cancel{10}^{2}}{\cancel{15}_{3}} = \frac{2}{3} = 0.67\ ml \text{ or } 0.7\ ml$$

or

DA: no conversion factor

$$ml = \frac{1\ ml \times \cancel{10}^{2}\ mg}{\cancel{15}_{3}\ mg \times 1} = \frac{2}{3} \text{ or } 0.7\ ml$$

Answer: Morphine 10 mg = 0.67 or 0.7 ml (use a tuberculin syringe or a 3-ml syringe)

PRACTICE PROBLEMS II Subcutaneous Injections

Answers can be found on page 183.

Use the formula you chose for calculating oral drug dosages in Chapter 7.

1. Which needle gauge and length should be used for a subcutaneous injection:
    a 25 g/⅝ inch or 26 g/⅜ inch? _____

2. Order: heparin 4000 U, SC.
Drug available:

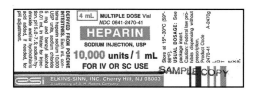

   a. How many milliliters of heparin would you give? _____

   b. At what angle would you administer the drug? _____

3. Order: heparin 7500 U, SC.
Drug available:

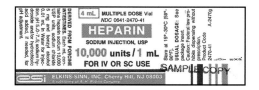

How many milliliters of heparin would you give? _____

4. Order: atropine SO₄ gr ¹⁄₁₀₀, SC.
Drug available:

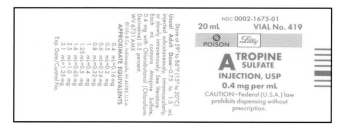

How many milliliters of atropine would you give? _____

5. Order: epoetin alfa (Epogen) 50 units/kg SC.
Drug available: Epogen 10,000 units/ml.
Client weighs 65 kg.

   a. What is the correct dosage? _____

   b. How many milliliters would you give? _____

6. Order: filgrastim (Neupogen) 6 mcg/kg SC bid.
Drug available: Neupogen 300 mcg/ml.
Client weighs 198 pounds.

   a. How many kilograms does the client weigh? _____

   b. How many micrograms (mcg) would you give? _____

   c. How many milliliters would you give? _____

   d. Explain how the drug should be drawn up. _____

INSULIN INJECTIONS

Insulin is prescribed and measured in USP units. Most insulins are manufactured in concentrations of 100 units per milliliter. Insulin should be administered with an insulin syringe, which is calculated to correspond with the U 100 insulin. Insulin bottles and syringes are color-coded. The U 100 insulin bottle and the U 100 syringe are color-coded orange.

The insulin syringe may be marked on one side in even units (10, 20, 30) and on the other side in odd units (5, 15, 25, etc.).

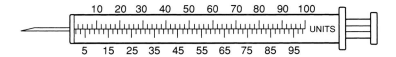

Insulin is easy to prepare and administer as long as the nurse uses the *same insulin concentration with the same calibrated insulin syringe,* e.g., a U 100 insulin bottle and a U 100 insulin syringe. For example, if the prescribed insulin dosage is 30 units, withdraw 30 units from a bottle of U 100 insulin using a U 100-calibrated insulin syringe.

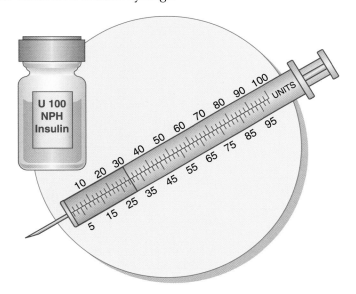

Administering insulin with a tuberculin syringe is *not* suggested and *should be avoided.*

TYPES OF INSULIN

Insulin is categorized as fast-acting, intermediate-acting, long-acting, and commercial premixed insulin. The following drug labels are arranged according to insulin action.

Insulins are clear (regular or crystalline insulin) or cloudy (NPH, Lente) because of the substances (protamine and zinc) used to prolong the action of

A, Fast-acting insulins

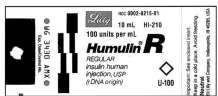

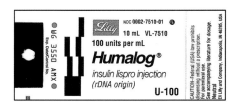

B, Intermediate acting insulins

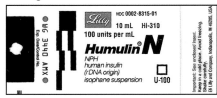

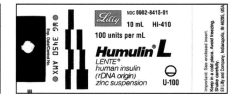

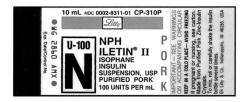

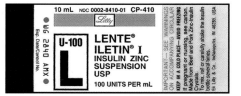

C, Long-acting insulin

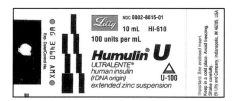

D, Selected combinations of insulins

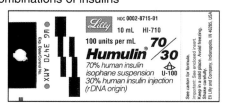

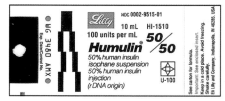

E, Selected insulins for pen injections

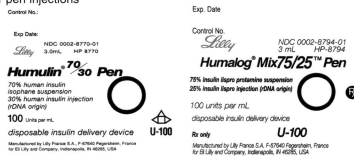

insulin in the body. Only clear (regular) insulin can be given intravenously, as well as subcutaneously. Insulin that contains protamine and zinc can be administered only subcutaneously.

A new fast-acting insulin that was approved for use in 1996 is lispro insulin (Humalog). Lispro insulin acts faster than regular insulin and thus can be administered 5 minutes before mealtime, whereas regular insulin is given 30 minutes before meals. Lispro insulin is formed by reversing two amino acids in human regular insulin (Humulin).

The new long-acting insulin is Lantus, an insulin glargine that is an analog of human insulin. Lantus is the first long-acting recombinant DNA (rDNA) human insulin for clients with type 1 and 2 diabetes mellitus. It is usually administered at bedtime; incidence of nocturnal hypoglycemia is not as common as with other insulins. Some clients complain of more pain at the injection site when Lantus is used as compared with NPH insulin. It is administered with an insulin pen.

The use of commercially premixed combination insulins has become popular for the client with diabetes who mixes fast-acting and intermediate-acting insulins. Examples of combination insulins are Humulin 70/30, Novolin 70/30, Humulin 50/50, and Humalog 75/25. The Humalog 75/25 contains 75% of lispro protamine insulin and 25% lispro "rapid" insulin. It is available in a prefilled disposable pen. The 70/30 vial contains 70% NPH insulin and 30% regular insulin, and the 50/50 vial contains 50% NPH insulin and 50% regular insulin. Humulin 70/30 may come in vials or prefilled disposable pens. The exterior of the insulin pen resembles a fountain pen. Some people need less than 30% regular insulin and more of NPH; they will need to mix the two insulins together.

The sources of insulins are beef, pork, beef-pork, and human (Humulin). Some individuals are allergic to beef insulin, so pork insulin is used because it has biologic properties similar to those of human insulin. Humulin insulins are more commonly used.

Insulin is administered subcutaneously at a 45-, 60-, or 90-degree angle into the subcutaneous tissue. The angle for administering insulin depends on the amount of fatty tissue in the client. For a very thin person, a 45-degree angle is suggested. A 90-degree angle should be used on obese or average-sized persons. When a 90-degree angle is used, the skin should be pinched upward so the insulin is deposited into the fatty tissue.

MIXING INSULINS

Regular insulin is frequently mixed with insulins containing protamine, such as NPH, and zinc, such as Lente.

EXAMPLE   Problem and method for mixing insulin.

PROBLEM 1: Order: Regular insulin U 10 and Lente insulin U 40, SC.
Drug available: Regular insulin U 100 and Lente insulin U 100, both in multidose vials. The insulin syringe is marked U 100.

Methods:

1. Cleanse the rubber tops or diaphragms of the insulin bottles.

2. Draw up 40 U of air* and inject into the Lente insulin bottle. Do not allow the needle to come into contact with the Lente insulin solution. Withdraw the needle.

3. Draw up 10 U of air and inject into the regular insulin bottle.

4. Withdraw 10 U of regular insulin. Regular insulin is withdrawn before Lente and NPH.

5. Withdraw 40 U of Lente insulin.

6. Administer the two insulins immediately after mixing. Do not allow the insulin mixture to stand, because unpredicted physical changes might occur. Unpredicted changes are more common with protamine insulins such as NPH than with Lente insulin.

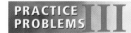
Insulin

Answers can be found on page 184.

1. Order: NPH insulin 35 U, SC.
   Drug available: NPH insulin U 100 and U 100 insulin syringe.
   Indicate on the insulin syringe the amount of insulin that should be withdrawn.

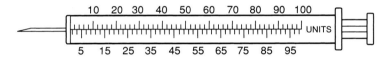

2. Order: Lente insulin 50 U, SC.
   Drug available: Lente U 100 and U 100 insulin syringe.
   Indicate on the insulin syringe the amount of insulin that should be withdrawn.

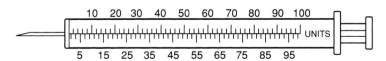

3. Order: regular insulin U 8 and NPH insulin U 52.
   Drug available: regular insulin U 100 and NPH insulin U 100.
   The insulin syringe is U 100.
   Explain the method for mixing the two insulins.

---

*You may draw up 50 units of air; inject 40 units into the NPH bottle and 10 units into the regular insulin bottle.

Indicate on the U 100 insulin syringe how much regular insulin should be withdrawn and how much NPH insulin should be withdrawn.

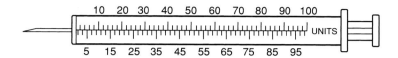

4. Order: regular insulin U 15 and Lente insulin U 45.
   Drug available: regular insulin U 100 and Lente insulin U 100.
   The insulin syringe is U 100.
   Explain the method for mixing the two insulins.

   _____

   Indicate on the U 100 insulin syringe how much regular insulin and how much Lente insulin should be withdrawn.

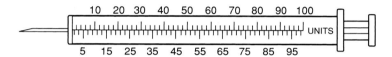

Insulin Pen Injectors

As stated before, an insulin pen resembles a fountain pen. The pen contains disposable needles and an insulin-filled cartridge. Pens come in two types: prefilled and reusable. Actually, the purpose of the insulin pen is to deliver an insulin dose more accurately than the traditional U 100 syringe and vial. Insulin pen injectors have been used in Europe and are now frequently used in the United States.

When the insulin pen is used, the amount of insulin that is desired is obtained by turning the dial to the number of insulin units needed. The capacity of the prefilled or reusable insulin pens is 150 to 300 units or 1.5 to 3 ml of the combination of insulins. The new long-acting insulin product, Lantus, can be administered with the insulin pen injector. However, both Humalog and Lantus are more expensive.

The use of insulin pens may increase the client's compliance with the insulin regimen. For work or travel, the client may find use of the insulin pen more convenient. With the insulin pens, many clients state there is less injection pain than with the traditional insulin syringe.

Intranasal Insulin

Insulin is being administered intranasally by a few patients with diabetes in the United States. A study is being conducted to determine the efficacy and safety of an inhaled insulin (Exubera) for persons with type 1 diabetes mellitus. The individuals participating in the study have not used more than 150 units of insulin per day.

However, this route of insulin administration has a rapid onset and short duration of action. At present, this method is primarily used to provide meal-time insulin supplements. Intermediate-acting insulin may still be needed. The intranasal insulin dose is usually greater than the subcutaneous dose, since only part of the insulin is absorbed through the nasal membrane. Intranasal insulin is expensive.

Insulin Jet Injectors

Insulin jet injectors administer insulin without a needle; the insulin goes directly through the skin into the fatty tissue. Because the insulin is given under high pressure, stinging, burning, pain, and bruising may occur. This method of insulin administration is not recommended for children or older adults. Also, this method is more expensive than the subcutaneous technique.

Insulin Pumps

There are two types of insulin pumps: the implantable and the portable. The implantable insulin pump is surgically implanted in the abdomen and delivers a basal insulin infusion and bolus doses with meals either intravenously or intraperitoneally. With the implantable insulin pumps, there are fewer hypoglycemic reactions and the blood glucose levels are mostly controlled.

The portable (external) insulin pumps, also called *continuous subcutaneous insulin infusion (CSII),* have been available since 1983. The portable (external) insulin pump keeps the blood glucose (sugar) levels as close to normal as possible. The insulin pump is a battery-operated device that administers regular insulin, which is stored in a reservoir syringe placed inside the device. The device is the size of a "call pager" and weighs about 3.5 ounces. Infusions are programmed by the client to: (1) infuse insulin at a set basal rate of units per hour, (2) deliver bolus infusions to cover meals (the client pushes a button to deliver a bolus dose at meals), (3) change delivery rates at specific times of the day (e.g., from 3:00 AM to 9:00 AM) to avoid early morning hyperglycemia, and (4) override the set basal rate to allow for unexpected changes in activity, such as early morning exercise.

Insulin is delivered from the device through plastic tubing that is attached to a metal or plastic needle and placed subcutaneously by the client. The needle can be inserted into the abdomen, upper thigh, or upper arm. Only regular insulin is used; NPH and Lente are not used because of unpredictable control of blood sugars. The pump can deliver small amounts of insulin such as 0.1 or 0.2 units much more accurately than a traditional insulin syringe.

The ongoing insulin delivery system helps to decrease the risk of a severe hypoglycemic reaction and maintains glucose control. However, glucose levels should still be monitored at least daily with or without an insulin pump. The person with type 1 diabetes mellitus receive the most benefit from the use of insulin pump. This method should reduce the number of long-term diabetic complications compared with the use of multiple injec-

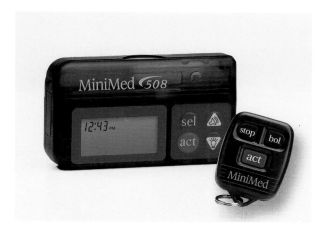

FIGURE 8-15 Portable insulin pump. (From MiniMed, Inc., Sylmar, CA.)

tions of regular and modified types of insulins. Portable (external) insulin pumps are expensive.

Figure 8-15 shows an example of an insulin pump.

 Additional information on "Understanding Insulin Administration" and practice problems are available on the CD-ROM in the "Calculating Dosages" section.

INTRAMUSCULAR INJECTIONS

The IM injection is a common method of administering injectable drugs. The muscle has many blood vessels (more than fatty tissue), so medications given by intramuscular injections are absorbed more rapidly than those given by SC injections. The volume of solution for an IM injection is 0.5 to 3.0 ml, with the average being 1 to 2 ml. A volume of drug solution greater than 3 ml causes increased muscle tissue displacement and possible tissue damage. Occasionally, 5 ml of certain drugs, such as magnesium sulfate, may be injected in a large muscle, such as the dorsogluteal. Dosages greater than 3 ml are usually divided and given at two different sites.

Needle gauges for IM injections containing thick solutions are 19 and 20, and for thin solutions, 20 to 21. IM injections are administered at a 90-degree angle. The needle length depends on the amount of adipose (fat) and muscle tissue; the average needle length is 1½ inches.

The common sites for IM injections are the deltoid, dorsogluteal, ventrogluteal, and vastus lateralis muscles. Figure 8-16 displays the sites for each muscle used with IM injection. Table 8-2 gives the volume for drug administration, common needle size, client's position, and angle of injection for the four IM injection sites.

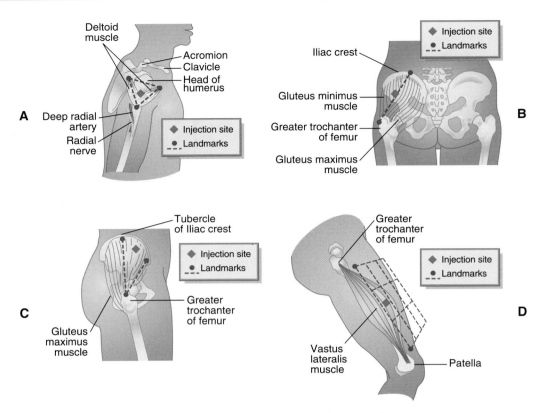

FIGURE 8-16 Intramuscular injection sites. **A**, Deltoid; **B**, dorsogluteal; **C**, ventrogluteal; **D**, vastus lateralis. (From Kee, J., & Hayes, E. [2003]. *Pharmacology: A Nursing Process Approach* [4th ed.]. Philadelphia: W. B. Saunders.)

The discussion on intramuscular injection is divided into three subsections: (1) drug solutions for injection, (2) reconstitution of powdered drugs, and (3) mixing of injectable drugs. An example is given for each type, and practice problems follow.

Drug Solutions for Injection

Commercially premixed drug solutions are stored in vials and ampules for immediate use. At times, there may be enough drug solution left in a vial for another dose, and the vial may be saved. The balance of a drug solution in an ampule is *always* discarded after the ampule has been opened and used.

EXAMPLES   Two problems are given as examples for calculating IM dosage. Choose one of the four methods for calculating drug dosage.

Table 8-2

Intramuscular Injection Sites in the Adult

	Deltoid	Dorsogluteal	Ventrogluteal	Vastus Lateralis
Volume for drug administration	*Usual:* 0.5–1 ml *Maximum:* 2.0 ml	*Usual:* 1.0–3 ml *Maximum:* 3 ml; 5 ml gamma-globulin	*Usual:* 1–3 ml *Maximum:* 3–4 ml	*Usual:* 1–3 ml *Maximum:* 3–4 ml
Common needle size	23–25 gauge; ⅝–1½ inches	18–23 gauge; 1¼–3 inches	20–23 gauge; 1¼–2½ inches	20–23 gauge; 1¼–1½ inches
Client's position	Sitting; supine; prone	Prone	Supine; lateral	Sitting (dorsal flex foot); supine
Angle of injection	90° angle, angled slightly toward the acromion	90° angle to flat surface; upper outer quadrant of the buttock *or* outer aspect of line from the posterior iliac crest to the greater trochanter of the femur	80°–90° angle; angle the needle slightly toward the iliac crest	80°–90° angle For thin person: 60°–75° angle

PROBLEM 1: Order: gentamycin 60 mg, IM.
Drug available: gentamycin 80 mg/2 ml in a vial.

Methods: BF: $\dfrac{D}{H} \times V = \dfrac{60}{80} \times 2 = \dfrac{120}{80} = 1.5$ ml

or

RP: H : V ::   D : X
       80 mg : 2 ml :: 60 mg : X ml
              80 X = 120
              $X = \dfrac{120}{80} = 1.5$ ml

or

DA: no conversion factor

$ml = \dfrac{2\ ml \ \times \ \overset{3}{\cancel{60}}\ mg}{\underset{4}{\cancel{80}}\ mg \ \times \quad 1} = \dfrac{6}{4} = 1.5$ ml

Answer: gentamycin 60 mg = 1.5 ml

PROBLEM 2: Order: Naloxone 0.5 mg, IM, STAT.
Drug available:

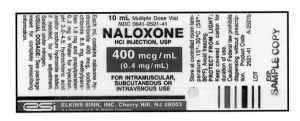

Methods: BF: $\dfrac{D}{H} \times V = \dfrac{0.5}{0.4} \times 1 = 0.4\overline{)0.5\,00}\;\;\dfrac{1.25}{}$ ml

or

RP: H :V :: D :X
   0.4 : 1 :: 0.5 : X

(0.4) X = 0.5
      X = 1.25 ml

or

DA: ml $= \dfrac{1\ \text{ml} \times 1\overset{10}{0\!\!\!/0\!\!\!/0}\ \text{mcg} \times 0.5\ \text{mg}}{\underset{4}{4\!\!\!/0\!\!\!/0}\ \text{mcg} \times 1\ \text{mg} \times 1} = \dfrac{10 \times 0.5}{4} = \dfrac{5}{4} = 1.25$ ml

Answer: Naloxone 0.5 mg = 1.25 ml

Reconstitution of Powdered Drugs

Certain drugs lose their potency in liquid form. Therefore manufacturers package these drugs in powdered form, and they are reconstituted before administration. To reconstitute a drug, look on the drug label or in the drug information insert (circular or pamphlet) for the type and amount of diluent to use. Sterile water, bacteriostatic water, and normal saline solution are the primary diluents. If the type and amount of diluent are not specified on the drug label or in the drug information insert, call the pharmacy.

The powdered drug occupies space and therefore increases the volume of drug solution. Usually, manufacturers determine the amount of diluent to mix with the drug powder to yield 1 to 2 ml per desired dose. After the powdered drug has been reconstituted, the unused drug solution should be dated, initialed, and refrigerated. Most drugs retain their potency for 48 hours to 1 week when refrigerated. Check the drug information insert or drug label for how long the reconstituted drug may be used.

EXAMPLES   PROBLEM 1: Order: oxacillin sodium 500 mg, IM, q6h.
Drug available:

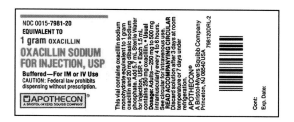

According to the label on the bottle, the amount of powdered drug in the vial is 1 g. The drug label states:

Add 5.7 ml of sterile water (diluent) to the vial. Each 250 mg = 1.5 ml or 1 g = 6 ml.

Methods: Change grams to milligrams or change milligrams to grams (see Table 5-1). 1 gram = 1000 mg *or* 500 mg = 0.500 g (0.5 g).
Move the decimal point three spaces to the left.

Milligrams

BF: $\dfrac{D}{H} \times V = \dfrac{500}{1000} \times 6\ ml = \dfrac{3000}{1000} = 3\ ml$

or

$\dfrac{D}{H} \times V = \dfrac{\overset{2}{\cancel{500}}}{\underset{1}{\cancel{250}}} \times 1.5\ ml = 3\ ml$

or

Grams

RP: H : V :: D : V
1 g : 6 ml :: 0.5 g : X
X = 3.0
X = 3.0 ml

or

DA: $ml = \dfrac{6\ ml \times 1\ \cancel{g} \times \overset{1}{\cancel{500}}\ \cancel{mg}}{1\ \cancel{g} \times \underset{2}{\cancel{1000}}\ \cancel{mg} \times 1} = \dfrac{6}{2} = 3\ ml$

Answer: oxacillin sodium 500 mg = 3 ml

PROBLEM 2: Order: nafcillin sodium 250 mg, IM, q6h.
Drug available:

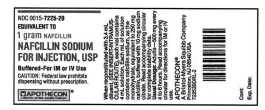

The drug label says to add 3.4 ml of sterile or bacteriostatic water. Each 4 ml contains 1 gram (1000 mg) of nafcillin.

Methods: BF: $\dfrac{D}{H} \times V = \dfrac{250}{1000} \times 4\ ml = \dfrac{1000}{1000} = 1\ ml$ nafcillin

or

RP:
$$H\ :\ V\ ::\ D\ :\ X$$
$$1000\ mg : 4\ ml\ ::\ 250\ mg : X$$
$$1000\ X = 1000$$
$$X = \dfrac{1000}{1000}$$
$$= 1\ ml\ of\ nafcillin$$

or

DA: $ml = \dfrac{4\ ml \times\ 1\ \cancel{g}\ \times 2\overset{1}{\cancel{5}}0\ \cancel{mg}}{1\ \cancel{g}\ \times 1\underset{4}{\cancel{0}00\ \cancel{mg}} \times\ 1} = \dfrac{4}{4} = 1\ ml\ of\ nafcillin$

Answer: nafcillin 250 mg = 1 ml

MIXING OF INJECTABLE DRUGS

Drugs mixed together in the same syringe must be compatible to prevent precipitation. To determine drug compatibility, check drug references or check with a pharmacist. When in doubt about compatibility, do *not* mix drugs.

The three methods of drug mixing are (1) mixing two drugs in the same syringe from two vials, (2) mixing two drugs in the same syringe from one vial and one ampule, and (3) mixing two drugs in a pre-filled cartridge and from a vial.

METHOD 1 Mixing Two Drugs in the Same Syringe from *Two Vials*

1. Draw air into the syringe to equal the amount of solution to be withdrawn from the first vial, and inject the air into the first vial. Do *not* allow the needle to come into contact with the solution. Remove the needle.
2. Draw air into the syringe to equal the amount of solution to be withdrawn from the second vial. Invert the second vial and inject the air.
3. Withdraw the desired amount of solution from the second vial.
4. Change the needle unless you will use the entire volume in the first vial.
5. Invert the first vial and withdraw the desired amount of solution.

or

1. Draw air into the syringe to equal the amount of solution to be withdrawn and inject the air into the first vial. Withdraw the desired drug dose.
2. Insert a 25-g needle into the rubber top (not in the center) of the second vial. This acts as an air vent. Injecting air into the second vial is *not* necessary.
3. Insert the needle in the center of the rubber-top vial (beside the 25-g needle–air vent), invert the second vial, and withdraw the desired drug dose.

METHOD 2 Mixing Two Drugs in the Same Syringe from *One Vial and One Ampule*

1. Remove the amount of desired solution from the vial.
2. Aspirate the amount of desired solution from the ampule.

METHOD 3 Mixing Two Drugs in a *Pre-filled Cartridge from a Vial*

1. Check the drug dose and the amount of solution in the pre-filled cartridge. If a smaller dose is needed, expel the excess solution.
2. Draw air into the cartridge to equal the amount of solution to be withdrawn from the vial. Invert the vial and inject the air.
3. Withdraw the desired amount of solution from the vial. Make sure the needle remains in the fluid, and do *not* take more solution than needed.

EXAMPLES | Mixing drugs in the same syringe.

PROBLEM 1: Order: meperidine (Demerol) 60 mg and atropine SO_4 gr $^1/_{150}$, IM. The two drugs are compatible.
Drugs available:

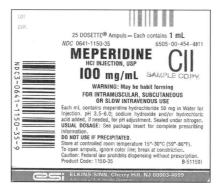

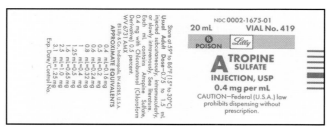

Note: Meperidine is in an ampule, and atropine sulfate is in a vial.

How many milliliters of each drug would you give? Explain how to mix the two drugs.

Methods: meperidine

$$BF: \frac{D}{H} \times V = \frac{60}{100} \times 1 = 0.6 \text{ ml}$$

or

RP: H : V ::   D : X
100 mg : 1 ml :: 60 mg : X ml
100 X = 60
X = 0.6 ml

or

DA: no conversion factor

$$ml = \frac{1\ ml \times 60\ mg}{100\ mg \times 1} = \frac{60}{100} = 0.6\ ml$$

atropine SO_4
gr $1/150$ = 0.4 mg (see Tables 2-1 and 5-1).

Answer: meperidine (Demerol) 60 mg = 0.6 ml
atropine gr $1/150$ = 1 ml

Procedure: Mix two drugs in a syringe for IM injection:

1. Remove 1 ml of atropine solution from the vial.

2. Withdraw 0.6 ml of meperidine (Demerol) from the ampule into the syringe containing atropine solution.

3. Syringe contains atropine 1 ml and meperidine 0.6 ml = total 1.6 ml.

PROBLEM 2: Order: meperidine 25 mg, Vistaril 25 mg, and Robinul 0.1 mg, IM. All three drugs are compatible.
Drugs available: meperidine (Demerol) is in a 2-ml Tubex cartridge labeled 50 mg/ml. Hydroxyzine (Vistaril) is in a 50 mg/ml ampule. Glycopyrrolate (Robinul) is in a 0.2 mg/ml vial.

How many milliliters of each drug would you give?
Explain how the drugs could be mixed together.

Methods:

a. meperidine 25 mg. Label: 50 mg/ml

$$BF: \frac{D}{H} \times V = \frac{25}{50} \times 1 = 0.5\ ml$$

or

RP: H : V ::   D : X
50 mg : 1 ml :: 25 mg : X ml

50 X = 25
X = ½ ml or 0.5 ml

or

$$DA: ml = \frac{1\ ml \times \overset{1}{25}\ mg}{\underset{2}{50}\ mg \times 1} = \frac{1}{2}\ ml\ or\ 0.5\ ml\ meperidine$$

b. Vistaril 25 mg. Label: 50 mg/ml ampule.

$$\text{BF:} \quad \frac{D}{H} \times V = \frac{25}{50} \times 1 = 0.5 \text{ ml}$$

or

RP: H : V ::   D : X
     50 mg : 1 ml :: 25 mg : X ml
          50 X = 25
               X = ½ ml or 0.5 ml

or

DA: same as above 0.5 ml Vistaril

c. Robinul 0.1 mg. Label: 0.2 mg/ml.

$$\text{BF:} \quad \frac{D}{H} \times V = \frac{0.1}{0.2} \times 1 = 0.5 \text{ ml}$$

or

RP: H : V ::   D : X
     0.2 mg : 1 ml :: 0.1 mg : X ml
          0.2 X = 0.1
               X = 0.5 ml

or

$$\text{DA: ml} = \frac{1 \text{ ml} \times 0.1 \text{ mg}}{0.2 \text{ mg} \times 1} = \frac{0.1}{0.2} = \frac{1}{2} \text{ or } 0.5 \text{ ml Robinul}$$

Answer: meperidine (Demerol) 25 mg = 0.5 ml; Vistaril 25 mg = 0.5 ml; Robinul 0.1 mg = 0.5 ml

Procedure: Mix three drugs in the cartridge:

1. Check drug dose and volume on pre-filled cartridge. Expel 0.5 ml of meperidine and any excess of drug solution from cartridge.

2. Draw 0.5 ml of air into the cartridge and inject into the vial containing the Robinul.

3. Withdraw 0.5 ml of Robinul from the vial into the pre-filled cartridge containing meperidine.

4. Withdraw 0.5 ml of Vistaril from the ampule into the cartridge.

PRACTICE PROBLEMS IV Intramuscular Injections

Answers can be found on page 185.

1. Order: tobramycin (Nebcin) 50 mg, IM, q8h.

Drug available:

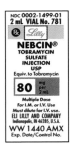

How many milliliters of tobramycin would you give? _____

2. Order: methylprednisolone (Solu-Medrol) 75 mg, IM, qd.
   Drug available: 125 mg/2 ml in vial.

   How many milliliters would you give? _____

3. Order: vitamin B$_{12}$ (cyanocobalamin) 30 mcg (μg), IM, qd.
   Drug available:

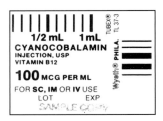

How many milliliters of cyanocobalamin would you give? _____

4. Order: Naloxone 0.2 mg, IM, STAT.
   Drug available:

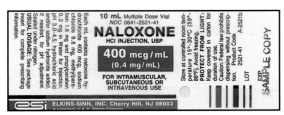

How many milliliters would you give? _____

5. Order: cefepime HCl (Maxipime) 500 mg, IM, q12h.
   Drug available:

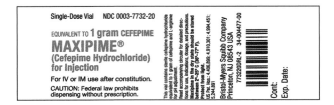

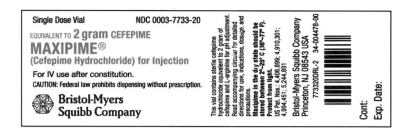

a. Which single-dose vial of Maxipime would you select? _____

Explain. _____

b. How many milliliters (ml) of diluent should you use for reconstitution of

the drug? _____

Note: The drug label does not indicate the amount of diluent to use. This may be found in the drug information insert. Usually, if you inject 2.6 ml of diluent, the amount of drug solution may be 3.0 ml. If you inject 3.4 or 3.5 ml of diluent, the amount of drug solution should be 4.0 ml.

c. How many milliliters of drug solution should the client receive? _____

6. Order: prochlorperazine (Compazine) 4 mg, IM, q8h, as needed.
Drug available:

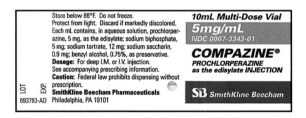

How many milliliters should the client receive? _____

7. Order: secobarbital (Seconal) 125 mg, IM, 1 hour before surgery.
Drug available: Seconal 50 mg/ml.

How many milliliters would you give? _____

8. Order: Thiamine HCl 75 mg, IM, qd.
Drug available: 100 and 200 mg/ml vials.

a. Which vial would you use? _____

b. How many milliliters would you give? _____

9. Order: hydroxyzine (Vistaril) 25 mg, deep IM, STAT.
Drug available: Vistaril 100 mg/2 ml in a vial.

How many milliliters would you give? _____

10. Order: cefonicid (Monocid) 750 mg, IM, qd.
Drug available:

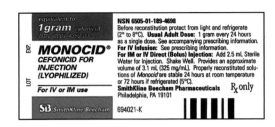

Change grams to milligrams (3 spaces to the right) or milligrams to gram (3 spaces to the left).

$$1.000 \text{ g} = 1000 \text{ mg or } 1000 \text{ mg} = 1 \text{ g}$$

a. How many gram(s) is 750 mg, IM, qd? _____

    b. How many milliliters (ml) of diluent should be injected into the vial (see

    drug label)? _____

    c. How many milliliters of cefonicid (Monocid) should the client receive per

    day? _____

11. Order: meperidine (Demerol) 35 mg and promethazine (Phenergan) 10 mg, IM.
Drugs available: meperidine 50 mg/ml in an ampule; promethazine 25 mg/ml in an ampule.

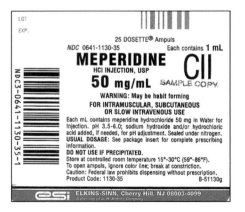

    a. How many milliliters of meperidine would you give? _____

    b. How many milliliters of promethazine would you give? _____

    c. Explain how the two drugs would be mixed.

_____

12. Order: meperidine (Demerol) 50 mg and atropine SO$_4$ 0.3 mg, IM.

Drugs available:

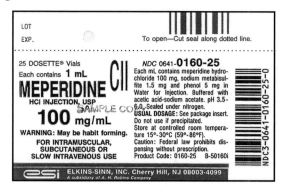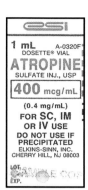

a. How many milliliters of meperidine would you give?_____

b. How many milliliters of atropine would you give? _____

c. Explain how the two drugs should be mixed.

_____

13. Order: tobramycin 50 mg, IM, q8h.
Drug available:

1 box • 25 vials • 2 mL   NDC 0003-**2725-10**

Equivalent to 80 mg TOBRAMYCIN/2 mL (40 mg/mL)
TOBRAMYCIN
Sulfate Injection USP
For INTRAMUSCULAR or INTRAVENOUS use
Must dilute for IV use
⬜**APOTHECON**®
A BRISTOL-MYERS SQUIBB COMPANY

TOBRAMYCIN Sulfate Injection USP
Each mL contains 40 mg tobramycin (as sulfate), 0.1 mg edetate disodium, 3.2 mg
sodium metabisulfite, and 5 mg phenol, as a preservative, in Water for Injection.
pH 3.0-6.5; sulfuric acid and, if necessary, sodium hydroxide have been added for
pH adjustment. Sealed under nitrogen.
Usual Dosage: Read accompanying package insert for dosage and IV dilution.
Store at controlled room temperature 15°-30° C (59°-86° F).
Caution: Federal law prohibits dispensing without prescription.

APOTHECON®
A Bristol-Myers Squibb Co.
Princeton, NJ 08540
Made in USA   C1640 **/** P2510

How many milliliters of tobramycin would you withdraw? _____

14. Order: heparin 2500 U, SC, q6h.
Drug available:

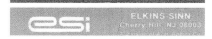

    a. Which drug vial would you use? _____

    b. How many milliliters of heparin would you give? _____

15. Order: chlordiazepoxide HCl (Librium) 50 mg, IM, STAT.
Drug available: 5 ml of dry Librium (100 mg) powder in ampule.
Add 2 ml of special intramuscular diluent to the ampule. When diluted, the powder content may increase the volume.

How many milliliters would be equivalent to 50 mg? _____

Explain. _____

16. Order: cefamandole (Mandol) 500 mg, IM, q6h.
Drug available:

    a. Change milligrams to grams (see Chapter 1).

    _____

    b. How many milliliters of diluent would you add (see drug label)?

    _____

    c. What size syringe would you use? _____

    d. How many milliliters = 1 g; how many milliliters = 500 mg? _____

17. Order: ticarcillin (Ticar), 400 mg, IM, q6h.
Drug available:

Drug label reads to add 2 ml of diluent. Total volume of solution is

_____

How many milliliters of ticarcillin should be withdrawn? _____

18. Order: morphine gr ⅙, IM, STAT.
    Drug available:

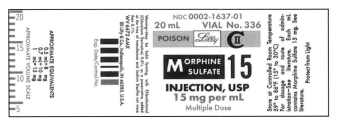

Change grains to milligrams (see Chapter 1 or Tables 2-1 and 5-1).

_____

How many milliliters of morphine would you give?_____

19. Order: ceftazidime (Fortaz) 500 mg, IM, q8h.
    Add 2.0 ml of diluent = 2.6 ml drug solution. Check the drug information
    insert.
    Drug available:

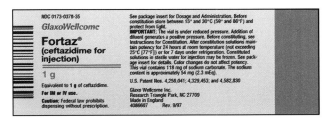

 a. How many gram(s) of ceftazidime (Fortaz) should the client receive per

    day? _____

 b. How many milliliters (ml) of ceftazidime would you give per dose?

    _____

20. Order: ampicillin 0.25 g, IM, q6h.
    Drug available:

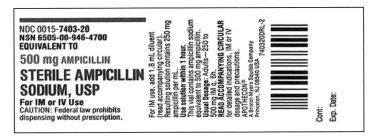

 a. To change grams to milligrams, move the decimal point 3 spaces to the

    _____

b. How many milliliters of diluent would you add to the vial? _____

c. How many milliliters should the client receive per dose? _____

21. Order: diazepam 8 mg, IM, STAT and repeat in 4 hours if necessary.
    Drug available:

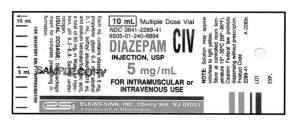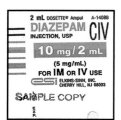

a. Which ampule or vial of diazepam would you select? _____

b. How many milliliters (ml) of diazepam should the client receive?

_____

22. Order: benztropine mesylate (Cogentin) 1.5 mg, IM, qd.
    Drug available:

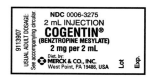

How many milliliters (ml) of Cogentin should the client receive?

_____

23. Order: interferon alfa-2b (Intron A) 10 million IU IM TIW (3 × week).
    Drug available: interferon alfa-2b (Intron A) 25 million IU/5 ml vials.

a. How many milliliters would you give per dose? _____

b. Explain how the drug should be drawn up._____

24. Order: vitamin K (AquaMEPHYTON) 2.5 mg IM × 1.
    Drug available:

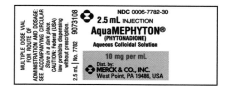

How many milliliters would you give? _____

Questions 25 through 29 relate to additional dimensional analysis. Refer to Chapter 5.

25. Order: droperidol 2 mg, IM, STAT.
    Drug available: droperidol 5 mg/2 ml.
    Factors: 5 mg/2 ml; 2 mg/1
    Conversion factor: *none; order and drug available are both in milligrams.*

    How many milliliters of droperidol should be given?_____

26. Order: morphine sulfate ⅙ gr, IM, PRN.
    Drug available:

    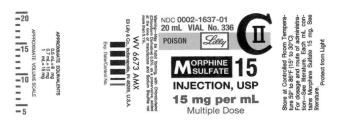

    Conversion factor: 1 gr = 60 mg

    How many milliliters of morphine would you give?_____

27. Order: cefobid 500 mg, IM, q6h.
    Add 2.0 ml of diluent to equal 2.4 ml solution. Drug available:

    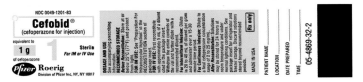

    How many milliliters of diluent would you add? _____

    Cefobid 1 g = _____ ml; 500 mg = _____ ml

    Conversion factor: 1 g = 1000 mg

    How many milliliters of Cefobid would you give? _____

28. Order: oxacillin 300 mg, IM, q8h.
    Drug available:

    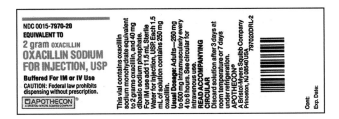

    a. Drug label and drug order _____

    b. Conversion factor:_____

    c. How many milliliters of oxacillin would you give? _____

29. Order: cefazolin (Ancef) 0.25 g, IM, q12h.
Drug available:

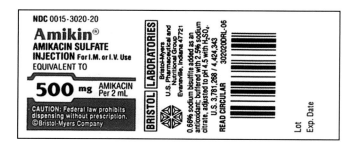

Note: Change grams to milligrams; drug label is in milligrams.

a. Label states to add _____ ml or _____ diluent.

b. How many milliliters of Ancef would you give?_____

Questions 30 through 32 relate to drug dosage per body weight.

30. Order: amikacin (Amikin) 15 mg/kg/day, q8h, IM.
Drug available:

Client weighs 140 pounds.

a. How many kilograms does the client weigh? _____.

b. How many milligrams should the client receive daily?_____

c. How many milligrams should the client receive q8h (three divided doses)? _____

d. How many milliliters should the client receive q8h? _____

31. Order: netilmicin sulfate (Netromycin) 2.0 mg/kg, q8h, IM.
Patient weighs 174 pounds.
Drug available: netilmicin 100 mg/ml.

a. How many kilograms does the client weigh? _____.

b. How many milligrams should the client receive daily?_____

c. How many milligrams should the client receive q8h? _____

d. How many milliliters should the client receive q8h? _____

32. Order: kanamycin (Kantrex) 15 mg/kg/day, q12h.
Drug available (drug is also available in 1 g = 3 ml vial):

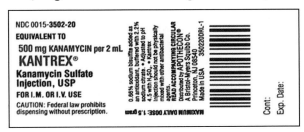

Client weighs 67 kg.

a. How many milligrams should the client receive per day? _____

b. How many milligrams should the client receive every 12 hours?

_____

c. How many milliliters should the client receive per dose? _____

d. How many milliliters from the 1 g = 3 ml vial should the client receive

per dose? _____

ANSWERS

I Needles
1. The 21-gauge needle, because it is the smaller gauge number.
2. The 26-gauge needle, because it is the larger gauge number.
3. The 20-gauge needle, because it has the larger lumen (small gauge). A needle with a 20 gauge and 1½-inch length is used for IM injection.
4. The 25-gauge needle, because it has the smaller lumen (larger gauge). It is used for SC injections. The needle is not long enough for an IM injection.
5. The 21-gauge needle with 1½-inch length (21 g/1½ inch). Muscle is under subcutaneous or fatty tissue, so a longer needle is needed.

II Subcutaneous Injections
1. *Both* needle gauge and length combinations could be used.
2. **a.** 0.4 ml
b. 45- to 60-degree angle. The angle depends on the amount of fatty tissue in the client.
3. ¾ ml or 0.75 ml
4. Change grains (apothecary system) to milligrams (metric system). See Table 2-1. gr $\frac{1}{100}$ = 0.6 mg.

$$\text{BF: } \frac{D}{H} \times V = \frac{0.6}{0.4} \times 1 = \frac{0.6}{0.4} = 1.5 \text{ ml}$$

or

RP: H   :   V   ::   D   :   X
      0.4 mg : 1 ml :: 0.6 mg : X ml
              0.4 = 0.6
              $X = \dfrac{0.6}{0.4} = 1.5$ ml

or

DA: ml = $\dfrac{1\ ml \times 0.6\ \cancel{mg}}{0.4\ \cancel{mg} \times 1} = \dfrac{0.6}{0.4} = 1.5$ ml

5. a. 50 units/kg × 65 kg = 3250 units

  b. $\dfrac{D}{H} \times V = \dfrac{3250}{10,000} \times 1 = 0.325$ ml

  or

      H   :   V   ::   D   : X
    10,000 U : 1 ml :: 3250 U : X
            10,000 X = 3250
                  X = 0.325 ml

  Answer: Epogen 3250 units = 0.325 ml

6. a. 198 lb ÷ 2.2 kg = 90 kg

  b. 90 kg × 6 mcg/kg = 540 mcg

  c. $\dfrac{D}{H} \times V = \dfrac{540\ mcg}{300\ mcg} \times 1$ ml
        = 1.8 ml

  Answer: Neupogen 540 mcg (μg) = 1.8 ml

  d. Drug can be prepared in two syringes, one with 1 ml, and the other with 0.8 ml. With subcutaneous injections, one (1) ml is given per site unless the person weighs more than 200 lb or the dose has been approved by the health care provider.

III Insulin

1. Withdraw 35 U of NPH insulin to the 35 mark on the insulin syringe. Both the insulin and the syringe have the same concentration: U 100.

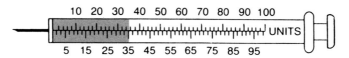

2. Withdraw 50 U of Lente insulin to the 50 mark on the insulin syringe. Both the insulin and the syringe have the same concentration: U 100.

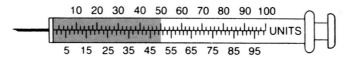

3. Inject 52 U of air into the NPH insulin bottle. Do not allow the needle to touch the insulin solution. Inject 8 U of air into the regular insulin bottle, and withdraw 8 U of regular insulin. Withdraw 52 U of NPH insulin. Total amount of insulin should be 60 U. Do *not* allow the insulin mixture to stand.

Administer immediately, because NPH contains protamine, and unpredicted physical changes could occur with a delay in administration.

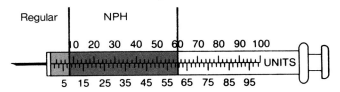

4. Inject 45 U of air into the Lente insulin bottle. Inject 15 U of air into the regular insulin bottle, and withdraw 15 U of regular insulin. Withdraw 45 U of Lente insulin. Total amount of insulin should be 60 U. Insulin mixture can stand for a short period because it is Lente insulin.

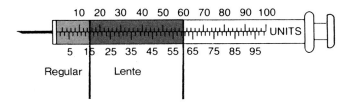

IV Intramuscular Injections

1. BF: $\dfrac{D}{H} \times V = \dfrac{50}{80} \times 2\ ml = \dfrac{100}{80} = 1.25\ ml$

or

RP: H : V :: D : X

80 mg : 2 ml :: 50 mg : X ml

$$80\ X = 100$$

$$X = \dfrac{100}{80} = 1.25\ ml$$

or

DA: no conversion factor

$$ml = \dfrac{2\ ml \times \overset{5}{\cancel{50}}\ mg}{\underset{8}{\cancel{80}}\ mg \times 1} = \dfrac{10}{8} = 1.25\ ml$$

Answer: tobramycin 50 mg = 1.25 ml

2. $\dfrac{D}{H} \times V = \dfrac{\overset{3}{\cancel{75}}}{\underset{5}{\cancel{125}}} \times 2\ ml = \dfrac{6}{5} = 1.2\ ml$

or

  H : V :: D : X

125 mg : 2 ml :: 75 mg : X ml

$$125\ X = 150$$

$$X = 1.2\ ml$$

Answer: methylprednisolone 75 mg = 1.2 ml

3. 0.3 ml of vitamin B_{12} (cyanocobalamin)
4. 0.5 ml of Naloxone (Narcan)
5. **a.** Select the Maxipime 1-gram vial. The Maxipime 2-gram vial is for intravenous use according to the drug label and cannot be used for intramuscular injection.
   b. The amount of diluent is 3.4 ml; 2.6 ml of diluent could also be used.
   c. Change 500 mg to 0.5 g or 1 g to 1000 mg
   $$\frac{D}{H} \times V = \frac{0.5 \text{ g}}{1 \text{ g}} \times 4 \text{ ml} = 2 \text{ ml of cefepime twice a day}$$

6. BF: $\dfrac{D}{H} \times V = \dfrac{4}{5} \times 1 \text{ ml} = \dfrac{4}{5}$

   0.8 ml of compazine
   or
   RP: H : V ::   D : X
       5 mg : 1 ml :: 4 mg : X
               5 X = 4
                 X = 0.8 ml

   or

   DA: ml $= \dfrac{1 \text{ ml} \times 4 \text{ mg}}{5 \text{ mg} \times 1} = \dfrac{4}{5} = 0.8 \text{ ml}$

7. 2.5 ml of secobarbital
8. **a.** 100-mg vial
   b. 0.75 ml of thiamine
9. ½ or 0.5 ml of hydroxyzine
10. **a.** 750 mg of cefonicid (Monocid) is equivalent to 0.75 g.
    b. Drug label indicates that 2.5 ml of diluent should be added to the drug powder, which yields 3.1 ml of drug solution.
    c. $\dfrac{D}{H} \times V = \dfrac{0.75 \text{ g}}{1 \text{ g}} \times 3.1 \text{ ml}$
    $= 2.33 \text{ ml or } 2.3 \text{ ml of cefonicid solution}$

11. **a.** meperidine 35 mg = 0.7 ml
    b. promethazine 10 mg = 0.7 ml
    c. Procedure: 1. Obtain 0.7 ml of meperidine from the ampule and 0.4 ml of promethazine from the ampule.
                2. Discard the remaining solutions within the ampules.
12. **a.** meperidine 50 mg = ½ or 0.5 ml
    b. atropine 0.3 mg = 0.75 or 0.8 ml
    Atropine
    BF: $\dfrac{D}{H} \times V = \dfrac{0.3}{0.4} \times 1 \text{ ml} = 0.75 \text{ or } 0.8 \text{ ml}$

    or
    Atropine
    RP: H : V ::   D : X
        0.4 mg : 1 ml :: 0.3 mg : X ml
                 0.4 X = 0.3
                     X $= \dfrac{0.3}{0.4} = 0.75 \text{ or } 0.8 \text{ ml}$

or

Meperidine

$$\text{DA: ml} = \frac{1 \text{ ml} \times \overset{1}{\cancel{50}} \text{ mg}}{\underset{2}{\cancel{100}} \text{ mg} \times 1} = \frac{1}{2} \text{ or } 0.5 \text{ ml}$$

c. 1. The two drugs are compatible.
   2. Inject 0.75 (0.8) ml of air into the atropine vial.
   3. Inject 0.5 ml of air into the meperidine vial and withdraw 0.5 ml of meperidine.
   4. Withdraw 0.8 ml of atropine from the atropine vial. Discard both vials.

13. BF: $\dfrac{D}{H} \times V = \dfrac{\overset{5}{\cancel{50}} \text{ mg} \times 2 \text{ ml}}{\underset{8}{\cancel{80}} \text{ mg}} = \dfrac{10}{8} = 1.25 \text{ ml}$

or

RP: H : V :: D : X
    80 mg : 2 ml :: 50 mg : X ml
            80 X = 100
                 X = 1.25 ml

Answer: tobramycin 50 mg = 1.25 ml

14. **a.** Use either heparin vial; 5000 U/ml or 10,000 U/ml
    b. 0.5 ml of heparin (U 5000); 0.25 ml of heparin (U 10,000)

15. Librium 50 mg = 1 ml (100 mg = 2 ml)
    After adding 2 ml of diluent, withdraw the entire drug solution to determine the total volume of drug solution. Expel half of the solution; the remaining drug solution is equivalent to chlordiazepoxide (Librium) 50 mg.

16. **a.** Change milligrams to grams (smaller to larger number) by moving the decimal point three spaces to the *left*. 500. mg = 0.5 g.

    Because the drug weight on the label is in grams, the conversion is to grams. However, the drug can be converted to milligrams by changing grams to milligrams (moving the decimal point three spaces to the *right*): 1 g = 1.000 mg = 1000 mg.

    b. Drug label states to add 3 ml of diluent and, after it is reconstituted, the drug solution will be 3.5 ml. Mandol 1 g = 3.5 ml.

    c. A 5-ml syringe is preferred: however, a 3-ml syringe can be used because less than 3 ml of the drug solution is needed.

    d. BF: $\dfrac{D}{H} \times V = \dfrac{0.5}{1} \times 3.5 \text{ ml} = 1.75 \text{ or } 1.8 \text{ ml}$

    or

    RP: H   :   V   ::   D   :   X
        1000 mg : 3.5 ml :: 500 mg : X ml
                1000 X = 1750
                      X = 1.75 or 1.8 ml

    or

    $$\text{DA: ml} = \frac{3.5 \text{ ml} \times 0.5 \text{ \cancel{g}}}{1 \text{ \cancel{g}} \times 1} = 1.75 \text{ or } 1.8 \text{ ml}$$

    Answer: cefamandole (Mandol) 500 mg = 1.8 ml

17. Change 400 milligrams to grams

400 mg = 0.400 g or 0.4 g

$$\frac{D}{H} \times V = \frac{0.4}{1} \times 2.6 = 1 \text{ ml}$$

or

H : V :: D : X
1 g : 2.6 ml :: 0.4 mg : X ml
X = 2.6 × 0.4
X = 1 ml

ticarcillin 400 mg or 0.4 g = 1.0 ml

18. 1 gr = 60 mg; gr ⅙ = 10 mg

$$\frac{D}{H} \times V = \frac{\overset{2}{\cancel{10}}}{\underset{3}{\cancel{15}}} \times 1 \text{ ml} = \frac{2}{3} = 0.66 \text{ or } 0.7 \text{ ml}$$

or

H : V :: D : X
15 mg : 1 ml :: 10 mg : X ml
15 X = 10
X = 0.66 or 0.7 ml

19. **a.** Change milligrams to grams; move the decimal point three spaces to the left: 500. mg = 0.5 g

0.5 g × 3 (q8h) = 1.5 g per day

b. Add 2 ml of diluent to yield 2.6 ml (check drug information insert):

$$\frac{D}{H} \times V = \frac{0.5 \text{ g}}{1 \text{ g}} \times 2.6 \text{ ml} = 1.3 \text{ ml per dose}$$

20. **a.** right, 0.25 g = 250 mg
    b. 1.8 ml (after dilution, 2 ml)
    c. 1 ml = 250 mg of ampicillin

21. **a.** Either the ampule or the vial could be used. The diazepam 5 mg/ml is a multiple-dose vial that contains 10 ml of drug solution.

    b. BF: Ampule: $\dfrac{8 \text{ mg}}{10 \text{ mg}} \times 2 \text{ ml} = 1.6 \text{ ml of diazepam}$

    Vial: $\dfrac{8 \text{ mg}}{5 \text{ mg}} \times 1 \text{ ml} = 1.6 \text{ ml of diazepam}$

    or

    DA: Ampule: ml = $\dfrac{2 \text{ ml} \times \overset{4}{\cancel{8}} \text{ mg}}{\underset{5}{\cancel{10}} \text{ mg} \times 1} = \dfrac{8}{5} = 1.6 \text{ ml}$

    or

    DA: Vial: ml = $\dfrac{1 \text{ ml} \times 8 \text{ mg}}{5 \text{ mg} \times 1} = \dfrac{8}{5} = 1.6 \text{ ml}$

22. $\dfrac{D}{H} \times V = \dfrac{1.5 \text{ mg}}{\underset{1}{\cancel{2}} \text{ mg}} \times \overset{1}{\cancel{2}} \text{ ml} = 1.5 \text{ ml of Cogentin}$

23. BF: $\dfrac{D}{H} \times V = \dfrac{10}{25} \times 5 = 0.4 \times 5 = 2$ ml

or

RP: H   : V   ::   D   : X

     25 million units : 5 ml :: 10 million units : X ml

                         25 X = 50

                            X = 2 ml

Answer: Intron A 2 ml three times a week

24. BF: $\dfrac{D}{H} \times V = \dfrac{2.5}{10} \times 1 = 0.25$ ml

or

RP: H   : V ::   D   : X

    10 mg : 1 ml :: 2.5 mg : X

           10 X = 2.5

             X = 0.25 ml

or

DA: no conversion factor

$$\text{ml} = \dfrac{1\ \text{ml} \times \overset{1}{\cancel{2.5}}\ \cancel{\text{mg}}}{\underset{4}{\cancel{10}}\ \cancel{\text{mg}} \times 1} = \dfrac{1}{4} \text{ or } 0.25 \text{ ml}$$

Answer: AquaMEPHYTON 2.5 mg = 0.25 ml

25. $\text{ml} = \dfrac{2\ \text{ml} \times 2\ \cancel{\text{mg}}}{5\ \cancel{\text{mg}} \times 1} = \dfrac{4}{5} = 0.8$ ml

0.8 ml of droperidol

26. $\text{ml} = \dfrac{1\ \text{ml} \times \overset{4}{\cancel{60}}\ \cancel{\text{mg}} \times \frac{1}{6}\ \cancel{\text{gr}}}{\underset{1}{\cancel{15}}\ \cancel{\text{mg}} \times 1\ \cancel{\text{gr}} \times 1} = 4 \times \frac{1}{6} = \dfrac{4}{6} = \dfrac{2}{3}$ ml or 1.75 ml

27. **a.** 2 ml of diluent (sterile or bacteriostatic water)

    b. 1 g = 2.4; 500 mg = 1.2 ml

    c. $\text{ml} = \dfrac{2.4\ \text{ml} \times 1\ \cancel{\text{g}} \times \overset{1}{\cancel{500}}\ \cancel{\text{mg}}}{1\ \cancel{\text{g}} \times \underset{2}{\cancel{1000}}\ \cancel{\text{mg}} \times 1} = \dfrac{2.4}{2} = 1.2$ ml

     Give 1.2 ml of Cefobid

28. **a.** Factors: drug label: 2 g = 12 ml (add 11.5 ml) **or** 250 mg = 1.5 ml **or** 0.25 g = 1.5 ml

                 drug order: 300 mg/1

    b. Conversion factor: 1 g = 1000 mg

    c. $\text{ml} = \dfrac{1.5\ \text{ml} \times 1\ \cancel{\text{g}} \times \overset{3}{\cancel{300}}\ \cancel{\text{mg}}}{0.25\ \cancel{\text{g}} \times \underset{10}{\cancel{1000}}\ \cancel{\text{mg}} \times 1} = \dfrac{4.5}{2.5} = 1.8$ ml of oxacillin per dose

     or

$$\text{ml} = \dfrac{\overset{6}{\cancel{12}}\ \text{ml} \times 1\ \cancel{\text{g}} \times \overset{3}{\cancel{300}}\ \cancel{\text{mg}}}{2\ \cancel{\text{g}} \times \underset{\underset{5}{10}}{\cancel{1000}}\ \cancel{\text{mg}} \times 1} = \dfrac{18}{10} = 1.8 \text{ ml of oxacillin}$$

29. 0.25 g = 0.025 mg (250 mg)
    a. Drug label: add 2 ml diluent = 2.2 ml of drug solution.
    b. Give 1.1 ml of Ancef.

30. **a.** 140 ÷ 2.2 = 63.6 kg
    b. 15 mg × 63.6 × 1 = 954 mg daily
    c. 954 ÷ 3 = 318 mg of amikacin q8h

    d. BF: $\dfrac{D}{H} \times V = \dfrac{318}{500} \times 2 = \dfrac{636}{500} = 1.27$ or 1.3 ml

    or

    RP: H : V ::   D : X
          500 mg : 2 ml :: 318 mg : X ml
                 500 X = 636
                     X = 1.27 or 1.3 ml

    or

    DA: ml $= \dfrac{2 \text{ ml} \times 318 \text{ mg}}{500 \text{ mg} \times 1} = \dfrac{636}{500} = 1.3$ ml per dose

    Answer: give 1.27 or 1.3 ml of amikacin q8h (three times a day)

31. **a.** 174 ÷ 2.2 = 79.1 kg
    b. 2 mg × 79.1 = 158 mg daily
    c. 158 ÷ 3 = 52 mg or 50 mg q8h

    d. BF: $\dfrac{D}{H} \times V = \dfrac{\overset{5}{\cancel{50}}}{\underset{10}{\cancel{100}}} \times 1 \text{ ml} = \dfrac{5}{10} = 0.5$ ml

    or

    RP: H : V ::   D : X
          100 mg : 1 ml :: 50 mg : X ml
                100 X = 50
                  X = 0.5 ml

    or

    DA: ml $= \dfrac{1 \text{ ml} \times \overset{1}{\cancel{50}} \text{ mg}}{\underset{2}{\cancel{100}} \text{ mg} \times 1} = \dfrac{1}{2}$ or 0.5 ml

    Answer: netilmicin 50 mg = 0.5 ml

32. **a.** 15 mg/67 kg/day = 15 × 67 = 1005 mg/day.
    b. 500 mg (1005 mg ÷ 2 = 500 mg)

    c. $\dfrac{\overset{1}{\cancel{500}}}{\underset{1}{\cancel{500}}} \times 2 = 2$ ml per dose of Kantrex

    d. 1 g = 1000 mg $\dfrac{D}{H} \times V = \dfrac{\overset{1}{\cancel{500}}}{\underset{2}{\cancel{1000}}} \times 3 = \dfrac{3}{2} = 1.5$ ml

Intravenous Preparations with Clinical Applications

OBJECTIVES

- Name catheter sites for intravenous access.
- Examine the three methods for calculating intravenous (IV) flow rate and select one of the methods for IV calculation.
- Calculate drops per minute of prescribed IV solutions for IV therapy.
- Determine the drop factor according to the manufacturer's product specification.
- Calculate the drug dosage for IV medications.
- Calculate the flow rate for IV drugs being administered in a prescribed amount of solution.
- Explain the types and uses of electronic IV delivery devices.
- Calculate the rate of direct IV injection.

OUTLINE

INTRAVENOUS ACCESS SITES
 Intermittent Infusion Devices
DIRECT INTRAVENOUS INJECTIONS
CONTINUOUS INTRAVENOUS ADMINISTRATION
 Intravenous Sets
CALCULATION OF INTRAVENOUS FLOW RATE
 Safety Considerations
 Mixing Drugs Used for Continuous Intravenous Administration
INTERMITTENT INTRAVENOUS ADMINISTRATION
 Secondary Intravenous Sets
 Electronic Intravenous Delivery Devices
FLOW RATES FOR IV PUMPS
 Calculating Flow Rates for Intravenous Drugs and Electrolytes

Intravenous (IV) therapy is used for administering fluids containing water, dextrose, fat emulsions, vitamins, electrolytes, and drugs. Approximately 90% of all hospitalized clients, some outpatients, and some home-care clients receive IV therapy. Drugs are administered intravenously for direct absorption and fast action. Many drugs cannot be absorbed through the gastrointestinal tract, and the IV route provides bioavailability. Certain drugs that need to be absorbed immediately are administered by direct intravenous injection—often diluted, over several minutes. However, many drugs administered intravenously are irritating to the veins because of the drugs' pH or osmolality and must be diluted and administered slowly.

Advantages of IV drug therapy are (1) rapid drug distribution into the bloodstream, (2) rapid onset of action, and (3) no drug loss to tissues. There are many complications of IV therapy, some of which are sepsis, thrombosis, phlebitis, air emboli, infiltration, and extravasation. The nurse must monitor for signs of these complications during the course of IV therapy.

Three methods are used to administer IV fluid and drugs: (1) direct IV drug injection, (2) continuous IV infusion, and (3) intermittent IV infusion. Continuous IV administration replaces fluid loss, maintains fluid balance, and is a vehicle for drug administration. Intermittent IV administration is primarily used for giving IV drugs.

Nurses play an important role in preparing and administering IV solutions and drugs. Nursing functions and responsibilities include (1) knowledge of IV sets and their drop factors, (2) calculating IV flow rates, (3) verifying compatibility of the IV solution and the drug, (4) mixing drugs and diluting in IV solution, (5) regulating IV infusion devices, and (6) maintaining patency of IV accesses.

INTRAVENOUS ACCESS SITES

The successful administration of IV drugs and fluids depends on a patent vascular access. The most common site for short-term therapy is the peripheral site, in which a short catheter or needle is inserted in a vein in the hand or arm. Feet and legs can be used, but the risk of a deep vein thrombus is always present. For individuals without adequate peripheral sites or those requiring long-term IV therapy, a central venous site is chosen. Central venous sites are the superior vena cava and the inferior vena cava. The superior vena cava is accessed from the internal jugular vein and the right or left subclavian vein, whereas the inferior vena cava is accessed from the femoral vein. The insertion requires a minor surgical procedure: percutaneous vein cannulation with the introduction of a catheter. The catheter may be single-lumen or multilumen. A long-line peripheral catheter can also be used to access the superior vena cava. The long-line catheter is inserted in a large vein (the basilic vein) and advanced through the subclavian vein to the superior vena cava. In some states, peripherally inserted central catheters (PICCs) are inserted by registered nurses.

Clients who need vascular access for long-term use, such as chemotherapy, antibiotic therapy, or nutritional support, are given much longer catheters, which are tunneled under the skin after the vein is cannulated. The catheter and its drug infusion port exit from the subcutaneous tissue to a site on the chest. Examples of these devices are the Hickman, Groshong, Neostar, and Cook catheters.

Another type of catheter for long-term use has an implantable infusion port that is inserted in the subcutaneous tissue under the skin. These devices are called *vascular access ports* and they have a larger drug port or septum than other catheters. Care must be taken to use a noncoring needle that slices the port instead of making holes so that the septum will close instead of leak after the needle has been removed (Fig. 9-1).

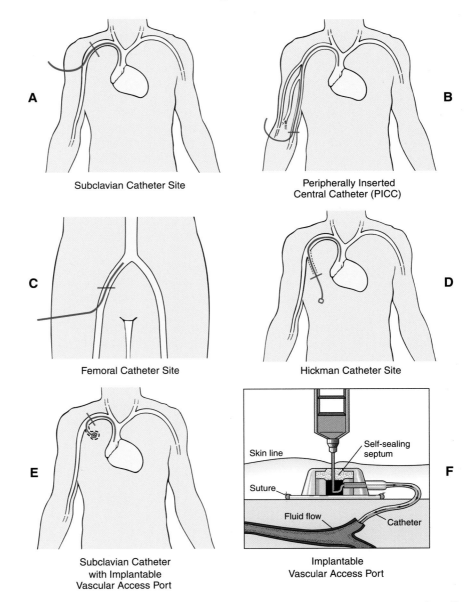

FIGURE 9-1 Central venous access sites: **A,** Subclavian catheter. **B,** Peripherally inserted central catheter (PICC). **C,** Femoral catheter. **D,** Hickman catheter. **E,** Subclavian catheter with implantable vascular access port. **F,** Implantable vascular access port. (**F** redrawn from Winter, B. [1984]. Implantable vascular access devices. *Oncology Nursing Forum* 11[6], 25-30.)

Intermittent Infusion Devices

When IV access sites are used not for continuous infusion but rather for intermittent therapy, they must be irrigated periodically to maintain patency. An intermittent infusion device can be attached to the end of the vascular access device, catheter, or needle, to close the connection that was attached to the IV tubing (Fig. 9-2). These devices have ports (stoppers) where needleless syringes can be inserted when drug therapy is resumed. This practice can eliminate the need for a constant low-rate infusion to keep the vein open (KVO) and reduce excessive fluid intake. The use of intermittent infusion devices can allow the client more mobility and can be cost-effective because less IV tubing, IV solution, and regulating equipment are needed.

IV sites should be irrigated every 8 to 12 hours or before and after each drug infusion, depending on institutional policy, to maintain patency. Table 9-1 gives suggested flushing/irrigation times. Pre-filled single-use syringes of saline solution are available to flush infusion devices. The intent of the pre-filled single-use syringes is to prevent the cross-contamination that can occur with a multidose vial. The volume of the flush used for vascular access devices is twice the volume of the catheter plus any connected devices such as a three-way stopcock or an extension set. Heparinized saline solution flushes are generally used for venous access devices that are tunneled or implanted.

DIRECT INTRAVENOUS INJECTIONS

Medications that are given by the IV injection route are calculated in the same manner as medications for intramuscular (IM) injection. This route is often referred to as *IV push*. Clinically, it is the preferred route for clients with poor muscle mass or decreased circulation, or for a drug that is poorly absorbed from the tissues. Medications administered by this route have a rapid onset of action, and calculation errors can have serious, even fatal, consequences. Drug information inserts must be read carefully, and attention must be paid to the amount of drug that can be given per minute. If the drug is

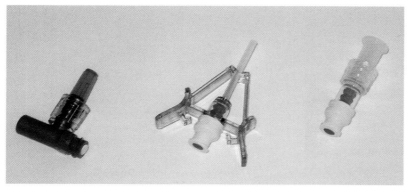
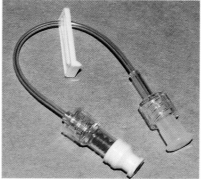

FIGURE 9-2 Needleless infusion devices. Medication in a needleless syringe can be inserted into a needleless infusion device.

Table 9-1

Venous Access Devices: Flushing for Peripheral and Central Venous*

Type	Length (inches)	Flush Before Use	Flush After Drug Use	Volume
Peripheral	1-2	NSS	NSS	1-3
Central venous				
Single-lumen	8	NSS	HSS	1-3
Multilumen	8	NSS	HSS	1-3
External-tunneled Hickman, Cook, or Groshong	35	NSS	HSS or NSS Flush q12h if not used	10
Peripherally inserted central catheter (PICC)	20	NSS	NSS Flush q12h if not used	10
Implanted vascular access device	35	NSS	HSS or NSS Flush q12h if not used	10

HSS, Heparinized saline solution; *NSS,* normal saline solution.
*If the adapter/cap is pressurized, then normal saline solution is used and not a heparin solution. Check with your institution.

pushed into the bloodstream at a faster rate than specified in the drug literature, adverse reactions to the medication are likely to occur.

Calculating the amount of time needed to infuse a drug given by direct IV infusion can be determined by using ratio and proportion.

REMEMBER

When giving drugs by direct IV infusion, always verify the compatibility of the IV solution and the drug. Consider the length of the injection port on the tubing from the IV site, and remember that the tubing usually needs to be flushed after direct IV infusion to ensure that part of the drug has not been left in the tubing. Drug dose is not complete until the drug has entered the client.

EXAMPLES

Set up a ratio and proportion using the recommended amount of drug per minute on one side of the equation; these are the known variables. On the other side of the equation are the desired amount of drug and unknown desired minutes. a. amount of milliliters (ml); b. number of minutes

PROBLEM 1: Order: Dilantin 200 mg, IV, STAT.
Drug available: Dilantin 250 mg/5 ml. IV infusion not to exceed 50 mg/min.

a. BF: $\dfrac{D}{H} \times V = \dfrac{\overset{4}{\cancel{200}}}{\underset{5}{\cancel{250}}} \times 5 = \dfrac{20}{5} = 4$ ml

or

RP: H : V ::   D   : X
250 mg : 5 ml :: 200 mg : X ml
250 X = 1000
X = 4 ml

or

$$\text{DA: ml} = \frac{5 \text{ ml} \times \overset{4}{\cancel{200}} \text{ m\cancel{g}}}{\underset{5}{\cancel{250}} \text{ m\cancel{g}} \times 1} = \frac{20}{5} = 4 \text{ ml}$$

200 mg = 4 ml (discard 1 ml of the 5 ml).

b. known drug : known minutes :: desired drug : desired minutes
   50 mg   :   1 min   ::   200 mg   :   X
50 X = 200
X = 4 min

PROBLEM 2: Order: Lasix 120 mg, IV, STAT.
Drug available: Lasix 10 mg/ml. IV infusion not to exceed 40 mg/min.
a. RP: H : V ::   D   :X
10 mg : 1 ml :: 120 mg : X
10 X = 120
X = 12 ml of Lasix

or

$$\text{DA: ml} = \frac{1 \text{ ml} \times \overset{12}{\cancel{120}} \text{ m\cancel{g}}}{\underset{1}{\cancel{10}} \text{ m\cancel{g}} \times 1} = 12 \text{ ml of Lasix}$$

b. known drug : known minutes :: desired drug : desired minutes
   40 mg   :   1 min   ::   120 mg   :   X
40 X = 120
X = 3 min

When dosing instructions give the amount of drug and specify infusion time, the amount of drug can be divided by the number of minutes to give the per minute amount to be infused.

EXAMPLE

PROBLEM 3: Order: Amrinone (Inocor) 65 mg, IV bolus over 3 minutes.
Drug available: Inocor 100 mg/20 ml
a.   H   : V ::   D :X
100 mg : 20 ml :: 65 mg : X
100 X = 1300
X = 13 ml

or

$$\text{DA: ml} = \frac{\overset{1}{\cancel{20}} \text{ ml} \times 65 \text{ m\cancel{g}}}{\underset{5}{\cancel{100}} \text{ m\cancel{g}} \times 1} = \frac{65}{5} = 13 \text{ ml}$$

b. $\dfrac{13 \text{ ml}}{3 \text{ min}} = 4.2 \text{ ml/min}$

Ⅰ **Direct IV Injection**

Answers can be found on page 221.

a. **Determine the amount in milliliters of drug solution to administer.**
b. **Determine the number of minutes that are required for the direct IV drug dose to be administered for each of the practice problems.**

1. Order: protamine sulfate 50 mg, IV, STAT.
Drug available:

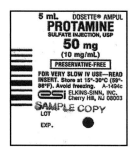

IV infusion not to exceed 5 mg/min.

a. Amount in milliliters (ml) _____

b. Number of minutes to administer _____

2. Order: dextrose 50% in 50 ml, IV, STAT.
Drug available: dextrose 50% in 50 ml
IV infusion not to exceed 10 ml/min.

a. Number of minutes to administer 50% of 50 ml _____

3. Order: calcium gluconate 4.5 mEq, IV, STAT.
Drug available:

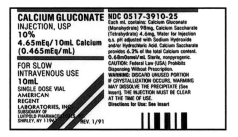

IV infusion not to exceed 1.5 ml/min. **Note:** 4.65 mEq/10 ml.

a. Amount in milliliters _____

b. Number of minutes _____

4. Order: prednisolone 50 mg, IV, q12h.
Drug available: prednisolone 50 mg in 5 ml.
IV infusion not to exceed 10 mg/min.

    a. Amount in milliliters _____

    b. Number of minutes _____

5. Order: morphine sulfate 6 mg, IV, q3h, PRN.
Drug available:

Infusion not to exceed 10 mg/4 mins.

    a. Amount in milliliters _____

    b. Number of minutes _____

6. Order: digoxin 0.25 mg, IV, qd.
Drug available:

Infuse slowly over 5 minutes

    a. Amount in milliliters _____

    b. How many ml/min should be infused? _____

7. Order: Haldol 2 mg, IV, q4h, PRN.
Drug available: Haldol 5 mg/ml.
IV infusion not to exceed 1 mg/min.

    a. Amount in milliliters _____

    b. Number of minutes _____

8. Order: Ativan 6 mg, IV, q6h, PRN.
Drug available: Ativan 4 mg/ml.
IV infusion not to exceed 2 mg/min.

    a. Amount in milliliters _____

    b. Number of minutes _____

9. Order: diltiazem (Cardizem) 20 mg IV over 2 minutes.
Drug available:

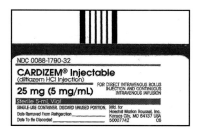

a. How many milliliters (ml) would you give? _____

b. How many milliliters (ml) would you infuse per minute? _____

10. Order: granisetron (Kytril) 10 μg/kg, 30 minutes before chemotherapy.
Infuse 1 mg over 60 seconds.
Patient weighs 140 pounds.
Drug available:

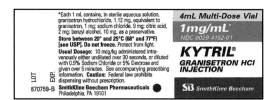

a. How many kilograms (kg) does the client weigh? _____

b. How many milligrams (mg) should the client receive? _____

c. For how many seconds should the drug dose be infused? _____

NOTE

When a drug is being pushed through IV tubing, the type of fluid used for infusion must be compatible with the drug, or precipitation can result. Incompatibilities can be avoided if IV tubing is flushed with a drug-compatible solution, either sterile normal saline solution or sterile water, before and after administration.

CONTINUOUS INTRAVENOUS ADMINISTRATION

When IV solutions are required, the health care provider orders the amount of solution per liter or milliliter to be administered for a specific time, such as for 24 hours. The nurse calculates the IV flow rate according to the drop factor, the amount of fluids to be administered, and the infusion time.

Intravenous Sets

There are various IV infusion sets. The drop factor, or the number of drops per milliliter, is usually printed on the package. Sets that deliver large drops per milliliter (10–20 gtt/ml) are referred to as *macrodrip sets,* and those that deliver small drops per milliliter (60 gtt/ml) are called *microdrip* or *minidrip sets.*

Examples of sets that deliver macrodrip (large drops) or microdrip (small drops) are listed in Table 9-2. Figures 9-3, 9-4, and 9-5 illustrate sizes of IV drops, IV bags and bottles, and IV tubing.

All microdrip sets deliver 60 gtt/ml. To determine the drop factor (gtt/ml), check the box or package of the IV set. This information is needed to calculate and regulate IV flow rate. In most instances, the nurse has a choice of using either a macrodrip or a microdrip set. If the IV rate is to infuse at 100 ml/hr or faster, a macrodrip set is generally used. If the infusion rate is slower than 100 ml/hr, the microdrip set is preferred. Slow drip rates of less

Table 9-2

Intravenous Sets

Drops (gtt) per Milliliter	
Macrodrip Sets	**Microdrip Sets**
10 gtt/ml 15 gtt/ml 20 gtt/ml	60 gtt/ml

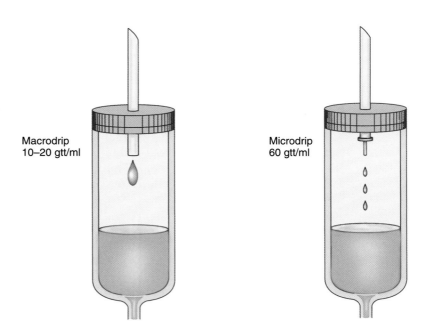

Macrodrip
10–20 gtt/ml

Microdrip
60 gtt/ml

FIGURE 9-3 Macrodrip and microdrip sizes.

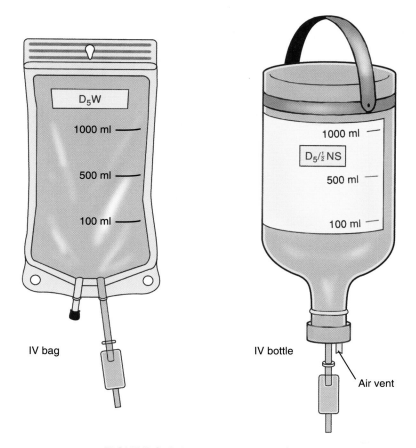

FIGURE 9-4 Intravenous containers.

than 100 ml/hr make macrodrip adjustment difficult. For example, at 50 ml/hr, the macrodrip rate would be 8 gtt/min.

At times, IV fluids are given at a slow rate to *keep vein open* (KVO), also called *to keep open* (TKO). Reasons for ordering KVO include (1) a suspected or potential emergency situation requiring rapid administration of fluids and drugs and (2) maintaining an open line to give IV drugs at specified hours. For KVO, a microdrip set (60 gtt/ml) and a 250-ml IV bag can be used. KVO is usually regulated to deliver 10 to 20 ml/hr or according to the institution's protocol.

CALCULATION OF INTRAVENOUS FLOW RATE

Three different methods can be used to calculate IV flow rate (drops per minute or gtt/min). The nurse should select one of the methods, memorize it, and use it to calculate dosages.*

---

*The two-step method is the method most commonly used for calculating IV flow rate.

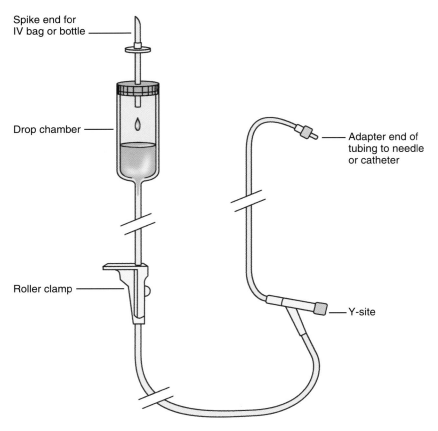

FIGURE 9-5 Intravenous tubing.

THREE-STEP METHOD

a. $\dfrac{\text{Amount of solution}}{\text{Hours to administer}} = \text{ml/hr}$

b. $\dfrac{\text{ml per hour}}{60 \text{ minutes}} = \text{ml/min}$

c. ml per minute $\times$ gtt per ml of IV set = gtt/min

TWO-STEP METHOD

a. Amount of fluid $\div$ Hours to administer = ml/hr

b. $\dfrac{\text{ml per hour} \times \text{gtt/ml (IV set)}}{60 \text{ minutes}} = \text{gtt/min}$

ONE-STEP METHOD

$$\dfrac{\text{Amount of fluid} \times \text{gtt/ml (IV set)}}{\text{Hours to administer} \times \text{minutes per hour (60)}} = \text{gtt/min}$$

Safety Considerations

All IV infusions should be checked every hour to ensure the rate of infusion and to assess for potential problems. Common problems associated with IV infusions are kinked tubing, extravasation of IV fluids, and "runaway" IV rates. IVs with electronic IV delivery devices also need to be monitored. Mechanical problems or incorrect settings can cause incorrect fluid administration. Fluid overload, thrombus formation, and infiltration at the IV site are complications of IV therapy that can be avoided with frequent monitoring of the IV infusion. See Appendix A for more detailed information on safe nursing practice for IV drug administration.

Mixing Drugs Used for Continuous Intravenous Administration

Drugs such as multiple vitamins and potassium chloride can be added to the IV solution bag for continuous IV infusion. It is suggested that the drug or drugs be added to the bag or bottle immediately before administering the IV fluid. Inject the drug into the rubber stopper on the IV bag or bottle and rotate bag or bottle several times to ensure dispersal of the drug. A medication label must be placed on the IV solution bag indicating the drug added, the date, time, and date of expiration. If drugs are injected into the IV bag before use, the bag should be refrigerated to maintain drug potency. Figure 9-6 shows that a drug mixed in the pharmacy is attached to a small IV fluid bag and is sent to the hospital unit.

NOTE

DO NOT add the drug while the infusion is running unless the bag is rotated. A drug solution injected into an upright infusing IV solution causes the drug to concentrate into the lower portion of the IV bag and not be dispersed. The client will receive a concentrated drug solution and this can be harmful (e.g., if the drug is potassium chloride).

There are various nutrient (dextrose) and electrolytes in commercially prepared IV solutions. The commonly used solutions are dextrose in water, dextrose with one-half normal saline solution, normal saline solution (0.9%),

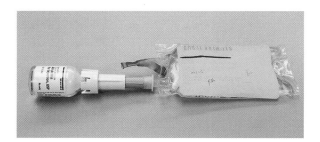

FIGURE 9-6 Medication mixed and attached to an IV bag.

Table 9-3

Abbreviations for IV Solutions

IV Solution	Abbreviation(s)
5% dextrose in water	D_5W, 5% D/W
10% dextrose in water	$D_{10}W$, 10% D/W
0.9% sodium chloride, normal saline solution	0.9% NaCl, NSS, PSS
0.45% sodium chloride, ½ normal saline solution	0.45% NaCl, ½ NSS, ½ PSS
5% dextrose in 0.9% sodium chloride	D_5NSS, 5% D/NSS, 5% D/0.9% NaCl, D_5 PSS
5% dextrose in 0.45% sodium chloride, 5% dextrose in ½ normal saline solution	D_5½ NSS, 5% D/½ NSS, D_5 PSS, ½ PSS
Lactated Ringer's solution	LRS

one-half normal saline solution, and lactated Ringer's solution. These types of solutions are abbreviated as listed in Table 9-3.

EXAMPLES

Two problems for determining IV flow rate are given. Each problem is solved with each of the three methods for calculating IV flow rate.

PROBLEM 1: Order: 1000 ml of D_5½ NSS (5% dextrose in ½ normal saline solution) in 6 hours.
Available: 1 L (1000 ml) of D_5½ NSS solution bag: IV set labeled 10 gtt/ml.
How many drops per minute (gtt/min) should the client receive?

Three-Step Method: a. $\dfrac{1000 \text{ ml}}{6 \text{ hr}} = 166.6$ or 167 ml/hr

b. $\dfrac{167 \text{ ml}}{60 \text{ min}} = 2.7$ or 2.8 ml/min

c. 2.8 ml/min × 10 gtt/ml = 28 gtt/min

Two-Step Method: a. 1000 ml ÷ 6 hr = 167 ml/hr

b. $\dfrac{167 \text{ ml/hr} \times \overset{1}{\cancel{10}} \text{ gtt/ml}}{\underset{6}{\cancel{60}} \text{ min}} = \dfrac{167}{6} = 28$ gtt/min

10 and 60 cancel to 1 and 6.
If ml/hr is given, use only part **b** of the two-step method for calculating IV flow rate.

One-Step Method: $\dfrac{1000 \text{ ml} \times \overset{1}{\cancel{10}} \text{ gtt/ml}}{6 \text{ hr} \times \underset{6}{\cancel{60}} \text{ min}} \times \dfrac{1000}{36} = 27\text{–}28$ gtt/min

10 and 60 cancel to 1 and 6.
For the purpose of avoiding errors, the use of a hand calculator is strongly suggested.

Answer: 28 gtt/min.

PROBLEM 2: Order: 1000 ml of D_5W (5% dextrose in water), 1 vial of MVI (multiple vitamin), and 20 mEq of KCl (potassium chloride) every 8 hours.
Available: 1000 ml D_5W solution bag
  1 vial of MVI = 5 ml
  40 mEq/20 ml of KCl in an ampule
  IV set labeled 15 gtt/ml

How many milliliters (ml) of KCl would you withdraw as equivalent to 20 mEq of KCl?
How would you mix KCl in the IV bag?
How many drops per minute should the client receive?

Procedure: MVI: Inject 5 ml of MVI into the rubber stopper on the IV bag.
  KCl: Calculate the prescribed dosage for KCl by using the basic formula, ratio and proportion, or dimensional analysis.

$$\frac{D}{H} \times V = \frac{20}{40} \times 20 = \frac{400}{40} = 10 \text{ ml}$$

or

$$H \quad : \quad V \quad :: \quad D \quad : \quad X$$
$$40 \text{ mEq} : 20 \text{ ml} :: 20 \text{ mEq} : X \text{ ml}$$
$$40 X = 400$$
$$X = 10 \text{ ml}$$

or

$$DA: \text{ml} = \frac{V \times D}{H \times 1}$$

$$\text{ml} = \frac{20 \text{ ml} \times \overset{1}{\cancel{20}} \cancel{\text{mEq}}}{\underset{2}{\cancel{40}} \cancel{\text{mEq}} \times 1} = \frac{20}{2} = 10 \text{ ml}$$

Withdraw 10 ml of KCl and inject it into the rubber stopper on the IV bag. Make sure the KCl solution is dispersed throughout the IV solution by rotating the IV bag.

Three-Step Method: **a.** $\dfrac{1000 \text{ ml}}{8 \text{ hr}} = 125 \text{ ml/hr}$

  b. $\dfrac{125 \text{ ml}}{60 \text{ min}} = 2.0\text{--}2.1 \text{ ml/min}$

  c. $2.1 \times 15 = 31\text{--}32 \text{ gtt/min}$

Two-Step Method: **a.** $1000 \div 8 = 125 \text{ ml/hr}$

  b. $\dfrac{125 \text{ ml/hr} \times \overset{1}{\cancel{15}} \text{ gtt/ml}}{\underset{4}{\cancel{60}} \text{ min}} = \dfrac{125}{4} = 31\text{--}32 \text{ gtt/min}$
  15 and 60 cancel to 1 and 4.
  IV flow rate should be 31 to 32 gtt/min.

One-Step Method: $\dfrac{1000 \text{ ml} \times \overset{1}{\cancel{15}} \text{ gtt/ml}}{8 \text{ hr} \times \underset{4}{\cancel{60}} \text{ min}} = \dfrac{1000}{32} = 32 \text{ gtt/min}$
  15 and 60 cancel to 1 and 4.
  IV flow rate should be 31 to 32 gtt/min.

NOTE

Medication volume can be added to the total volume if strict intake and output are being recorded. In general, an IV bag contains more fluid than labeled on the bag; some estimates are as much as 50 ml. If an electric infusion device is used, the client will receive the amount programmed into the device. When the volume of the medication exceeds 20 ml, the amount should be added to the total volume to be infused. If the volume is less than 20 ml, it will not greatly change the hourly rate.

PRACTICE PROBLEMS II Continuous Intravenous Administration

Answers can be found on page 223.

Select *one* of the three methods for calculating IV flow rate. The two-step method is preferred by most nurses.

1. Order: 1000 ml of D_5W to run for 12 hours.

   a. Would you use a macrodrip or microdrip IV set? _____

   b. Calculate the drops per minute (gtt/min) using one of the three methods.

   _____

2. Order: 3 L of IV solutions for 24 hours: 2 L of 5% D/½ NSS and 1 L of D_5W.

   a. One liter is equal to _____ ml.

   b. Each liter should run for _____ hours.

   c. The institution uses an IV set with a drop factor of 15 gtt/ml. How many

   drops per minute (gtt/min) should the client receive?_____

3. Order: 250 ml of D_5W for KVO.

   a. What type of IV set would you use? _____

   Why? _____

   b. How many drops per minute should the client receive? _____

4. Order: 1000 ml of 5% D/0.2% NaCl with 10 mEq of KCl for 10 hours. Available: Macrodrip IV set with a drop factor of 20 gtt/ml and microdrip set; KCl 20 mEq/20 ml vial.

   a. How many milliliters (ml) of KCl should be injected into the IV bag?

   _____

   b. How is KCl mixed in the IV solution?_____

   c. How many drops per minute (gtt/min) should the client receive with both

   the macrodrip set and the microdrip set?_____

5. A liter (1000 ml) of IV fluid was started at 9 AM and was to run for 8 hours. The IV set delivers 15 gtt/ml. Four hours later, only 300 ml have been absorbed.

   a. How much IV fluid is left? _____

   b. Recalculate the flow rate for the remaining IV fluids. _____

6. The client is to receive D_5W, 100 ml/hr.
   Available: Microdrip set (60 gtt/ml).

   How many drops per minute should the client receive? _____

7. Order: 1000 D_5W with 40 mEq KCl at 125 ml/hr.
   Drug available:

   a. Which concentration of KCl would you choose? _____

   b. How many milliliters (ml) of KCl should be injected into the IV bag?

   _____

   c. How many hours will the IV last? _____

8. Order: 1000 $D_5/\frac{1}{2}$ NSS with 20 mEq KCl at 100 ml/hr.
   Available: Macrodrip set (10 gtt/ml)
   Drug available:

   a. Which concentration of KCl would you choose? _____

   b. How many milliliters (ml) of KCl should be injected into the IV bag?

   _____

   c. How many hours will the IV last? _____

   d. How many drops per minute (gtt/min) should the client receive?

   _____

INTERMITTENT INTRAVENOUS ADMINISTRATION

Giving drugs via the intermittent IV route has many advantages. The IV route allows for rapid therapeutic concentration of the drug and control over the onset of action and peak concentrations. Blood serum concentrations can be achieved via the IV route if the oral route is unavailable because of the client's condition, such as gastrointestinal malabsorption or neurological deficits that prevent swallowing. The IV route can be used on an outpatient basis and can ensure compliance with drug therapy. The IV route also allows for the rapid correction of electrolyte imbalances. IV medications can be given at intervals within a 24-hour period for days or weeks. These medications are administered in a small volume of fluid (50 to 250 ml of D_5W or saline solution). The drug solution is usually delivered to the client in 15 minutes to 1 hour, depending on the medication. A separate delivery set or secondary set is used for intermittent therapy if the client is also receiving continuous infusion through the same IV site.

Secondary Intravenous Sets

Two sets available for administering IV drugs are (1) the calibrated cylinder (chamber) with tubing, such as Buretrol, Volutrol, and Soluset, and (2) the secondary set, which is similar to a regular IV set except that the tubing is shorter (Fig. 9-7). The secondary set is primarily used for infusing small volumes, such as 50-, 100-, and 250-ml bags or bottles. The chambers of the Buretrol, Volutrol, and Soluset devices each hold 150 ml of solution. Medication is injected into the chamber and diluted with solution. These methods for administering IV drugs are referred to as *IV piggyback* (IVPB). Usually, drugs administered by Buretrol, Volutrol, or Soluset are prepared by the nurse.

Normally, drugs for IV infusion are diluted before infusion. Clinical agencies frequently have their own protocols for dilutions; if not, the drug information insert should have infusion guidelines. If the information is not available, the hospital pharmacy should be contacted. Guidelines and protocols help in preventing drug and fluid incompatibility.

The current trend in IV medication administration is the use of premixed IV drugs in 50- to 500-ml bags. These premixed IV medications can be prepared by the manufacturer or by the hospital pharmacy. The problems of contamination and drug errors are decreased with the use of premixed IV medication. Each IV drug bag has separate tubing to prevent admixture. Cost is higher but risk is lower with the use of premixed IV drug bags. Because not all medication can be premixed in the solution, nurses will continue to prepare some drugs for IV administration.

NOTE

When using a calibrated cylinder such as the Buretrol, add 15 ml of IV solution to flush the drug out of the IV line after the drug infusion is completed. The flush volume is added to the client's intake.

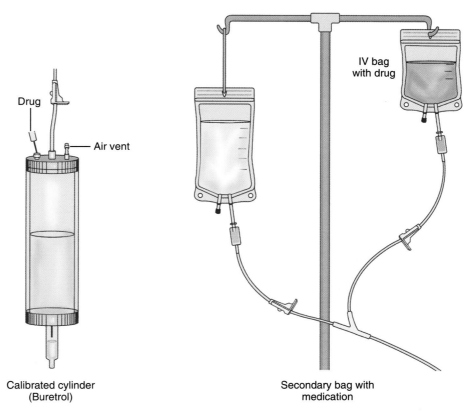

Drug

Air vent

Calibrated cylinder
(Buretrol)

IV bag
with drug

Secondary bag with
medication

FIGURE 9-7 Secondary intravenous sets.

Electronic Intravenous Delivery Devices

IV Delivery Pumps

An IV delivery pump pushes with pressure to infuse the fluid. The two types of IV delivery pumps are the linear peristaltic pump and the volumetric pump (Fig. 9-8). The linear peristaltic pump and the volumetric pump have different pushing mechanisms. With the peristaltic pump, ridges move in wavelike motion against the IV tubing. The pressure on the IV tubing moves the fluid along.

The volumetric pump is more accurate. It requires a specific administration set that functions as a reservoir. The pump fills the reservoir and empties every cycle to deliver the programmed fluid rate. The increments of fluid delivered can be as low as one tenth to one hundredth of a milliliter with micropumps.

Pumps have safety features such as air-in-line, occlusion, and infusion complete alarms, as well as low battery or low power alerts. IV pumps are recommended for use with all central venous lines, arterial lines, and hyperalimentation. For clients who need multiple infusions, multichanneled pumps

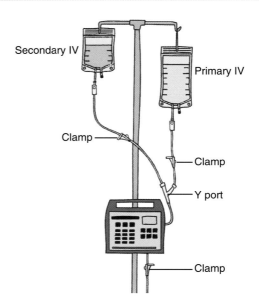

Secondary IV

Primary IV

Clamp

Clamp

Y port

Clamp

FIGURE 9-8 Infusion pump.

are available; and they have two or more programmable pumps, each of which can be set for a different infusion rate (Fig. 9-9). Every model pump has different features and parameters, and nurses must be familiar with the capabilities of the infusion devices they use.

Syringe Pumps

Syringe pumps are primarily used when a small volume of medication is given. The syringe with medication is fitted into the pump, and the plunger is pushed by a piston-controlled mechanism, which delivers the medication at a controlled rate (Fig. 9-9, *A*). Some pumps can operate with syringes of various sizes, from a 5 ml to a 60 ml. Syringe pumps are therapy-specific and are commonly used in oncology, obstetrics, and anesthesia. Syringe pumps usually do not have the same alarms as IV delivery pumps and require closer monitoring.

Patient-Controlled Analgesia (PCA)

Patient-controlled analgesia (PCA) devices enable the client to self-administer IV analgesics (Fig. 9-9, *D*). These programmable pumps are designed to deliver the analgesic at a loading dose or a continual dose, and allow a client to administer a bolus dose at set intervals. The pump can be programmed to lock out bolus doses that are not within the preset time frame to prevent overdose. Morphine is commonly used as the analgesic with a dilution of 1 mg/ml. Clients' therapy is documented every 2 to 4 hours, with assessments and recordings of the amount of drug infused.

Additional information on "Patient-Controlled Analgesia" is available on the CD-ROM in the "Calculating Dosages" section.

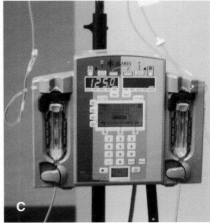

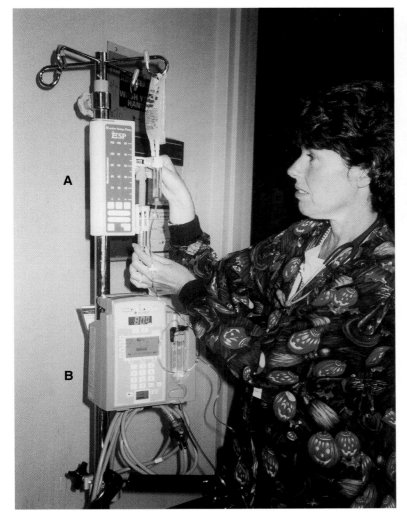

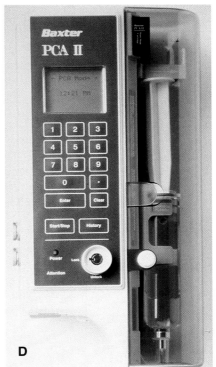

FIGURE 9-9 **A,** Syringe pump. **B,** Single infusion pump.
C, Dual-channel infusion pump. **D,** Patient-controlled analgesia
(PCA) pump.

FLOW RATES FOR IV PUMPS

IV pumps are designed to deliver a wide variety of fluids over a broad range
of infusion rates from multiple fluid container types. Pumps deliver a specific
volume of fluid at a specific rate, measured in milliliters per hour (ml/hr).
They deliver general IV fluids and electrolytes, blood and blood products,
lipids, cardiovascular drugs, hyperalimentation, anesthetics, antibiotics, and
analgesics. The pumps use electronic monitoring to detect partial or full oc-

clusions, especially at low flow rates. In addition, accidental free flow of fluids is eliminated. The pumps are designed to notify the nurse of empty fluid containers and any upstream occlusion, such as a clamp that is not released. Pumps can deliver IV rates from 0.1 to 999.9 ml/hr.

Calculating Flow Rates for Intravenous Drugs and Electrolytes

Drugs that are given by intermittent infusion must be diluted and infused slowly. The pH and the osmolality determine the dilution. A slower infusion time allows for the medication to be diluted in the blood vessel, thereby preventing phlebitis and high concentrations of the drug in plasma and tissues that might cause time-related overdose, toxic effects, or allergic reactions. Drug-dosing instructions indicate the amount and type of solution and the length of infusion time. The nurse must calculate the drug dose from the physician's order, then calculate the flow rate from the drug-dosing information.

When calibrated cylinders, such as Voltrol, Buretrol, or Soluset, are used for drug infusion, the tubing must be flushed after each infusion to make sure the entire drug dose was given. The rinse can range from 10 to 25 ml and is added to the IV intake. When a minibag is used, the IV tubing should be drained so the client receives the complete dose.

Secondary Sets

Secondary sets (calibrated cylinders and 50- to 250-ml IV bags) use drops per minute (gtt/min). The one-step method for calculating drops per minute (gtt/min) is used when IV drugs are administered with secondary sets.

One-Step Method for IV Drug Calculation with Secondary Set

$$\frac{\text{Amount of solution} \times \text{gtt/ml of the set}}{\text{Minutes to administer}} = \text{gtt/min}$$

Infusion Pumps

Infusion pumps use units of milliliters per hour. Use the following method to calculate milliliters per hour.

$$\text{Amount of solution} \div \frac{\text{Minutes to administer}}{\text{60 minutes/hour}} = \text{ml/hr}$$

NOTE

Medication volume that exceeds 5 ml should be added to the dilution volume in intermittent drug therapy. Because smaller volumes of fluid are used for IV infusion, drug dosage may be decreased if the volume of medication is not included in the dilution volume. The amount of solution in the formula should include both volumes.

EXAMPLES

PROBLEM 1: Order: Tagamet 200 mg, IV, q6h.
Drug available:

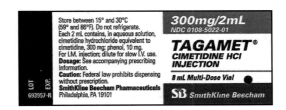

Set and solution: Buretrol set with drop factor of 60 gtt/ml; 500 ml of D₅W.
Instruction: Dilute drug in 100 ml of D₅W and infuse over 20 minutes.

Drug Calculation:

$$\text{BF: } \frac{D}{H} \times V = \frac{200}{300} \times 2 = \frac{400}{300}$$

$$X = 1.3 \text{ ml of Tagamet}$$

or

RP: H : V ::   D : X
   300 mg : 2 ml :: 200 mg : X ml
          300 X = 400

$$X = \frac{400}{300} = 300\overline{)400.0}^{\,1.3}$$

$$X = 1.3 \text{ ml of Tagamet}$$

or

$$\text{DA: ml} = \frac{2 \text{ ml} \times \overset{2}{\cancel{200}} \text{ m\cancel{g}}}{\underset{3}{\cancel{300}} \text{ m\cancel{g}} \times 1} = \frac{4}{3} = 1.3 \text{ ml}$$

Flow Rate Calculation:

$$\frac{\text{Amount of solution} \times \text{gtt/ml}}{\text{Minutes to administer}} = \frac{100 \text{ ml} \times \overset{3}{\cancel{60}} \text{ gtt}}{\underset{1}{\cancel{20}}} = 300 \text{ gtt/min}$$

Answer: Inject 1.3 ml of Tagamet into 100 ml of D₅W in the Buretrol chamber.
Regulate IV flow rate to 300 gtt/min.
It would be impossible to count 300 gtt/min. Instead of using the Buretrol, the
nurse could use a secondary set with a larger drop factor or a regulator. If the
Buretrol is the only available secondary IV set, the 300 gtt/min rate should be
approximated.

PROBLEM 2: Order: Mandol 500 mg, IV, q6h.
Drug available:

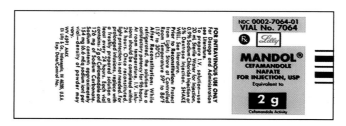

Add 6.6 ml of diluent = 8 ml of drug solution (2 g = 8 ml).
Set and solution: secondary set with 100 ml D$_5$W and a drop factor of 15 gtt/ml.
Instruction: Dilute in 100 ml of D$_5$W and infuse over 30 minutes.

Drug Calculation: (2.0 g = 2.000 mg).

$$\text{BF:} \quad \frac{D}{H} \times V = \frac{500}{2000} \times 8 = \frac{4000}{2000} = 2 \text{ ml of Mandol}$$

or

RP: H   :   V   ::   D   :   X
    2000 mg : 8 ml :: 500 mg : X ml

$$2000\, X = 4000$$
$$X = 2 \text{ ml of Mandol}$$

or

$$\text{DA: ml} = \frac{\overset{4}{8} \text{ ml} \times 1 \text{ g} \times \overset{1}{500} \text{ mg}}{\underset{1}{2} \text{ g} \times \underset{2}{1000} \text{ mg} \times 1} = \frac{4}{2} = 2 \text{ ml of Mandol}$$

Flow Rate Calculation:

$$\frac{\text{Amount of solution} \times \text{gtt/ml}}{\text{Minutes to administer}} = \frac{100 \text{ ml} \times \overset{1}{15}}{\underset{2}{30}} = \frac{100}{2} = 50 \text{ gtt/min}$$

Answer: Inject 2 ml of Mandol into the 100 ml D$_5$W bag.
Regulate IV flow rate to 50 gtt/min.

PROBLEM 3: Order: oxacillin 1 g, IV, q6h.
Drug available:

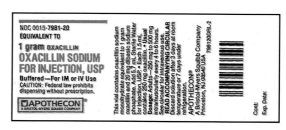

Add 5.7 ml of diluent = 6 ml per 1 g.
Set: Use an infusion pump.
Instruction: Dilute in 50 ml of D_5W and infuse over 15 minutes.

Drug Calculation: oxacillin 1 g = 6 ml of drug solution

Infusion Pump Rate: Amount of solution $\div$ $\dfrac{\text{Minutes to administer}}{60 \text{ minutes}}$ = ml/hr

$$56 \text{ ml} \div \frac{15 \text{ min}}{60 \text{ min}} = 56 \times \frac{\overset{4}{\cancel{60}}}{\underset{1}{\cancel{15}}} = 224 \text{ ml/hr}$$

Note: Amount of solution is 50 ml of D_5W + 6 ml of medication = 56 ml.

Answer: Rate on infusion pump should be set at 224 ml/hr to deliver oxacillin 1 g in 15 minutes.

PROBLEM 4: Order: albumin 25 g, IV.
Available: albumin 25 g in 50 ml.
Set: Use an infusion pump.
Instruction: Administer over 25 minutes, or 2 ml/min.

Drug Calculation: Not applicable.

Infusion Pump Rate:

$$50 \text{ ml} \div \frac{25 \text{ min}}{60 \text{ min}} = 50 \times \frac{60}{25} = \frac{3000}{25} = 120 \text{ ml/hr}$$

Answer: Infusion rate should be set at 120 ml/hr.

PROBLEM 5: Order: potassium phosphate 10 mM IV in 100 ml NSS over 90 minutes.
Drug available:

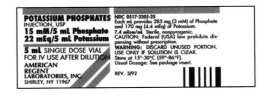

Set: Use infusion pump.

Drug Calculation:
BF: $\dfrac{D}{H} \times V = \dfrac{10}{15} \times 5 = \dfrac{50}{15} = 3.3$ ml of potassium phosphate

or

RP: H : V ::   D : X
    15 mM : 5 ml :: 10 mM : X ml
            15 X = 50
              X = 3.3 ml or potassium phosphate

or

$$DA: ml = \frac{5\ ml \times \overset{2}{\cancel{10}}\ mM}{\underset{3}{\cancel{15}}\ mM \times 1} = \frac{10}{3} = 3.3\ ml$$

Infusion Pump Rate:

$$Amount\ of\ solution \div \frac{Minutes\ to\ administer}{60\ minutes} = ml/hr$$

$$100\ ml \div \frac{90\ min}{60\ min} = 100 \times \frac{60}{90} = 66.6\ or\ 67\ ml/hr$$

Answer: Rate on the infusion pump should be 67 ml/hr to deliver potassium phosphate 10 mM in 90 minutes.

NOTE

When the electrolyte potassium is administered, the maximum infusion rate is 10 mEq/hr.

PRACTICE PROBLEMS III **Intermittent Intravenous Administration**

Answers can be found on page 224.

Calculate the fluid rate by using a calibrated cylinder (Buretrol), secondary set, or an infusion pump, as indicated in each question.

1. Order: cephapirin (Cefadyl) 500 mg, IV, q6h.
Drug available:

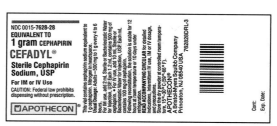

Drug label: add _____ ml of diluent _____; 1 g = _____ ml; 100 mg = 1 ml.

What type of syringe should be used? _____
Set and solution: Buretrol set with a drop factor of 60 gtt/ml; 500 ml of D_5W.
Instruction: Dilute drug in 75 ml of D_5W and infuse over 30 minutes.

Drug calculation:

_____

Flow rate calculation:

_____

2. Order: oxacillin 400 mg, IV, q6h.

Drug available:

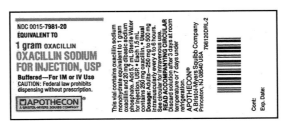

Drug label: add _____ ml of diluent _____;

250 mg = _____ ml; 1 g = _____ ml.

Set and solution: secondary set with a drop factor of 15 gtt/ml; 500 ml of D₅W.

Instruction: Dilute drug in 100 ml of D₅W and infuse over 40 minutes.

Drug calculation:

_____

Flow rate calculation:

_____

3. Order: ticarcillin (Ticar) 500 mg, IV, q6h.
Drug available:

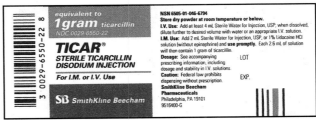

Set and solution: Buretrol set with a drop factor of 60 gtt/ml; infusion pump; 500 ml of D₅W.
Instruction: Dilute drug in 75 ml of D₅W and infuse over 40 minutes.

Drug calculation: Add _____ ml to ticarcillin vial (see drug label).

_____

Flow rate calculation (gtt/min):
How many drops per minute should the client receive with use of the Buretrol set?

_____

Infusion pump rate (ml/hr):
With an infusion pump, how many ml/hr should be administered?

_____

4. Order: piperacillin 2.5 g, IV, q6h.
   Drug available: piperacillin 4 g vial in powdered form; add 7.8 ml of diluent to yield 10 ml of drug solution (4 g = 10 ml).
   Set and solution: Buretrol set with a drop factor of 60 gtt/ml; infusion pump; 500 ml of D₅W.
   Instruction: Dilute drug in 100 ml of D₅W and infuse over 30 minutes.

   Drug calculation:

   _____

   Flow rate calculation (gtt/min):
   How many drops per minute should the client receive with use of the Buretrol set?

   _____

   Infusion pump rate (ml/hr):
   With an infusion pump, how many ml/hr should be administered?

   _____

5. Order: methicillin (Staphcillin) 1 g, IV, q6h.
   Drug available: Staphcillin 4 g in powdered form in vial; add 5.7 ml of diluent to yield 8 ml.
   Set and solution: secondary set with a drop factor of 15 gtt/ml; 100-ml bag of D₅W; infusion pump.
   Instruction: Dilute drug in 100 ml of D₅W and infuse over 40 minutes.

   Drug calculation:

   _____

   Explain the procedure for diluting the drug and adding it to the IV bag.

   _____

   Flow rate calculation (gtt/min):
   How many drops per minute should the client receive with use of a secondary set?

   _____

   Infusion pump rate (ml/hr):
   With an infusion pump, how many ml/hr should be administered?

   _____

6. Order: Vibramycin 100 mg, IV, q12h.
   Drug available: doxycycline (Vibramycin) 100-mg vial in powdered form; add 10 ml of diluent.
   Set and solution: secondary set with a drop factor of 15 gtt/ml; 100 ml of D₅W; infusion pump.
   Instruction: Dilute 10 ml in 90 ml of D₅W and infuse over 60 minutes.
   Dilution should be 1 mg = 1 ml.

   Drug calculation:

   _____

Flow rate calculation (gtt/min):
How many drops per minute should the client receive with use of the Buretrol set?

_____

Infusion pump rate (ml/hr):
With an infusion pump, how many ml/hr should be administered?

_____

7. Order: potassium chloride 20 mEq in 150 ml D$_5$W infused over 2 hours.
   Drug available:

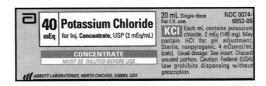

Set and solution: secondary set with drop factor of 15 gtt/ml; 150-ml bottle D$_5$W; infusion pump.

Drug calculation:

_____

Infusion pump rate (ml/hr):
How many ml/hr should be administered?

_____

8. Order: magnesium sulfate 5 g in 100 ml D$_5$W infused over 3 hours.
   Drug available:

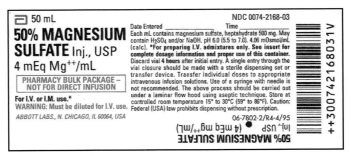

Set and solution: secondary set with drip factor of 15 gtt/ml; 10-ml bag D$_5$W; infusion pump.

Drug calculation:

a. 1 ml = _____ mg (see drug label).

b. 5 g = _____ ml.

Infusion pump rate (ml/hr):
How many ml/hr should be administered?

_____

9. Order: calcium gluconate 10%, 16 mEq in 100 ml D$_5$W infused over 30 minutes. Drug available:

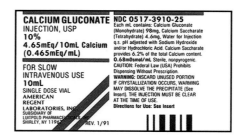

Set and solution: secondary set with a drip factor of 15 gtt/ml; 100-ml bag D$_5$W; infusion pump.

Drug calculation:

_____

Infusion pump rate (ml/hr):
How many ml/hr should be administered?

_____

10. Order: ranitidine (Zantac) 50 mg, IV, q6h.
Set: infusion pump.
Drug available: premixed drug in bag (Zantac 50 mg in 0.45% NaCl [½ NSS]).

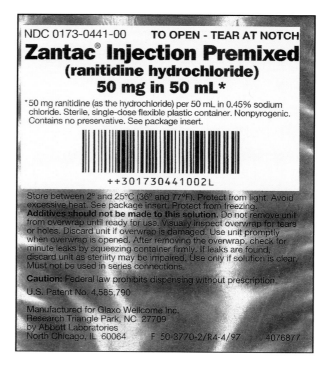

Instruction: Infuse over 15 minutes.

Infusion pump rate:
How many ml/hr should be administered?

11. Order: cefepime (Maxipime) 750 mg, IV, q12h.
Set and solution: Infusion pump; 100 ml D₅W.
Drug available:

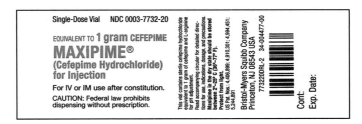

Instruction: Add 8.7 ml of diluent to Maxipime to yield 10 ml of drug solution. Dilute in 100 ml of D₅W; infuse over 30 minutes.

Drug calculations:

Infusion pump rate (ml/hr):

12. Order: rifampin (Rifadin) 600 mg, IV, qd.
Set and solution: Infusion pump; 500 ml D₅W.
Drug available: Rifadin, 600 mg sterile powder
Instruction: Add 10 ml of diluent to the rifampin vial. Dilute rifampin in 500 ml of D₅W; infuse over 3 hours.

Infusion pump rate (ml/hr):

 Additional practice problems for "IV Dosage" are available on the CD-ROM in the "Calculating Dosages" section.

ANSWERS

I   Direct IV Injection
1. **a.** 5 ml drug solution
   b. known drug : known minutes :: desired drug : desired minutes
       5 mg : 1 min :: 50 mg : X
                     5 X = 50
                       X = 10 minutes

2. a. known drug : known minutes :: desired drug : desired minutes

   10 ml : 1 min :: 50 ml :   X

          10 X = 50

           X = 5 minutes

3. a. 10 ml

 b. known drug : known minutes :: desired drug : desired minutes

   1.5 ml : 1 min :: 10 ml :   X

         1.5 X = 10

           X = 6.6 minutes or 7 minutes

4. a. 5 ml

 b. known drug : known minutes :: desired drug : desired minutes

   10 mg : 1 min :: 50 mg :   X

          10 X = 50

           X = 5 minutes

5. a. RP: H : V :: D : X

   10 mg : 1 ml :: 6 mg : X

      10 X = 6

        X = 0.6 ml morphine

 b. known drug : known minutes :: desired drug : desired minutes

   10 mg : 4 min :: 6 mg :   X

         10 X = 24

          X = 2.4 minutes

6. a. 1 ml

 b. known drug : known minutes :: desired drug : desired minutes

   1 ml : 5 min :: X ml : 1 min

         5 X = 1

          X = 0.2 ml/minutes

7. a. DA: ml = $\dfrac{1 \text{ ml} \times 2 \text{ mg}}{5 \text{ mg} \times 1}$ = $\dfrac{2}{5}$ = 0.4 ml of Haldol

 b. known drug : known minutes :: desired drug : desired minutes

   1 mg : 1 min :: 2 mg :   X

          X = 2 minutes

8. known drug : known minutes :: desired drug : desired minutes

 a. BF: $\dfrac{D}{H} \times V = \dfrac{6 \text{ mg}}{4 \text{ mg}} \times 1$ = 1.5 ml of Ativan

 b. known drug : known minutes :: desired drug : desired minutes

   2 mg : 1 min :: 6 mg :   X

         2 X = 6

          X = 3 minutes

9. RP: H : V :: D : V

  25 mg : 5 ml :: 20 mg : X ml

     25 X = 100

       X = 4 ml

 or

DA: $V = \dfrac{V \times D}{H \times 1}$

$$ml = \dfrac{5\ ml \times \overset{4}{\cancel{20}}\ mg}{\underset{5}{\cancel{25}}\ mg \times 1} = \dfrac{20}{5} = 4\ ml$$

$$\dfrac{\text{Amount of drug}}{\text{Number of minutes}} = \dfrac{4\ ml}{2\ min} = 2\ ml/min$$

Answer: Infuse 2 ml of cardizem per minute.

10. **a.** 140 lb ÷ 2.2 = 64 kg

   b. 10 μg × 64 kg = 640 μg

   c. Change micrograms (μg) to milligrams by moving the decimal point three spaces to the *left:*
   640 μg = 0.640 mg or 0.6 mg.

   known drug : known seconds :: desired drug : desired seconds
   　1 mg 　 : 　60 seconds 　 :: 　　.6 mg 　 : 　　　X
   　　　　　　　　　　　　X = 36 seconds

   Answer: Infuse 0.6 mg of granisetron (Kytril) over 36 seconds.

II Continuous Intravenous Administration

1. **a.** Microdrip set, because the patient is to receive 83 ml/hr

   b. Three-step method: (a) $\dfrac{1000}{12} = 83\ ml/hr$

   　　　　　　　　　(b) $\dfrac{83}{60} = 1.38\ ml/min$

   　　　　　　　　　(c) 1.4 ml/min × 60 gtt/ml = 84 gtt/min

   Using a microdrip set (60 gtt/ml); IV should run at 84 gtt/min.

2. **a.** 1 L = 1000 ml

   b. Each liter should run for 8 hours.

   c. Two-step method: 1000 ÷ 8 = 125 ml/hr

   $$\dfrac{125 \times \overset{1}{\cancel{15}}}{\underset{4}{\cancel{60}}} = \dfrac{125}{4} = 31\text{–}32\ gtt/min$$

   With a 15 gtt/ml drop set, IV should run at 31 to 32 gtt/min.

3. **a.** Microdrip set with drop factor of 60 gtt/ml

   b. One-step method: $\dfrac{250 \times \overset{1}{\cancel{60}}}{24 \times \underset{1}{\cancel{60}}} = 10\ gtt/min$

   With a microdrip set, IV should run at 10 gtt/min. KVO usually means 24 hours.

4. **a.** 10 ml of KCl

   b. Use a 10-ml syringe; withdraw 10 ml of KCl and inject into the rubber stopper part of the IV bag.

   c. Microdrip set: 100 gtt/min
   Macrodrip set: drop factor of 20 gtt/ml; 34 gtt/min

5. **a.** 700 ml of IV fluid is left and 4 hours are left.
   b. Recalculate using 700 ml and 4 hours to run.

   Three-step method: (a) $\dfrac{700}{4} = 175$ ml/hr

   (b) $\dfrac{175}{60} = 2.9$ ml/min

   (c) $2.9 \times 15 = 44$ gtt/min

6. 100 gtt/min

   Two-step method: $\dfrac{100 \times \overset{1}{\cancel{60}}\ \text{gtt/ml}}{\underset{1}{\cancel{60}}\ \text{min}} = 100$ gtt/min

7. **a.** KCl 40 mEq/20 ml
   b. 20 ml
   c. $\dfrac{1000\ \text{ml}}{125\ \text{ml/hr}} = 8$ hours

8. **a.** KCl 20 mEq/10 ml
   b. 10 ml
   c. $\dfrac{1000\ \text{ml}}{100\ \text{ml/hr}} = 10$ hours

   d. $\dfrac{100\ \text{ml} \times \overset{1}{\cancel{10}}\ \text{gtt/ml}}{\underset{6}{\cancel{60}}\ \text{min}} = \dfrac{100}{6} = 16$ to 17 gtt/min

   or

   $\dfrac{1000\ \text{ml} \times \overset{1}{\cancel{10}}\ \text{gtt/ml}}{\underset{1}{\cancel{10}}\ \text{hr} \times 60\ \text{min}} = \dfrac{1000}{60} = 16$ to 17 gtt/min

III Intermittent Intravenous Administration

1. Add 10 ml of sterile or bacteriostatic water (1 g = 10 ml).
   Drug calculation: Change 500 mg to grams because the drug label is in grams. Move the decimal point three spaces to the *left:* 500. mg = 0.5 g.

   BF: $\dfrac{D}{H} \times V = \dfrac{0.5}{1} \times 10\ \text{ml} = \dfrac{5}{1} = 5$ ml Cefadyl

   or

   RP: H : V :: D : X
       1 g:10 ml :: 0.5 g:X ml
           1 X = 10 × 0.5
             X = 5 ml Cefadyl

   or

   DA: ml $= \dfrac{\overset{1}{\cancel{10}}\ \text{ml} \times\quad \cancel{1\ \text{g}}\quad \times \overset{5}{\cancel{500}}\ \text{mg}}{\cancel{1\ \text{g}} \times \underset{\underset{1}{100}}{\cancel{1000}}\ \text{mg} \times\quad 1} = 5$ ml

   Use a 10-ml syringe to reconstitute the drug.

Flow rate calculation:

$$\frac{\text{Amount of solution} \times \text{gtt/ml (set)}}{\text{Minutes to administer}} = \frac{75 \text{ ml} \times \overset{2}{\cancel{60}} \text{ gtt/ml}}{\underset{1}{\cancel{30}} \text{ minutes}} = 150 \text{ gtt/min}$$

Regulate flow rate for 150 gtt/min.

2. Add 5.7 ml of sterile water.

   250 mg = 1.5 ml; 1 g = 6 ml (250 mg is ¼ of a gram; 4 × 1.5 = 6 ml)

   Drug calculation: Change 400 mg to grams because the drug label is in grams. Move the decimal point three spaces to the *left:* $\underset{\smile}{400}$. mg = 0.4 g.

$$\frac{0.4}{1} \times 6 \text{ ml} = 2.4 \text{ ml of oxacillin}$$

   or

   1 g : 6 ml :: 0.4 g : X ml

       1 X = 6 × 0.4

          X = 2.4 ml of oxacillin

   Flow rate calculation:

$$\frac{100 \text{ ml} \times 15 \text{ gtt/ml (set)}}{40 \text{ minutes}} = 37.5 \text{ or } 38 \text{ gtt/min}$$

   Regulate flow rate for 38 gtt/min.

3. *Drug calculation:* ticarcillin 500 mg = 2 ml

   Flow rate calculation: total solution: 75 ml D_5W + 2 ml of drug solution = 77 ml

   For Buretrol set:

$$\frac{77 \text{ ml} \times \overset{3}{\cancel{60}} \text{ gtt/ml (set)}}{\underset{2}{\cancel{40}} \text{ minutes}} = \frac{231}{2} = 115.5 \text{ or } 116 \text{ gtt/min}$$

   Infusion pump rate:

$$\text{Amount of solution} \div \frac{\text{Minutes to administer}}{60 \text{ min/hr}} = \text{ml/hr}$$

$$77 \text{ ml} \div \frac{\overset{2}{\cancel{40}} \text{ min to administer}}{\underset{3}{\cancel{60}} \text{ min/hr}} = 77 \times \frac{3}{2} = \frac{231}{2} = 116 \text{ ml/hr}$$

   Set pump rate at 116 ml/hr to deliver Ticar 500 mg in 40 minutes.

4. *Drug calculation:*

   BF: $\dfrac{D}{H} \times V = \dfrac{2.5 \text{ g}}{\underset{2}{\cancel{4}} \text{ g}} \times \overset{5}{\cancel{10}} \text{ ml} = \dfrac{12.5}{2} = 6.25 \text{ ml}$

   or

   RP: H : V :: D : X

       4 g : 10 ml :: 2.5 g : X ml

           4 X = 25

             X = 6.25 ml

   or

DA: ml = $\dfrac{10 \text{ ml} \times 2.5 \cancel{g}}{4 \cancel{g} \times 1} = \dfrac{25}{4} = 6.25$ ml

piperacillin 2.5 g = 6.25 ml

Flow rate calculation for Buretrol set:

$$\dfrac{100 \text{ ml} \times \overset{2}{\cancel{60}} \text{ gtt/ml}}{\underset{1}{\cancel{30}} \text{ min/hr}} = 200 \text{ gtt/minute}$$

Infusion pump rate: 100 ml + 6 ml medication = 106 ml

106 ml ÷ $\dfrac{\overset{1}{\cancel{30}} \text{ min to administer}}{\underset{2}{\cancel{60}} \text{ min/hr}} = 106 \times \dfrac{2}{1} = 212$ ml/hr

Set pump rate at 212 ml/hr to deliver piperacillin 2.5 g in 30 minutes.

5. *Drug calculation:* Staphcillin 4 g = 8 ml. Withdraw 2 ml from vial to yield Staphcillin 1 g.

Flow rate calculation for secondary set:

$$\dfrac{\overset{5}{\cancel{100}} \text{ ml} \times 15 \text{ gtt/ml (set)}}{\underset{2}{\cancel{40}} \text{ minutes}} = \dfrac{75}{2} = 37.5 \text{ or } 38 \text{ gtt/min}$$

Infusion pump rate:

100 ml × $\dfrac{\overset{2}{\cancel{40}} \text{ min to administer}}{\underset{3}{\cancel{60}} \text{ min/hr}} = 100 \times \dfrac{3}{2} = \dfrac{300}{2} = 150$ ml/hr

Set pump rate at 150 ml/hr to deliver Staphcillin 1 g in 40 minutes.

6. *Drug Calculation:* Mix 10 ml of diluent with Vibramycin 100 mg in vial.

Flow rate calculation: Expel 10 ml of IV solution. Inject 10 ml of drug solution into 90 ml of IV solution.

For secondary set:

$$\dfrac{100 \text{ ml} \times \overset{1}{\cancel{15}} \text{ gtt/ml}}{\underset{4}{\cancel{60}} \text{ minutes}} = \dfrac{100}{4} = 25 \text{ gtt/min}$$

Infusion pump rate:

100 ml ÷ $\dfrac{\overset{1}{\cancel{60}} \text{ minutes to administer}}{\underset{1}{\cancel{60}} \text{ min/hr}} = 100$ ml/hr

Set pump rate at 100 ml/hr to deliver Vibramycin 100 mg in 60 minutes.

7. *Drug calculation:*

BF: $\dfrac{D}{H} \times V = \dfrac{20}{40} \times 20 = \dfrac{400}{40} = 10$ ml KCl

or

RP: H : V :: D : X
    40 : 20 :: 20 : X
      40 X = 400
          X = 10 ml KCl

or

DA: ml = $\dfrac{20 \text{ ml} \times \overset{1}{\cancel{20}} \text{ mEq}}{\underset{2}{\cancel{40}} \text{ mEq} \times 1} = \dfrac{20}{2} = 10$ ml

Amount of solution: 150 ml + 10 ml = 160 ml

Infusion pump rate:

$$160 \text{ ml} \div \frac{120 \text{ min to administer}}{60 \text{ min/hr}} = 160 \times \frac{1}{2} = 80 \text{ ml/hr}$$

Set pump rate at 80 ml/hr to deliver KCl 20 mEq in 2 hours.

8. *Drug calculation:*

  a. 1 ml = 500 mg and 2 ml = 1 g.

  b. BF: $\dfrac{D}{H} \times V = \dfrac{5}{1} \times 2 = 10$ ml of $MgSO_4$

  or

  RP: H:V::D:X

      1:2::5:X

        X = 10

        X = 10 ml $MgSO_4$

  or

  DA: ml = $\dfrac{1 \text{ ml} \times \overset{2}{\cancel{1000}} \text{ mg} \times 5 \cancel{g}}{\underset{1}{\cancel{500}} \text{ mg} \times 1 \cancel{g} \times 1} = 10$ ml $MgSO_4$

Amount of solution: 10 ml + 100 ml = 110 ml

Infusion pump rate:

$$110 \text{ ml} \div \frac{\overset{3}{\cancel{180}} \text{ min to administer}}{\underset{1}{\cancel{60}} \text{ min/hr}} \text{ (3 hr)} = 110 \times \frac{1}{3} = 36.6 \text{ or } 37 \text{ ml/hr}$$

Set pump rate at 37 ml/hr to deliver $MgSO_4$ 5 g in 3 hours.

9. *Drug calculation:*

  BF: $\dfrac{D}{H} \times V = \dfrac{16 \text{ mEq}}{4.65 \text{ mEq}} \times 10 \text{ ml} = 34.4$ ml

  or

  RP: H : V ::   D : X

      4.65 mEq:10 ml :: 16 mEq:X ml

         4.65 X = 160

            X = 34.4 ml

  or

  DA: ml = $\dfrac{10 \text{ ml} \times 16 \cancel{\text{mEq}}}{4.65 \cancel{\text{mEq}} \times 1} = 34.4$ ml

Amount of solution: 34.4 ml + 100 ml = 134.4 ml

Infusion pump rate:

$$134.4 \text{ ml} \div \frac{30 \text{ min to administer}}{60 \text{ min/hr}} = 134.4 \times \frac{2}{1} = 268.8 \text{ or } 269 \text{ ml/hr (insert divisor)}$$

10. *Amount of solution:* $\div \dfrac{\text{min to administer}}{60 \text{ ml/hr}}$

  $$50 \text{ ml} \div \frac{15 \text{ min}}{60 \text{ min}} = 50 \text{ ml} \times \frac{\overset{4}{\cancel{60}} \text{ min}}{\underset{1}{\cancel{15}} \text{ min}} = 200 \text{ ml/hr}$$

Infusion pump rate: 200 ml/hr

11. 1 g = 1000 mg (use conversion table as needed) of Maxipime

   a. $\dfrac{D}{H} \times V = \dfrac{\overset{3}{\cancel{750}} \text{ ml}}{\underset{4}{\cancel{1000}} \text{ ml}} \times 10 \text{ ml} = \dfrac{30}{4} = 7.5$ ml drug solution

   b. *Pump rate:*

   7.5 drug solution + 100 ml $\div \dfrac{30 \text{ min to administer}}{60 \text{ min/hr}} = 107.5 \text{ ml} \times \dfrac{\overset{2}{\cancel{60}}}{\underset{1}{\cancel{30}}} = 215$ ml/hr pump rate

12. 10 ml of drug solution + 500 ml $\div \dfrac{180 \text{ min (3 hr)}}{60 \text{ min/hr}} = 510 \text{ ml} \times \dfrac{\overset{1}{\cancel{60}}}{\underset{3}{\cancel{180}}} = \dfrac{510}{3} = 170$ ml/hr

   Infusion pump rate: 170 ml/hr for 3 hours

PART IV

CALCULATIONS FOR SPECIALTY AREAS

Pediatrics

OBJECTIVES

- Use the two primary methods in determining pediatric drug dosages.
- State the reason for checking pediatric dosages before administration.
- Describe the dosage inaccuracies that can occur with pediatric drug formulas.
- Identify the steps in determining body surface area from a pediatric nomogram and with the square root method.

OUTLINE

FACTORS INFLUENCING PEDIATRIC DRUG ADMINISTRATION
    Oral
    Intramuscular
    Intravenous
PEDIATRIC DRUG CALCULATIONS
    Dosage per Kilogram Body Weight
    Dosage per Body Surface Area
PEDIATRIC DOSAGE FROM ADULT DOSAGE
    Body Surface Area Formula
    Age Rules
    Body Weight Rule

FACTORS INFLUENCING PEDIATRIC DRUG ADMINISTRATION

Drug dosages for children differ greatly from those for adults because of the physiological differences between the two groups. Neonates and infants have immature kidney and liver function, which delays metabolism and elimination of many drugs. Drug absorption in neonates is different as a result of slow gastric emptying. Decreased gastric acid secretion in children younger than 3 years contributes to altered drug absorption. Neonates and infants have a lower concentration of plasma proteins, which can cause toxic effects with drugs that are highly bound to proteins. They have less total body fat and more total body water. Therefore lipid-soluble drugs require smaller doses because less than normal fat is present, and water-soluble drugs can require larger doses because of a greater percentage of body water. As children grow, changes in fat, muscle, body water, and organ maturity can alter the pharmacokinetic effects of drugs. It is the nurse's responsibility to ensure that a safe drug dosage is given and to closely monitor signs and symptoms of adverse reactions to drugs. The purpose of learning how to calculate pediatric drug doses is to ensure that each child receives the correct dose within the therapeutic range.

Oral

Oral pediatric drug delivery often requires the use of a calibrated measuring device, because most drugs for small children are in liquid form. The measuring device can be a small plastic cup, an oral dropper, a measuring spoon, or an oral syringe (Fig. 10-1). Some liquid medications come with their own cali-

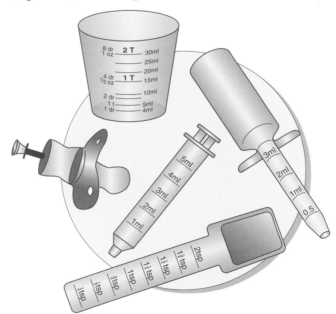

FIGURE 10-1 Calibrated measuring devices. (Modified from Kee, J., & Hayes, E. [2003]. *Pharmacology: A Nursing Process Approach* [4th ed.]. Philadelphia: W. B. Saunders.)

brated droppers. The type of measuring device chosen depends on the developmental level of the child. For infants and toddlers, the oral syringe and dropper provide better drug delivery than a small cup. A young child who is cooperative is able to use a small cup or measuring spoon. All liquid medications can be drawn up with a syringe to ensure accuracy and then transferred to a small cup or measuring spoon. It may be necessary to refill the cup or spoon with water or juice and have the child drink that as well to ensure that all of the prescribed medication has been administered. Avoid giving oral medications to a crying child or infant, who could easily aspirate the medication. Some chewable medications are available for administration to the older child. Because many drugs are enteric-coated or in time-release form, the child must be told which medications are to be swallowed and not chewed.

Intramuscular

Intramuscular sites are chosen on the basis of the age and muscle development of the child (Table 10-1). All injections should be given in a manner that minimizes physical and psychosocial trauma. The child must be adequately restrained, if necessary, and provided with a momentary distraction. The procedure must be performed quickly, with comfort measures immediately following.

NOTE

The usual needle length and gauge for pediatric clients are $\frac{1}{2}$ to 1 inch long and 22 to 25 gauge. Another method of estimating needle length is to grasp the muscle for injection between the thumb and the forefinger; half the distance would be the needle length.

Intravenous

For children, the maximum amount of intravenous (IV) fluids varies with body weight. Their 24-hour fluid status must be monitored closely to prevent overhydration. The amount of fluid given with IV medication must be con-

Table 10-1

Pediatric Guidelines for Intramuscular Injections According to Muscle Group*

Age	Amount by Muscle Group (ml)			
	Vastus Lateralis	Gluteus Maximus	Ventrogluteal	Deltoid
Birth to 4 months	0.5–1	Not safe	0.5–1	Not safe
Infants	0.5–1	Not safe	1	Not safe
Toddlers	0.5–2	0.5–1	0.5–1	0.5–1
Preschool and older children	2	0.5–2	2–3	0.5–1
Adolescents	2	2	2–5	1–1.5

*The safe use of all sites is based on normal muscle development and size of the child.

Table 10-2

Pediatric Guidelines for 24-Hour Intravenous Fluid Therapy

100 ml/kg up to 10 kg body weight
50 ml/kg for the next 5 kg body weight
10 ml/kg after 15 kg body weight

Example: Child's weight 25 kg

$$100 \text{ ml/kg} \times 10 \text{ kg} = 1000 \text{ ml}$$
$$50 \text{ ml/kg} \times 5 \text{ kg} = 250 \text{ ml}$$
$$10 \text{ ml/kg} \times 10 \text{ kg} = \underline{100 \text{ ml}}$$
$$1350 \text{ ml for 24 hours}$$

sidered in the planning of their 24-hour intake (Table 10-2). After the correct dosage of drug is obtained, it may need further dilution and to be given over a specified time, as mentioned in Chapter 9. Usually, the drug is diluted with 5 to 60 ml of IV fluid, depending on the drug or dosage, placed in a calibrated cylinder, and infused over 20 to 60 minutes, depending on the type of drug. After the drug has been infused, the cylinder is flushed with 3 to 20 ml of IV fluid to ensure that the child has received all of the medication and to prevent admixture. Refer to Chapter 9 for methods of calculating IV infusion rates.

The safety factors that must be considered when medications are administered to children are similar to those for adults. See Appendix A for more detailed information on safe nursing practice for drug administration.

PEDIATRIC DRUG CALCULATIONS

The two main methods in determining drug dosages for pediatric drug administration are body weight and body surface area (BSA). The first method uses a specific number of milligrams, micrograms, or units for each kilogram of body weight (mg/kg, mcg/kg, U/kg). Usually, drug data for pediatric dosage (mg/kg) are supplied by manufacturers in a drug information insert. BSA, measured in square meters (m^2), is considered a more accurate method than body weight. BSA takes into consideration the relation between basal metabolic rate and surface area, which correlates with blood volume, cardiac output, and organ growth and development. Although BSA has primarily been used to calculate the dosage of antineoplastic agents, manufacturers are beginning to include BSA parameters (mg/m^2, mcg/m^2, U/m^2) in drug information.

If the manufacturer does not supply data for pediatric dosing, the child's dosage can be determined from the adult dose. The BSA formula is used to calculate the pediatric dose. The BSA formula is considered more accurate than previously used formulas, such as Clark's, Young's, and Fried's rules. Drug calculations according to the BSA formula are safer than those done with formulas that rely solely on the child's age or weight. Although the BSA formula has improved the accuracy of drug dosing in infants and children, calculation of drug doses for neonates and preterm infants with this method does not guarantee complete accuracy.

NOTE

If the manufacturer states in the drug information insert that the medication is not for pediatric use, the alternative formulas should not be used for dosage calculation.

Dosage per Kilogram Body Weight

The following information is needed to calculate the dosage.
a. Physician's order with the name of the drug, the dosage, and the frequency of administration.
b. The child's weight in kilograms:

$$1 \text{ kg} = 2.2 \text{ lb}$$

c. The pediatric dosage as listed by the manufacturer or hospital formulary.
d. Information on how the drug is supplied.

EXAMPLES

PROBLEM 1
a. Order: amoxicillin (Amoxil) 60 mg, po, tid.
Child's weight: 12½ lb.
b. Change pounds to kilograms.

$$\frac{12.5}{2.2} = 5.7 \text{ kg}$$

c. Pediatric dosage for children who weigh 20 kg: 20-40 mg/kg/day in three equal doses.

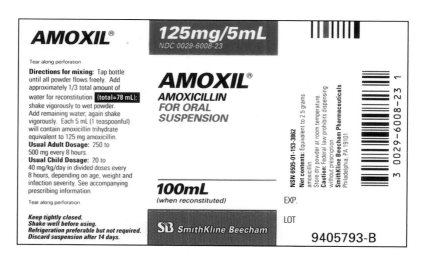

Step 1: Check dosing parameters by multiplying the child's weight by the minimum and maximum daily dose of the drug.

$$20 \text{ mg/kg/day} \times 5.7 \text{ kg} = 114 \text{ mg/day}$$

$$40 \text{ mg/kg/day} \times 5.7 \text{ kg} = 228 \text{ mg/day}$$

Step 2: Multiply the dosage by the frequency to determine the daily dose. The order for amoxicillin 60 mg, po, tid means that three doses will be given per day.

$$60 \text{ mg} \times 3 = 180 \text{ mg}$$

Because the daily dose of amoxicillin 180 mg falls within the recommended range, it is considered a safe dose.

d. Drug preparation:
Use the basic formula (BF), ratio and proportion (RP), or dimensional analysis (DA).
Basic Formula

$$\frac{D}{H} \times V = \frac{60 \text{ mg}}{125 \text{ mg}} \times 5 \text{ ml} = 2.4 \text{ ml}$$

or

Ratio and Proportion
125 mg : 5 ml :: 60 mg : X ml
$$125X = 300$$
$$X = 2.4 \text{ ml}$$

or

Dimensional Analysis

$$\text{ml} = \frac{5 \text{ ml} \quad \times 60 \text{ m\!\!\!/g}}{125 \text{ m\!\!\!/g} \times \quad 1} = \frac{300}{125} = 2.4 \text{ ml}$$

Answer: amoxicillin 60 mg, po = 2.4 ml

PROBLEM 2
a. Order: ampicillin 350 mg, IV, q6h. Mix with 20 ml D$_5$/¼ NSS, infuse over 20 minutes. Flush with 15 ml. Child weighs 61.5 lb.
b. Change pounds to kilograms.

$$\frac{61.5}{2.2} = 27.95 \text{ or } 28 \text{ kg}$$

c. Pediatric dose is 25 to 50 mg/kg/day in divided doses.
Step 1: Multiply weight by minimum and maximum daily dose:

$$25 \text{ mg} \times 28 \text{ kg} = 700 \text{ mg/day}$$

$$50 \text{ mg} \times 28 \text{ kg} = 1400 \text{ mg/day}$$

Step 2: Multiply the dose by the frequency:

$$350 \text{ mg} \times 4 = 1400 \text{ mg/day}$$

The dose is considered safe because it does not exceed the therapeutic range.

d. Drug available: When diluted, 500 mg = 2 ml. Use your selected formula to calculate the dosage.

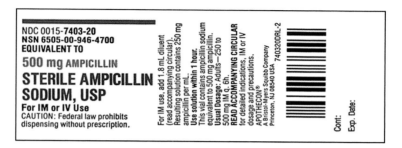

BF: $\dfrac{D}{H} \times V = \dfrac{350 \text{ mg}}{500 \text{ mg}} \times 2 \text{ ml} = 1.4 \text{ ml}$

or

RP: 500 mg : 2 ml :: 350 mg : X ml

500X = 700

X = 1.4 ml

or

DA: no conversion factor

$$ml = \dfrac{2 \text{ ml} \times \overset{7}{\cancel{350}} \text{ mg}}{\underset{10}{\cancel{500}} \text{ mg} \times 1} = \dfrac{14}{10} = 1.4 \text{ ml}$$

Answer: Each dose is 1.4 ml.

e. Amount of fluid to infuse medication:

1.4 ml + 20 ml (dilution) = 21.4 ml

f. Flow rate calculation (60 gtt/ml set):

$$\dfrac{\text{Amount of solution} \times \text{gtt/ml (set)}}{\text{Minutes to administer}} = \text{gtt/min}$$

$$\dfrac{21.4 \text{ ml} \times \overset{3}{\cancel{60}} \text{ gtt/ml}}{\underset{1}{\cancel{20}} \text{ minutes}} = 64.2 \text{ gtt/min}$$

g. Total fluid for medication infusion: 21.4 ml + 15 ml (flush) = 36.4 ml

REMEMBER

- The IV flush (3-20 ml) is part of the total IV fluids necessary for medication administration and must be included in client intake. The flush is started after IV medication infusion is completed, and it is infused at the same rate.
- For a 60 gtt/ml set, the drop per minute rate is the same as the milliliter per minute rate.

Dosage per Body Surface Area

The following information is needed to calculate the dosage:
a. Physician's order with name of drug, dosage, and time frame or frequency.
b. Child's height, weight in kilograms, and age.
c. Information on how the drug is supplied.
d. Pediatric dosage (in m²) as listed by manufacturer or hospital formulary.
e. BSA with square root.
f. BSA nomogram for children (Fig. 10-2).

EXAMPLES

PROBLEM 1
a. Order: methotrexate 50 mg, IV, × 1.
b. Child's height, weight, age: 134 cm, 32.5 kg, 9 yr.
c. Pediatric dose: 25-75 mg/m² wk.
d. Drug preparation: 2.5 mg/ml, 25 mg/ml.
e. BSA with square root (see BSA metric formula on page 100)

$$\sqrt{\frac{134 \times 32.5}{3600}} = 1.09$$

$$75 \text{ mg/m}^2 \times 1.09 = 81.75 \text{ or } 82 \text{ mg}$$

Compare answer with nomogram.

f. BSA nomogram for children: The child's height (134 cm) and weight (32.5 kg) intersect at 1.11 m² BSA.

Multiply the BSA, 1.11 m², by the minimum and maximum dose. (Substitute BSA for weight.)

$$25 \text{ mg/m}^2 \times 1.11 \text{ m}^2 = 28.0 \text{ mg}$$

$$75 \text{ mg/m}^2 \times 1.11 \text{ m}^2 = 83.0 \text{ mg}$$

This dose is considered safe because it is within the therapeutic range for the child's BSA.

g. Calculate drug dose: For determination of the amount of drug to be administered, either formula can be used:

$$\frac{D}{H} \times V = \frac{50 \text{ mg}}{25 \text{ mg}} \times 1 \text{ ml} = 2 \text{ ml}$$

or

$$25 \text{ mg} : 1 \text{ ml} :: 50 \text{ mg} : X \text{ ml}$$
$$25X = 50$$
$$X = 2 \text{ ml}$$

Answer: methotrexate 50 mg = 2 ml

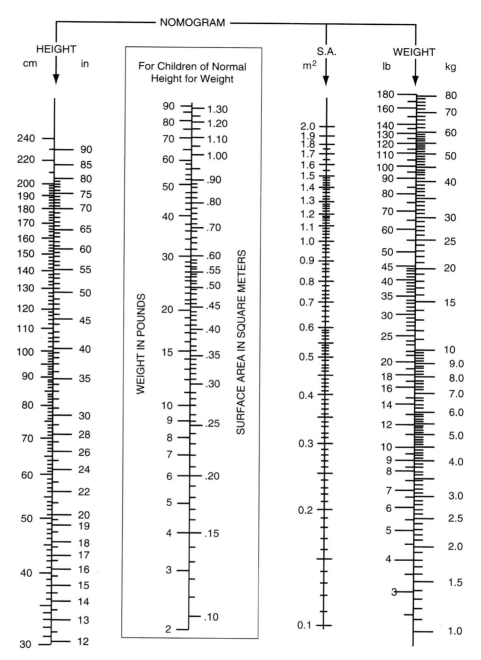

FIGURE 10-2 West Nomogram for Infants and Children. *Directions:* (1) Find height; (2) Find weight; (3) Draw a straight line connecting the height and weight. Where the line intersects on the S.A. (surface area) column is the body surface area in square meters (m²). (Modified from data of E. Boyd and C. D. West. In Behrman, R. E., Kliegman, R. M., and Jenson, H.B. [2000]. *Nelson Textbook of Pediatrics* [16th ed.]. Philadelphia: W. B. Saunders.)

SUMMARY PRACTICE PROBLEMS

In the following dosage problems for oral, IM, and IV administration, determine whether the ordered dose is safe and how much of the drug should be given. Answers are on page 250.

I. Oral

1. Child with rheumatic fever.
   Order: penicillin V potassium 250 mg, po, q8h.
   Child's weight: 45 lb.
   Pediatric dose: 25-50 mg/kg/day.
   Drug available:

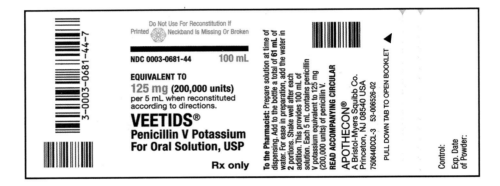

Do Not Use For Reconstitution If Printed Neckband Is Missing Or Broken

NDC 0003-0681-44   100 mL

EQUIVALENT TO
125 mg (200,000 units)
per 5 mL when reconstituted according to directions.

VEETIDS®
Penicillin V Potassium
For Oral Solution, USP

Rx only

To the Pharmacist: Prepare solution at time of dispensing. Add to the bottle a total of **61 mL** of water. For ease in preparation, add the water in 2 portions. Shake well after each addition. This provides 100 mL of solution. Each 5 mL contains penicillin V potassium equivalent to 125 mg V potassium equivalent to 125 mg (200,000 units) of penicillin V.
READ ACCOMPANYING CIRCULAR

APOTHECON®
A Bristol-Myers Squibb Co.
Princeton, NJ 08540 USA
750644DCCL-3   53-006526-02

PULL DOWN TAB TO OPEN BOOKLET

Control:
Exp. Date
of Powder:

2. Child with seizures.
   Order: Phenobarbital 25 mg, po, bid.
   Child's weight: 7.2 kg.
   Pediatric dose: 5-7 mg/kg/day.
   Drug available: phenobarbital 20 mg/5 ml.

3. Child with lower respiratory tract infection.
   Order: cefprozil (Cefzil) 100 mg, po, q12h.
   Child's weight: 17 lb; age: 6 months.
   Pediatric dose > mo: 15 mg/kg/q12h.
   Drug available:

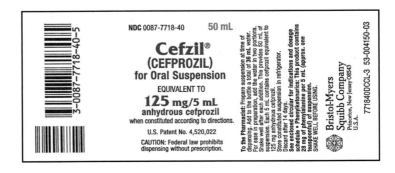

NDC 0087-7718-40   50 mL

Cefzil®
(CEFPROZIL)
for Oral Suspension
EQUIVALENT TO
125 mg/5 mL
anhydrous cefprozil
when constituted according to directions.

U.S. Patent No. 4,520,022

CAUTION: Federal law prohibits dispensing without prescription.

To the Pharmacist: Prepare suspension at time of dispensing. Add to the bottle a total of 36 mL water. For ease in preparation, add the water in two portions. Shake well after each addition. This provides 50 mL of suspension. Each 5 mL contains cefprozil equivalent to 125 mg anhydrous cefprozil. Store constituted suspension in refrigerator. Discard after 14 days.
See enclosed circular for indications and dosage schedule. • Phenylketonurics: This product contains 28 mg of phenylalanine per 5 mL (approx. one teaspoonful) of suspension.
SHAKE WELL BEFORE USING.

Bristol-Myers
Squibb Company
Princeton, New Jersey 08543
U.S.A.

771840DCCL-3 53-004150-03

4. Child with pain.
Order: codeine 7.5 mg, po, q4h, prn × 6 doses/day.
Child's height and weight: 43 inches, 50 lb.
Pediatric dose: 100 mg/m^2/day (see Fig. 10-2) or solve by square root.
Drug available: codeine 15 mg tablets.

5. Child with seizures.
Order: Zarontin 125 mg, po, bid.
Child's weight: 13 kg.
Pediatric dose: 20 mg/kg/day.
Drug available:

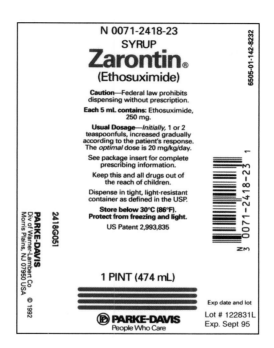

6. Child with seizures.
Order: Dilantin 40 mg, po, bid.
Child's weight: 6.7 kg.
Pediatric dose: 5-7 mg/kg/day.
Drug available: Dilantin 125 mg/5 ml.

7. Child with a urinary tract infection.
Order: Gantrisin 1.5 g, po, qid.
Child's weight: 30.4 kg.
Pediatric dose: 150-200 mg/kg/day.
Drug available: Gantrisin 500 mg tablets.

8. Infant with upper respiratory tract infection.
Order: Augmentin oral suspension 75 mg, po, q8h.
Child's weight: 8 kg.
Pediatric dose: 20-40 mg/kg/day.

Drug available:

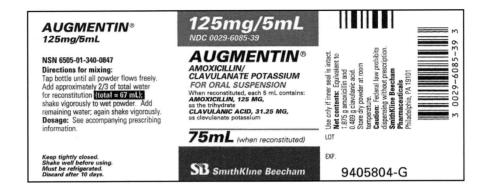

9. Child with poison ivy.
   Order: Benadryl 25 mg, po, q6h.
   Child's weight: 25 kg.
   Pediatric dose: 5 mg/kg/day.
   Drug available: Benadryl 12.5 mg/5 ml.

10. Child with cystic fibrosis exposed to influenza A.
    Order: Symmetrel 25 mg, po, tid.
    Child's weight: 14 kg.
    Pediatric dose: 4-8 mg/kg/day.
    Drug available: Symmetrel 50 mg/5 ml.

11. Order: cefaclor (Ceclor) 50 mg, qid.
    Child's weight: 15 lb.
    Pediatric dose: 20-40 mg/kg/day in three to four divided doses.
    Drug available:

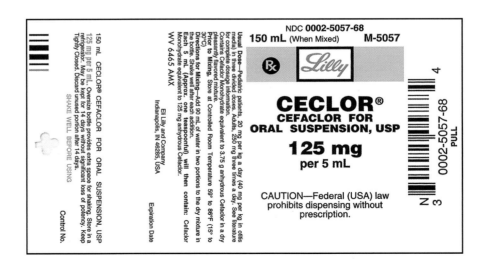

II. Intramuscular

12. Child with nausea after surgery.
Order: Phenergan 20 mg, IM, q6h.
Child's weight: 45 kg.
Pediatric dose: 0.25-0.5 mg/kg/dose, repeat 4-6 hr.
Drug available: Phenergan 25 mg/ml.

13. Child has strep throat (streptococcal pharyngitis).
Order: Bicillin C-R, 1,000,000 U, IM, × 1.
Child's weight: 44 lb.
Pediatric dose: 30-60 lb: 900,000-1,200,000 U daily.
Drug available: Bicillin C-R, 1,200,000 U/2 ml.

14. Child receiving preoperative medication (may solve by nomogram or square root).
Order: hydroxyzine (Vistaril) 25 mg, IM.
Child's height and weight: 47 inches, 45 lb.
Pediatric dose: 30 mg/m^2.
Drug available:

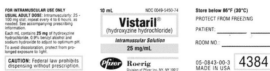

15. Child receiving preoperative medication.
Order: atropine 0.2 mg, IM.
Child's weight: 12 kg.
Pediatric dose: 24-40 lb/0.2 mg.
Drug available:

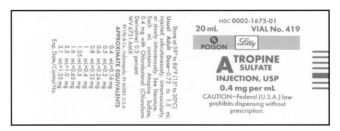

16. Child with cancer.
Order: methotrexate 50 mg, IM, q weekly (may solve by nomogram or square root).
Child's height and weight: 56 inches, 100 lb.
Pediatric dose: 25-75 mg/m^2/wk.
Drug available: methotrexate 2.5 mg/ml; 25 mg/ml; 100 mg/ml.

17. Order: A newborn is to receive AquaMEPHYTON (vitamin K) 0.5 mg IM immediately after delivery.
Pediatric dose: 0.5-1 mg.

Drug available:

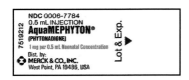 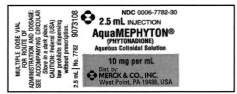

a. Which AquaMEPHYTON container would you select?
b. How many milliliters (ml) should the newborn receive?
c. Is drug dose within the safe range?

III. Intravenous

18. Adolescent with progressive hip pain secondary to rheumatoid arthritis.
Order: morphine sulfate 2.5 mg, IV piggyback, in 10 ml NSS over 5 minutes.
  Flush with 5 ml.
Child's weight: 50 kg.
Pediatric dose: 50-100 mcg/kg/dose for IV.
Drug available:

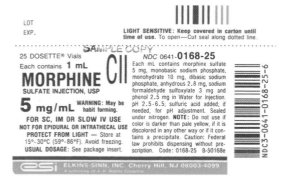

19. Treatment to reverse postoperative narcotic depression.
Order: Narcan (naloxone) 0.3 mg, IV push.
Child's weight: 32 kg.
Pediatric dose: 0.005-0.01 mg/kg.
Drug available:

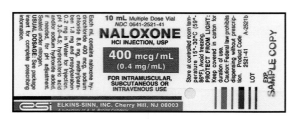

20. Infant with sepsis.
Order: Amikin 40 mg, IV, q12h, in D$_5$W 5 ml, over 20 minutes. Flush with
  3 ml.
Child's weight: 5.3 kg.

Pediatric dose: 15 mg/kg/day.
Drug available:

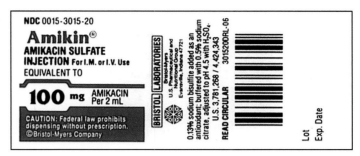

21. Child with head trauma.
    Order: Decadron 2 mg, IV, q6h, in D$_5$W 10 ml, over 15 minutes. Flush with
    5 ml.
    Child's weight and age: 10.1 kg, 16 months.
    Pediatric dose: 0.4 mg/kg/day in divided doses.
    Drug available:

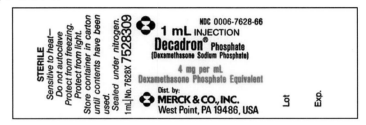

22. Child with pneumonia.
    Order: cefazolin (Ancef) 500 mg, IV, q6h, in D$_5$W 20 ml, over 30 minutes.
    Flush with 10 ml.
    Child's weight: 5.6 kg.
    Pediatric dose: 25-100 mg/kg/day in four divided doses.
    Drug available:

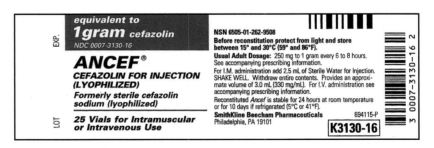

23. Child with sepsis.
    Order: gentamicin 10 mg, IV, q8h, in D$_5$W, 4 ml, over 30 minutes. Flush with
    3 ml.
    Child's height, weight, age: 21 inches, 4 kg, 1 month.
    Pediatric dose: >7 days old: 5-7.5 mg/kg/day, three divided doses.
    Drug available: gentamicin 10 mg/ml.

24. Child with postoperative wound infection.
Order: cefazolin 185 mg, IV, q6h, in D$_5$W 20 ml, over 20 minutes. Flush with 15 ml.
Child's weight: 15 kg.
Pediatric dose: 25-50 mg/kg/day.
Drug available:

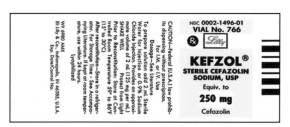

25. Child with wound infection after spinal fusion.
Order: nafcillin 250 mg, IV, q6h, in D$_5$W 20 ml, over 30 minutes. Flush with 15 ml.
Child's weight: 40 kg.
Pediatric dose: 25 mg/kg/day.
Drug available:

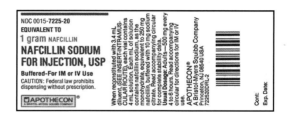

26. Child with congestive heart failure.
Order: digoxin 40 mcg, IV, bid, in NSS 2 ml, over 1 minute.
Child's weight and age: 6 lb, 1 month.
Pediatric dose: 2 weeks to 2 years: 25-50 mcg(μg)/kg.
Drug available: digoxin 0.1 mg/ml.

27. Child with lymphoma.
Order: Cytoxan 180 mg, IV, in D$_5$½ NSS, 300 ml, over 3 hours, no flush to follow.
Child's weight and height: 16 kg, 75 cm (may solve by nomogram or square root).
Pediatric dose: 300 mg/m²/day.
Drug available:

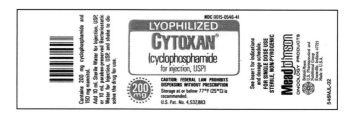

28. Child with severe respiratory tract infection.
Order: kanamycin (Kantrex) 60 mg, IV, q8h.
Child's weight and age: 26 lb, 12 months.
Pediatric dose parameters: 15 mg/kg/day q8-12h, not to exceed 1.5 g per day.
Drug available:

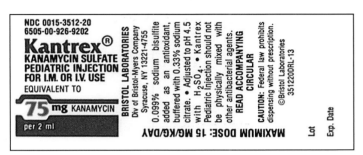

a. How many milliliters of kanamycin will the child receive every 8 hours?

_____

b. How many milliliters of kanamycin will the child receive per day?

_____

c. Is the drug dose within the safe range? _____

29. Child with severe systemic infection.
Order: tobramycin (Nebcin) 15 mg, IV, q6h.
Drug available:

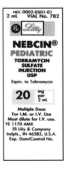

Child's weight and age: 10 kg, 18 months.
Pediatric dose parameters: 6-7.5 mg/kg/day in four divided doses.

a. How many milliliters of tobramycin would you give?

_____

b. Is the drug dose within the safe range?

_____

30. Child with acute lymphocytic leukemia.
Order: daunorubicin HCl 40 mg, IV, qd.
Pediatric dose parameters: >2 yr: 25-45 mg/m²/day.
Child's age, weight, and height: 10 years, 72 lb, 60 inches.

Drug available: daunorubicin 20 mg/4 ml.
Instruction: Mix in 100 ml D₅W; infuse in 45 minutes.

a. The BSA is _____

b. How many milliliters should be mixed in the D₅W? _____

c. Is the drug dose within the safe range? _____

31. Child, 7 years old, with pin worms.
Order: Pyrantel pamoate suspension 50 mg/ml.
Child's weight: 52 lb.
Pediatric dose: 11 mg/kg.

a. How much does the child weigh in kilograms? _____

b. What dosage should the child receive? _____

c. How many milliliters should the child receive? _____

IV. Neonates

32. Neonate with bradycardia, heart rate <60 beats/min.
Order: Epinephrine 0.25 mg IV now.
Pediatric dose: 0.1 mg/kg.
Neonate weight: 2.5 kg.
Drug available:

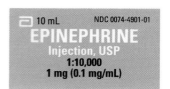

33. Neonate with respiratory depression after delivery, mother received Stadol during labor.
Neonate weight: 8 lb 8 oz.
Order: Naxolone 0.04 mg IM now.
Pediatric dose: 0.01 mg/kg.
Drug available: Naxolone 0.4 mg/ml.

34. Neonate with bacterial meningitis.
Neonate weight: 2.5 kg.
Order: Ampicillin 125 mg IV push over 2 minutes.
Pediatric dose parameters: 50 to 75 mg/kg/dose.
Drug available:

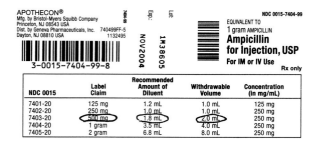

35. Neonate with IV fluids for sepsis.
    Neonate weight: 2.5 kg.
    Order: $D_{10}W$ 80 ml/kg for 24 hours.

    a. How much $D_{10}W$ should be given in 24 hours?

    b. How many milliliters per hour should be infused?

36. Neonate with sepsis.
    Neonate weight: 2.5 kg.
    Order: Gentamicin 10 mg IV over 24 hours.
    Pediatric dosage parameters: 4 to 5 mg/kg.
    Drug available: Gentamicin 40 mg/ml.

PEDIATRIC DOSAGE FROM ADULT DOSAGE

Body Surface Area Formula

The following information is needed to calculate the pediatric dosage with the BSA formula:

a. Physician's order with the name of the drug, the dosage, and the time frame or frequency.
b. The child's height and weight.
c. A BSA nomogram for children.
d. The adult drug dosage.
e. The BSA formula:

$$\frac{BSA\ (m^2)}{1.73\ m^2} \times Adult\ dose = Child's\ dose$$

EXAMPLE

PROBLEM 1
a. erythromycin 80 mg, po, qid.
b. Child's height is 34 inches and weight is 28.5 lb.

Note: *Height and weight do not have to be converted to the metric system.*

c. Height (34 inches) and weight (28.5 lb) intersect the nomogram at 0.57 m². See BSA nomogram, Figure 10-2.
d. The adult drug dosage is 1000 mg/24 hr.
e. BSA formula:

$$\frac{BSA\ (m^2)}{1.73\ m^2} \times Adult\ dose = \frac{0.57\ m^2}{1.73\ m^2} \times 100$$
$$= 0.33 \times 1000$$
$$= 330\ mg/24\ hr$$

Dose frequency:

$$330\ mg \div 4\ doses = 82.5\ \textbf{or}\ 80\ mg\ per\ dose$$

$$80\ mg \times 4\ times\ per\ day = 320\ mg/day$$

Dosage is safe.

Age Rules

Fried's rule and Young's rule are two methods for determining pediatric drug doses based on the child's age. Fried's rule is primarily used for children younger than 1 year of age, whereas Young's rule is used for children between 2 and 12 years of age. In current practice, these rules are infrequently used. Because the maturational development of infants and children is variable, age cannot be an accurate basis for drug dosing.

Fried's Rule:

$$\frac{\text{Age in months}}{150} \times \text{Adult dose} = \text{Infant dose}$$

Young's Rule:

$$\frac{\text{Child's age in years}}{\text{Age in years} + 12} \times \text{Adult dose} = \text{Child dose}$$

Body Weight Rule

Clark's rule is another method of deriving a pediatric dosage based on the child's weight in pounds and the average adult weight of 150 lb. Population studies have shown an increase in the average weight of adults; therefore 150 lb is not an accurate constant. Using the fixed constant in Clark's rule can lead to underdosing of infants. Clark's rule is being phased out as a method for determining drug dosage in children.

Clark's Rule:

$$\frac{\text{Child's weight in pounds}}{150 \text{ lb}} \times \text{Adult dose} = \text{Child dose}$$

NOTE

The age and weight rules should not be used if a pediatric dose is provided by the manufacturer.

ANSWERS SUMMARY PRACTICE PROBLEMS

I. Oral

1. Pounds to kilograms: $\frac{45 \text{ lb}}{2.2 \text{ lb/kg}} = 20.4 \text{ kg}$

Dosage parameters: 25 mg/kg/day × 20.4 kg = 510 mg/day
50 mg/kg/day × 20.4 kg = 1020 mg/day
Dosage frequency: 250 mg × 3 = 750 mg
Dosage is safe.

BF: $\dfrac{D}{H} \times V = \dfrac{250 \text{ mg}}{125 \text{ mg}} \times 5 \text{ ml} = 10 \text{ ml}$

or

RP: H : V ::   D   :X

        125 mg : 5 ml :: 250 mg : X

             125 X = 1250

                 X = 10 ml

2. Dosage parameters: 5 mg/kg/day $\times$ 7.2 kg = 36 mg/day

                          7 mg/kg/day $\times$ 7.2 kg = 50.4 mg/day

   Dose frequency: 25 mg $\times$ 2 = 50 mg

   Dosage is safe.

BF: $\dfrac{D}{H} \times V = \dfrac{25 \text{ mg}}{20 \text{ mg}} \times 5 \text{ ml} = 6.25 \text{ ml/dose}$

or DA: $\text{ml} = \dfrac{5 \text{ ml} \times \overset{5}{\cancel{25}} \text{ mg}}{\underset{4}{\cancel{20}} \text{ mg} \times 1} = \dfrac{25}{4} = 6.25 \text{ ml}$

3. Dosage parameters: 15 mg/kg, q12h $\times$ 8 kg = 120 mg, q12h

   Dosage frequency: 100 mg, q12h.

   Dosage is safe.

BF: $\dfrac{D}{H} \times V = \dfrac{100 \text{ mg}}{125 \text{ mg}} \times 5 \text{ ml} = 4 \text{ ml/dose}$

4. Height and weight intersect at 0.84 m² with nomogram.

   Dosage parameters: 100 mg/0.84 m²/day = 84 mg/day

   Dose frequency: 84 mg/day $\div$ 6 = 14 mg/dose

   Dosage is safe.

   BSA with the Square Root: BSA Pounds and Inches Formula, see page 99

$$\sqrt{\dfrac{43 \times 50}{3131}} = \sqrt{0.686} = 0.828 \text{ or } 0.83 \text{ m}^2$$

   Dosage parameters: 100 mg/0.83 m² = 83 mg/day (compare with nomogram)

   Dosage frequency: 83 mg/day/6 = 13.8 or 14 mg per dose

   Dosage is safe.

BF: $\dfrac{D}{H} \times V = \dfrac{7.5 \text{ mg}}{15 \text{ mg}} \times 1 = 0.50 \text{ or } \frac{1}{2} \text{ tablet}$

or

RP: H : V ::   D   :X

        15 mg : 1 ml :: 7.5 mg : X

             15 X = 7.5

               X = $\frac{1}{2}$ tablet

5. Dosage parameters: 20 mg/kg/day $\times$ 13 kg = 260 mg/day

   Dose frequency: 125 mg $\times$ 2 = 250 mg/day

   Dosage is safe.

BF: $\dfrac{D}{H} \times V = \dfrac{125 \text{ mg}}{250 \text{ mg}} \times 5 \text{ ml} = 2.5 \text{ ml}$

6. Dosage parameters: 5 mg/kg/day × 6.7 kg = 33.5 mg/day
   7 mg/kg/day × 6.7 kg = 46.9 mg/day
   Dose frequency: 40 mg × 2 = 80 mg/day
   Dosage exceeds the therapeutic range. Dosage is *not safe.*

7. Dosage parameters: 150 mg/kg/day × 30.4 = 4560 mg or 4.5 g
   200 mg/kg/day × 30.4 = 6080 mg or 6.1 g
   Dose frequency: 1.5 g × 4 = 6.0 g or 6000 mg
   Dosage is safe.

   BF: $\dfrac{D}{H} = \dfrac{1500 \text{ mg}}{500 \text{ mg}} = 3$ tablets/dose

   or

   DA: tab $= \dfrac{1 \text{ tab} \times \overset{2}{\cancel{1000}} \cancel{\text{mg}} \times 1.5 \cancel{\text{g}}}{\underset{1}{\cancel{500}} \cancel{\text{mg}} \times 1 \cancel{\text{g}} \times 1} = 3$ tablets

8. Dosage parameters: 20 mg/kg/day × 8 kg = 160 mg/day
   40 mg/kg/day × 8 kg = 320 mg/day
   Dose frequency: 75 mg × 3 = 225 mg
   Dosage is safe.

   BF: $\dfrac{D}{H} \times V = \dfrac{75 \text{ mg}}{125 \text{ mg}} \times 5 \text{ ml} = 3$ ml

   or

   RP: H : V :: D :X
   125 mg:5 ml::75 mg:X
   125X = 375
   X = 3 ml

9. Dosage parameters: 5 mg/kg/day × 25 kg = 125 mg/day
   Dose frequency: 25 mg × 4 = 100 mg/day
   Dosage is safe.

   BF: $\dfrac{D}{H} \times V = \dfrac{25 \text{ mg}}{12.5 \text{ mg}} \times 5 \text{ ml} = 10$ ml

   or

   DA: ml $= \dfrac{5 \text{ ml} \times \overset{2}{\cancel{25}} \cancel{\text{mg}}}{\underset{1}{\cancel{12.5}} \cancel{\text{mg}} \times 1} = 10$ ml

10. Dosage parameters: 4 mg/kg/day × 14 kg = 56 mg/day
    8 mg/kg/day × 14 kg = 112 mg/day
    Dose frequency: 25 mg × 3 = 75 mg
    Dosage is safe.

    BF: $\dfrac{D}{H} \times V = \dfrac{25 \text{ mg}}{50 \text{ mg}} \times 5 \text{ ml} = 2.5$ ml/dose

    11. a.   15 l
    Dosage parameters: 20 mg × 6.8 kg = 136 mg/day
    40 mg × 6.8 kg = 272 mg/day
    Dose frequency: 50 mg × 4 = 200 mg/day
    Dosage is safe.

b. BF: $\dfrac{D}{H} \times V = \dfrac{50}{125} \times 5 = \dfrac{250}{125} = 2$ ml

or

RP: H : V :: D : X

125 mg : 5 ml :: 50 mg : X ml

125X = 250

X = 2 ml

or

DA: ml $= \dfrac{5 \text{ ml} \times \overset{2}{\cancel{50}} \text{ mg}}{\underset{5}{\cancel{125}} \text{ mg} \times 1} = \dfrac{10}{5} = 2$ ml

II. Intramuscular

12. Dosage parameters: 0.25/kg/dose $\times$ 45 kg = 11.25 mg/dose

0.5/kg/dose $\times$ 45 kg = 22.5 mg/dose

Dose frequency: 20 mg IM/dose

Dosage is safe.

BF: $\dfrac{D}{H} \times V = \dfrac{20 \text{ mg}}{25 \text{ mg}} \times 1 = 0.8$ ml

or

DA: ml $= \dfrac{1 \text{ ml} \times \overset{4}{\cancel{20}} \text{ mg}}{\underset{5}{\cancel{25}} \text{ mg} \times 1} = \dfrac{4}{5} = 0.8$ ml

13. Dosage parameters: Child's weight is 44 lb, which falls in the 30 to 60 lb pediatric dose range.

Dose frequency: The one-time dose of 1,000,000 U falls within the pediatric dose range.

Dosage is safe.

BF: $\dfrac{D}{H} \times V = \dfrac{1{,}000{,}000 \text{ U}}{1{,}200{,}000 \text{ U}} \times 2 = 1.6$ ml

14. Height and weight intersect at 0.82 m² with the nomogram.

BSA with Square Root (Pounds and Inches Formula)

$$\sqrt{\dfrac{47 \text{ inches} \times 45 \text{ pounds}}{3131}} = \sqrt{0.675} = 0.82 \text{ m}^2 \text{ (same as the nomogram)}$$

Dosage parameters: 30 mg/m² $\times$ 0.82 m² = 24.6 mg or 25 mg

Dose frequency: 25 mg IM/dose

Dosage is safe.

BF: $\dfrac{D}{H} \times V = \dfrac{25 \text{ mg}}{25 \text{ mg}} \times 1 = 1.0$ ml

or

DA: ml $= \dfrac{1 \text{ ml} \times \overset{1}{\cancel{25}} \text{ mg}}{\underset{1}{\cancel{25}} \text{ mg} \times 1} = 1$ ml

15. Kilograms to pounds: 12 kg $\times$ 2.2 lb/kg = 26.4 lb

Dosage is safe.

BF: $\dfrac{D}{H} \times V = \dfrac{0.2}{0.4} \times 1 = 0.5$ ml

16. Height and weight intersect at 1.38 m² with the nomogram.
    Dosage parameters: 25 mg/m²/wk × 1.38 m² = 34.5 mg/wk
    75 mg/m²/wk × 1.38 m² = 103.5 mg/wk
    BSA with Square Root (Pounds and Inches Formula)

$$\sqrt{\frac{56 \text{ inches} \times 100 \text{ pounds}}{3131}} = \sqrt{1.788} = 1.34 \text{ m}^2$$

Dosage parameters: 25 mg × 1.34 = 33.5 mg/wk
75 mg × 1.34 = 100.5 mg/wk
Dose frequency: 50 mg/wk IM
Dosage is safe.

$$\frac{D}{H} \times V = \frac{50 \text{ mg}}{100 \text{ mg}} \times 1 \text{ ml} = 0.5 \text{ ml}$$

17. **a.** Preferred selection is AquaMEPHYTON 1 mg = 0.5 ml
    b. *AquaMEPHYTON 1 mg = 0.5 ml:*

$$\text{BF: } \frac{D}{H} \times V = \frac{0.5 \text{ mg}}{1.0 \text{ mg}} \times 0.5 \text{ ml} = \frac{0.25}{1.0} = 0.25 \text{ ml}$$

or

RP: H : V ::   D   :X
       1 mg:0.5 ml :: 0.5 mg:X
              X = 0.25 mg

AquaMEPHYTON 10 mg = 1 ml:

$$\text{BF: } \frac{D}{H} \times V = \frac{0.5 \text{ mg}}{10 \text{ mg}} \times 1.0 \text{ ml} = \frac{0.5}{10} = 0.05 \text{ ml}$$

For AquaMEPHYTON 1 mg = 0.5 ml, give 0.25 ml (use a tuberculin syringe).
For AquaMEPHYTON 10 mg = 1 ml, give 0.05 ml (use a tuberculin syringe; however, it would be difficult to give this small amount.)
    c. Drug dose is within the safe range.

III. Intravenous

18. Dosage parameters: 50 mcg/kg/dose × 50 kg = 2500 mcg/dose or 2.5 mg/dose
    100 mcg/kg/dose × 50 kg = 5000 mcg/dose or 5 mg/dose
    Dosage is safe.

$$\text{BF: } \frac{D}{H} \times V = \frac{2.5}{5} \times 1 = 0.5 \text{ ml}$$

or

$$\text{DA: ml} = \frac{1 \text{ ml} \times \overset{1}{\cancel{2.5}} \text{ mg}}{\underset{2}{\cancel{5}} \text{ mg} \times 1} = \frac{1}{2} \text{ or } 0.5 \text{ ml}$$

Amount of fluid to be infused: 0.5 ml + 10 ml = 10.5 ml

$$\frac{10.5 \text{ ml} \times \overset{12}{\cancel{60}} \text{ gtt/ml}}{\underset{1}{\cancel{5}} \text{ minutes}} = 125 \text{ gtt/min}$$

Total fluid for medication infusion plus flush: 10.5 ml + 5 ml = 15.5 ml.

19. Dosage parameters: 0.005 mg/kg/dose $\times$ 32 kg = 0.16 mg

0.01 mg/kg/dose $\times$ 32 kg = 0.32 mg

Dosage is safe.

BF: $\dfrac{D}{H} \times V = \dfrac{0.3}{0.4} \times 1 = 0.75$ ml

20. Dosage parameters: 15 mg/kg/day $\times$ 5.3 = 79.5 mg/day

Dose frequency: 40 mg IV $\times$ 2 = 80 mg

79.5 mg is rounded off to 80 mg. The dosage is safe.

BF: $\dfrac{D}{H} \times V = \dfrac{40 \text{ mg}}{100 \text{ mg}} \times 2 = 0.8$ ml

or

RP: $\qquad$ H $\quad$: V $\;::\;$ D $\;$: X

$\qquad$ 100 mg : 2 ml $::$ 40 mg : X

$\qquad\qquad$ 100X = 80

$\qquad\qquad\qquad$ X = 0.8 ml

Amount of fluid to be infused: 0.8 ml + 5 ml = 5.8 ml

$\dfrac{5.8 \text{ ml} \times \overset{3}{\cancel{60}} \text{ gtt/ml}}{\underset{1}{\cancel{20}} \text{ minutes}} = 17.4$ gtt/min

Total fluid for medication infusion plus flush: 5.8 ml + 3 ml = 8.8 ml.

21. Dosage parameters: 0.4 mg/kg/day $\times$ 10.1 kg = 4 mg/day

4 mg $\div$ 4 doses = 1 mg per dose

Dose frequency: 2 mg $\times$ 4 times/day = 8 mg per day

Dose exceeds therapeutic range of 1 mg per dose. Dosage is *not safe.*

22. Dosage parameters: 25-100 mg/kg/day in four divided doses.

25 mg $\times$ 5.6 kg = 140 mg/day

100 mg $\times$ 5.6 kg = 560 mg/day

560 mg $\div$ 4 = 140 mg/dose

Dose frequency: 500 mg $\times$ 4 = 2000 mg/day

Dose exceeds therapeutic range of 560 mg/day. Dosage is *not safe.*

23. Dosage parameters: 5 mg/kg/day $\times$ 4 kg = 20 mg/day

7.5 mg/kg/day $\times$ 4 kg = 30 mg/day

Dose frequency: 10 mg $\times$ 3 times/day = 30 mg

Dosage is safe.

BF: $\dfrac{D}{H} \times V = \dfrac{10 \text{ mg}}{10 \text{ mg}} \times 1 \text{ ml} = 1$ ml

or

DA: ml $= \dfrac{1 \text{ ml} \times \overset{1}{\cancel{10}} \text{ mg}}{\underset{1}{\cancel{10}} \text{ mg} \times \quad 1} = 1$ ml

Amount of fluid to be infused: 1 ml + 4 ml = 5 ml

$\dfrac{5 \text{ ml} \times \overset{2}{\cancel{60}} \text{ gtt/ml}}{\underset{1}{\cancel{30}} \text{ minutes}} = 10$ gtt/min

Total fluid for medication infusion plus flush: 5 ml + 3 ml = 8 ml

24. Dosage parameters: 25 mg/kg/day $\times$ 15 kg = 375 mg/day
   50 mg/kg/day $\times$ 15 kg = 750 mg/day
   Dose frequency: 185 mg $\times$ 4 = 740 mg/day
   Dosage is safe. 250 mg = 2 mg or 125 mg = 1 ml

   BF: $\dfrac{D}{H} \times V = \dfrac{185 \text{ mg}}{125 \text{ mg}} \times 1 \text{ ml} = 1.48$ or 1.5 ml

   or
   RP: H : V :: D : X
   125 mg : 1 ml :: 185 mg : X
   125X = 185
   X = 1.5 ml
   Amount of fluid to be infused: 1.5 ml + 20 ml = 21.5 ml

   $$\dfrac{21.5 \text{ ml} \times \overset{3}{\cancel{6}0} \text{ gtt/ml}}{\underset{1}{\cancel{2}0} \text{ minutes}} = 64.5 \text{ gtt/min}$$

   Total fluid for medication infusion plus flush: 21.5 ml + 15 ml = 36.5 ml

25. Dosage parameters: 25 mg/kg/day $\times$ 40 kg = 1000 mg
   Dose frequency: 250 mg $\times$ 4 = 1000 mg/day
   Dosage is safe. Mix with 3.4 ml diluent = 4 ml of drug solution.

   BF: $\dfrac{D}{H} \times V = \dfrac{250}{1000} \times 4 = 1 \text{ ml}$

   or
   DA: ml = $\dfrac{4 \text{ ml} \times \overset{1}{\cancel{1} \text{ g}} \times \overset{1}{\cancel{2}5\cancel{0}} \text{ mg}}{\underset{1}{\cancel{1} \text{ g}} \times \underset{4}{\cancel{1}0\cancel{0}0} \text{ mg} \times 1} = \dfrac{4}{4} = 1 \text{ ml}$

   Amount of fluid to be infused: 1 ml + 20 ml = 21 ml

   $$\dfrac{21 \text{ ml} \times \overset{2}{\cancel{6}0} \text{ gtt/ml (set)}}{\underset{1}{\cancel{3}0} \text{ minutes}} = 42 \text{ gtt/min}$$

   Total fluid for medication infusion plus flush: 21 ml + 15 ml = 36 ml

26. Dosage parameters: 25 mcg/kg/day $\times$ 2.72 kg = 68 mcg
   50 mcg/kg/day $\times$ 2.72 kg = 136 mcg
   Dose frequency: 40 mcg $\times$ 2 = 80 mcg
   0.1 mg = 100 mcg (μg)
   Dosage is safe.

   BF: $\dfrac{D}{H} \times V = \dfrac{40 \text{ mcg}}{100 \text{ mcg}} \times 1 = 0.4 \text{ ml}$

27. Height and weight intersect at 0.6 m^2 according to the nomogram.
   Dosage parameters: 300 mg/m^2/day $\times$ 0.6 m^2 = 180 mg/day
   BSA with the Square Root (Metric Formula)

   $$\sqrt{\dfrac{16 \text{ kg} \times 75 \text{ cm}}{3600}} = \sqrt{0.333} = 0.58 \text{ m}^2$$

   Dosage parameters: 300 mg $\times$ 0.58 m^2 = 174 mg
   Dosage is safe.

BF: $\dfrac{D}{H} \times V = \dfrac{180 \text{ mg}}{200 \text{ mg}} \times 10 \text{ ml} = 9 \text{ ml}$

or

DA: ml $= \dfrac{10 \text{ ml} \times \overset{9}{\cancel{180}} \text{ mg}}{\underset{10}{\cancel{200}} \text{ mg} \times 1} = \dfrac{90}{10} = 9 \text{ ml}$

Total amount of fluid to be infused: 9 ml + 300 ml = 309 ml

$\dfrac{309 \text{ ml}}{3 \text{ hr}} = 103 \text{ ml/hr or } 103 \text{ gtt/min with a } 60 \text{ gtt/ml set}$

28. a. BF: $\dfrac{60}{75} \times 2 \text{ ml} = \dfrac{120}{75} = 1.6 \text{ ml}$

    or
RP: 75 mg : 2 ml :: 60 mg : X
              75X = 120
                  X = 1.6 ml of kanamycin

  b. 4.8 ml/day
  c. Dosage parameters: 15 mg × 12 kg = 180 mg/day
                           60 mg × 3 (q8h) = 180 mg/day
  Drug dose per day is within the safe range.

29. a. BF: $\dfrac{15}{\underset{10}{\cancel{20}}} \times \overset{1}{\cancel{2}} \text{ ml} = \dfrac{15}{10} = 1.5 \text{ ml of Nebcin}$

    or
RP: 20 mg : 2 ml :: 15 mg : X
             20X = 30
               X = 1.5 ml of Nebcin

  b. Pediatric dosage parameters: 6 mg/10 kg/day = 60 mg/day
                               7.5 mg/10 kg/day = 75 mg/day
                             15 mg × 4 (q6h) = 60 mg/day
  Drug dose per day is within the safe range.

30. a. The BSA is 1.16.
  b. 8 ml of daunorubicin HCl mixed in 100 ml D$_5$W.
  c. Dosage parameters: 25 mg × 1.16 m^2 = 29 mg/day
                           45 mg × 1.16 m^2 = 52.2 mg/day
  Child is to receive 40 mg of daunorubicin HCl per day.
  Drug dose is within the safe range.

$$\dfrac{108 \text{ ml} \times \overset{1}{\cancel{15}} \text{ gtt/min (secondary set)}}{\underset{3}{\cancel{45}} \text{ minutes}} = 36 \text{ gtt/min}$$

31. a. Child weighs 23.6 kg
  b. 23.6 kg × 11 mg/kg = 259.6 or 260 mg
  c. 260 mg/50 mg/ml = 5.2 ml

IV. Neonates

32. $0.1 \text{ mg/kg} \times 2.5 \text{ kg} = 0.25 \text{ mg}$

BF: $\dfrac{0.25 \text{ mg}}{0.1 \text{ mg}} \times 1 \text{ ml} = 2.5 \text{ ml}$

or

DA: ml = $\dfrac{1 \text{ ml} \times 0.25 \text{ mg}}{0.1 \text{ mg} \times 1} = \dfrac{0.25}{0.1} = 2.5 \text{ ml}$

33. $\dfrac{8.8}{2.2} = 4 \text{ kg}$

$0.01 \text{ mg/kg} \times 4 \text{ kg} = 0.04 \text{ mg dose}$

BF: $\dfrac{D}{H} \times V = \dfrac{0.04 \text{ mg}}{0.4 \text{ ml}} \times 1 \text{ ml} = 0.1 \text{ ml}$

or

RP: H   : V   ::   D   : X
    0.4 mg : 1 ml :: 0.04 mg : X ml
           0.4X = 0.04
              X = 0.1 ml

34. a. Dosage parameters:
    $50 \text{ mg/kg} \times 2.5 \text{ kg} = 125 \text{ mg}$
    $75 \text{ mg/kg} \times 2.5 \text{ kg} = 187.5 \text{ mg}$

BF: $\dfrac{125 \text{ mg}}{500 \text{ mg}} \times 2 \text{ ml} = 0.5 \text{ ml}$

or

DA: ml = $\dfrac{2 \text{ ml} \times \overset{1}{125} \text{ mg}}{\underset{4}{500} \text{ mg} \times 1} = \dfrac{2}{4} = 0.5 \text{ ml}$

35. a. $80 \text{ ml/kg} \times 2.5 \text{ kg} = 200 \text{ ml } D_{10}W \text{ in 24 hours}$

b. $\dfrac{200 \text{ ml}}{24 \text{ hr}} = 8.3 \text{ ml/hr}$

36. a. Dosage parameters: $4 \text{ mg/kg} \times 2.5 \text{ kg} = 10 \text{ mg}$
                  $5 \text{ mg/kg} \times 2.5 \text{ kg} = 12.5 \text{ mg}$
Drug is safe.

b. BF: $\dfrac{D}{H} \times V = \dfrac{10 \text{ mg}}{40 \text{ mg}} \times 1 \text{ ml} = 0.25 \text{ ml}$

or

RP: H   : V   ::   D   : X
    40 mg : 1 ml :: 10 mg : X ml
          40X = 10
             X = 0.25 ml

Critical Care

OBJECTIVES

- Calculate the prescribed concentration of a drug in solution.
- Identify the units of measure designated for the amount of drug in solution.
- Describe the four determinants of infusion rates.
- Calculate the concentration of drug per unit time for a specific body weight.
- Recognize the variables needed for the basic fractional formula.
- Describe how the titration factor is used when infusion rates are changed.
- Recognize the methods of determining the total amount of drug infused over time.

OUTLINE

CALCULATING AMOUNT OF DRUG OR CONCENTRATION OF A SOLUTION
    Calculating Units per Milliliter
    Calculating Milligrams per Milliliter
    Calculating Micrograms per Milliliter
CALCULATING INFUSION RATE FOR CONCENTRATION AND VOLUME
    PER UNIT TIME
    Concentration and Volume per Hour and Minute with a Drug in Units
    Concentration and Volume per Hour and Minute with a Drug in
        Milligrams
    Concentration and Volume per Minute and Hour with a Drug in
        Micrograms
CALCULATING INFUSION RATES OF A DRUG FOR SPECIFIC BODY
    WEIGHT PER UNIT TIME
    Micrograms per Kilogram Body Weight
BASIC FRACTIONAL FORMULA
    Using Basic Formula to Find Volume per Hour or Drops per Minute
    Using Basic Formula to Find Desired Concentration per Minute
    Using Basic Formula to Find Concentration of Solution
TITRATION OF INFUSION RATE
TOTAL AMOUNT OF DRUG INFUSED OVER TIME

Medication administration has become increasingly individualized for critically ill clients. Nurses are responsible for safe and accurate delivery of these drugs. Administration of potent drugs in milligrams, micrograms, or units per body weight or unit time requires extreme accuracy in calculations. Physicians determine the amount of drug to be mixed in the intravenous (IV) solution and designate infusion rates or the dosage per kilogram of body weight per unit time. Some institutions have their own guidelines for preparation of medication in the critical care areas. Research studies have shown a high incidence of error in drug calculations among nurses and physicians. Many institutions have initiated policies of drug infusion standardization, especially for the concentration of solution, to limit infusion errors.

Because some institutions have their own guidelines for preparations and medication in the critical care areas, the medication often comes in premixed bags or bottles from the pharmacy ready for infusion. Still, in some facilities, these drugs are prepared by the nurse. The nurse must know what data are needed for each drug and apply those parameters to whatever IV equipment is available. Wide use of volumetric IV infusion pumps has improved the safety of individualized drug administration. The accuracy of the infusion rate with the pump has almost eliminated the need for drop counting, but nurses are still responsible for all other infusion rates. Each drug has its own dosing parameters. Some drugs are dosed in the concentration per hour or minute and others are administered in micrograms, milligrams, or units per kilogram of body weight. The nurse must be familiar with the specific dosing parameters to ensure the accuracy of infusion rates.

The mathematical skills needed to solve problems in this chapter include knowledge of proper and improper fractions, cancellation of units, ratio and proportion, and conversion to the metric system.

CALCULATING AMOUNT OF DRUG OR CONCENTRATION OF A SOLUTION

The first step in administering a medication is to determine the concentration of the solution, which is the amount of drug in each milliliter of solution. This is written as units per milliliter, milligrams per milliliter, or micrograms per milliliter and must be calculated for each problem. For all problems, remember to convert to like units before solving.

Calculating Units per Milliliter

EXAMPLE

PROBLEM: Infuse heparin 5000 U in D₅W 250 ml at 30 ml/hr. What will be the concentration of heparin in each milliliter of D₅W?

Method: units/ml

Set up a ratio and proportion. Solve for X.	$5000 \text{ U}:250 \text{ ml} :: X \text{ U}:ml$
	$250 \text{ X} = 5000$
	$X = 20 \text{ U}$

Answer: The D₅W with heparin will have a concentration of 20 U/ml of solution.

Calculating Milligrams per Milliliter

EXAMPLE

PROBLEM: Infuse lidocaine 2 g in 500 ml D$_5$W at 2 mg/min. What will be the concentration of lidocaine in each milliliter of D$_5$W?

Method: mg/ml

Convert grams to milligrams. Set up a ratio and proportion and solve for X.	2 g = 2000 mg 2000 mg:500 ml :: X mg:ml 500 X = 2000 X = 4 mg

Answer: The D$_5$W with lidocaine has a concentration of 4 mg/ml of solution.

Calculating Micrograms per Milliliter

EXAMPLE

PROBLEM: Infuse dobutamine 250 mg in 500 ml D$_5$W at 650 mcg/min. What is the concentration of dobutamine in each milliliter of D$_5$W?

Method: mcg/ml

Convert milligrams to micrograms. Set up a ratio and proportion and solve for X.	250 mg = 250,000 mcg 250,000 mcg:500 ml :: X mcg:ml 500 X = 250,000 X = 500 mcg/ml

Answer: The D$_5$W with dobutamine will have a concentration of 500 mcg/ml of solution.

PRACTICE PROBLEMS I Calculating Concentration of a Solution

Answers can be found on page 277.

1. Infuse heparin 10,000 U in 250 ml D$_5$W at 30 ml/hr.

_____

2. Infuse aminophylline 250 mg in 500 ml D$_5$W at 50 ml/hr.

_____

3. Order: regular insulin 100 U in 500 ml NSS at 30 ml/hr.

_____

4. Order: lidocaine 1 g in 100 ml D$_5$W at 30 ml/hr.

_____

5. Order: norepinephrine 4 mg in 500 ml D$_5$W at 15 ml/hr.

_____

6. Order: dopamine 500 mg in 250 ml D$_5$W at 10 ml/hr.

_____

7. Order: dobutamine 400 mg in 250 ml D$_5$W at 20 ml/hr.

_____

8. Order: Isuprel 2 mg in 250 ml D$_5$W at 10 ml/hr.

_____

9. Order: streptokinase 750,000 U in 50 ml D$_5$W over 30 minutes.

_____

10. Order: nitroprusside 50 mg in 500 ml D$_5$W at 50 mcg/min.

_____

11. Order: aminophylline 1 g in 250 ml D$_5$W at 20 ml/hr.

_____

12. Order: Pronestyl 2 g in 250 ml D$_5$W at 16 ml/hr.

_____

13. Order: heparin 25,000 U in 250 ml D$_5$W at 5 ml/hr.

_____

14. Order: aminophylline 1 g in 500 ml D$_5$W at 40 cc/hr.

_____

15. Order: nitroglycerin 50 mg in 250 ml D$_5$W at 50 mcg/min.

_____

16. Order: alteplase 100 mg in NSS 100 ml over 2 hours.

_____

17. Order: theophylline 800 mg in D$_5$W 500 ml at 0.5 mg/kg.

_____

18. Order: milrinone 20 mg in D$_5$W 100 ml at 0.50 mcg/kg/min.

_____

19. Order: streptokinase 1.5 million units in D$_5$W 100 ml over 60 minutes.

_____

20. Order: amiodarone 150 mg in D$_5$W 100 ml over 10 minutes.

_____

CALCULATING INFUSION RATE FOR CONCENTRATION AND VOLUME PER UNIT TIME

The second step for administering medication is to calculate the *infusion rate* of drug per *unit time*. Infusion rates can mean two things: the rate of volume (ml) given or the rate of concentration (units, mg, mcg) administered. *Unit time* means per hour or per minute. For drugs administered by continuous infusion, the four most important determinants are the concentration per hour and minute and the volume per hour and minute. Infusion rates of potent drugs are usually part of the physician's order and may be stated in concentration or volume per unit time.

Many hospitals have policies requiring that all potent drugs be delivered via volumetric infusion pump. New technology has produced pumps that are programmable and calculate the drug dosage. The information entered in the pump's control panel is (1) the name of the drug, (2) the amount of the drug, (3) the amount of the solution, and (4) the client's weight in kilograms. The nurse enters the ordered dose and the correct dosage parameters, i.e., mg/min, U/hr, mcg/min. The pump automatically delivers the appropriate dosage.

Not all facilities have infusion pumps with advanced technology; therefore the nurse must be able to calculate the infusion rates. For infusion pumps that deliver ml/hr, the volume per hour of the drug must be known. *Remember:* If an infusion device is unavailable, a microdrip IV administration set is the appropriate set to use because the drops per minute rate (gtt/min) corresponds to the volume per hour rate (ml/hr).

Complete infusion rates for volume and concentration are given in the examples and practice problems. In clinical practice, not all the data are needed for each drug. For heparin, the concentration per minute is not as vital as the concentration per hour, whereas for vasoactive drugs such as dobutamine, the concentration per minute is essential information and the concentration per hour is not. The same methods of calculation are used for both drugs, and the same information can be obtained. The nurse must have knowledge of pharmacology and clinical practice to determine the most useful data.

Concentration and Volume per Hour and Minute with a Drug in Units

EXAMPLES

PROBLEM: Infuse heparin 5000 U in D₅W 250 ml at 30 ml/hr. Concentration of solution is 20 units/ml. (Also note that volume/hour is given.) How many milliliters will be infused per minute?

Find volume per minute:

Method: ml/min

Set up a ratio and proportion. Use volume/hour, 30 ml/hr, or 30 ml/60 min as the known variable.

30 ml:60 min :: X ml: min
60 X = 30
X = 0.5 ml

Answer: The infusion rate for volume per minute is 0.5 ml/min and the hourly rate is 30 ml/hr.

What is the concentration per minute and hour?
Find concentration per minute:

Method: U/min

Multiply the concentration of solution by the volume per minute.	20 U/ml × 0.5 ml/min = 10 U/min

Find concentration per hour:

Method: U/hr

Multiply the volume per minute by 60 min/hr.	10 U/min × 60 min/hr = 600 U/hr

Answer: The concentration per minute of heparin is 10 U/min and the concentration per hour is 600 U/hr.

Concentration and Volume per Hour and Minute with a Drug in Milligrams

EXAMPLES   PROBLEM: Infuse lidocaine 2 g in D$_5$W 500 ml at 2 mg/min. Concentration of solution is 4 mg/ml. (Also note that concentration/minute is given.) How many milligrams will be infused per hour?

Find concentration per hour:

Method: mg/hr

Find the concentration/minute. Multiply concentration/minute × 60 min/hr.	lidocaine 2 mg/min 2 mg/min × 60 min = 120 mg/hr

Answer: The amount of lidocaine infused per hour is 120 mg/hr.

How many milliliters of lidocaine will be infused in 1 hour?
Find volume per hour:

Method: ml/hr

Calculate concentration of solution. Divide the concentration/hour by the concentration of solution.	lidocaine 4 mg/ml $\dfrac{120 \text{ mg/hr}}{4 \text{ mg/ml}} = 30$ ml/hr

Answer: The infusion rate in milliliters for lidocaine 2 mg/min is 30 ml/hr.

How many milliliters of lidocaine will be infused in 1 minute?

Divide the concentration/minute by the concentration of the solution.	$\dfrac{2 \text{ mg/min}}{4 \text{ mg/ml}} = 0.5 \text{ ml/min}$

Answer: The infusion rate for lidocaine 2 mg/min is 0.5 ml/min.

Concentration and Volume per Hour and Minute with a Drug in Micrograms

EXAMPLES

PROBLEM: Infuse dobutamine 250 mg in D_5W 500 ml at 650 mcg/min. Concentration of solution is 500 mcg/ml. (Also note that concentration/minute is given in the order.) How many micrograms will be infused in 1 hour?

Find concentration per hour:

Method: mcg/hr

Find the concentration/minute. Multiply concentration/minute by 60 min/hr.	dobutamine 650 mcg/min 650 mcg/min × 60 min/hr = 39,000 mcg/hr

Answer: The concentration of dobutamine infused per hour is 39,000 mcg/hr.

How many milliliters of dobutamine will be infused in 1 hour?
Find volume per hour:

Method: ml/hr

Calculate concentration of solution. Divide the concentration/hour by the concentration of solution.	dobutamine 500 mcg/ml $\dfrac{39,000 \text{ mcg/hr}}{500 \text{ mcg/ml}} = 78 \text{ ml/hr}$

Answer: The infusion rate for dobutamine 650 mcg/min is 78 ml/hr.

How many milliliters of dobutamine should be infused in 1 minute?
Find volume per minute:

Method: ml/min

Divide concentration/minute by concentration of solution.	$\dfrac{650 \text{ mcg/min}}{500 \text{ mcg/ml}} = 1.3 \text{ ml/min}$

Answer: The infusion rate for dobutamine is 1.3 ml/min.

PRACTICE PROBLEMS **11** **Calculating Infusion Rate**

Answers can be found on page 279.

Use the examples to find the following information:

- Concentration of the solution

- Infusion rates per unit time:

  a. Volume per minute

  b. Volume per hour

  c. Concentration per minute

  d. Concentration per hour

1. Order: heparin 1000 U in D_5W 500 ml at 50 ml/hr.

_____

2. Order: nitroprusside 100 mg in D_5W 500 ml at 60 ml/hr.

_____

3. Order: nitroprusside 25 mg in D_5W 250 ml at 50 mcg/min.

_____

4. Order: dopamine 800 mg in D_5W 500 ml at 400 mcg/min.

_____

5. Order: norepinephrine 2 mg in D_5W 250 ml at 45 ml/hr.

_____

6. Order: dobutamine 1000 mg in D_5W 500 ml at 12 ml/hr.

_____

7. Order: dobutamine 250 mg in D_5W 250 ml at 10 ml/hr.

_____

8. Order: lidocaine 2 g in D_5W 500 ml at 4 mg/min.

_____

9. Order: dopamine 400 mg in D_5W 250 ml at 60 ml/hr.

_____

10. Order: isoproterenol 4 mg in D_5W 500 ml at 65 ml/hr.

_____

11. Order: morphine sulfate 50 mg in 150 ml NSS at 3 mg/hr.

_____

12. Order: regular Humulin insulin 50 U in 250 ml NSS at 4 U/hr.

_____

13. Order: aminophylline 2 g in 250 ml D$_5$W at 20 ml/hr.

_____

14. Order: nitroglycerin 50 mg in 250 ml D$_5$W at 24 ml/hr.

_____

15. Order: heparin 25,000 U in 500 ml D$_5$W at 10 ml/hr.

_____

16. Order: amiodarone 900 mg in D$_5$W 500 ml at 33.3 ml/hr.

_____

17. Order: procainamide 1 g in D$_5$W 250 ml at 4 mg/min.

_____

18. Order: diltiazem 100 mg in 100 ml NSS at 10 mg/hr.

_____

19. Order: streptokinase 750,000 U in 250 ml NSS at 100,000 U/hr.

_____

20. Order: bretylium 1 g in 250 ml D$_5$W at 1 mg/min.

_____

CALCULATING INFUSION RATES OF A DRUG FOR SPECIFIC BODY WEIGHT PER UNIT TIME

The last method is calculating infusion rates for the amount of drug per unit time for a specific body weight. The weight parameter is an accurate means of dosing for a therapeutic effect. The metric system is used for all drug dosing, so pounds must be changed to kilograms. The physician orders the _desired dose per kilogram of body weight_ and the _concentration of the solution_. From this information, infusion rates can be calculated for administering an individualized dose. Accurate daily weights are essential for the correct dosage.

The previous methods for calculating _concentration of solution_ and _infusion rates_ for concentration and volume are used, with one addition. The _concentration per minute_ is obtained by multiplying the _body weight_ by the _desired dose per kilogram per minute,_ which must be done before the other infusion rates can be calculated. For many vasoactive drugs given as examples in this chapter, the most useful information clinically is the concentration per minute for the specific body weight, volume per minute, and volume per hour, because these parameters determine the infusion pump settings.

New volumetric infusion pumps now can deliver fractional portions of a milliliter from tenths to hundredths in addition to calculating dosages for infusion rates. If the infusion pumps available do not have this feature and the volume per hour is a fractional amount, it must be rounded off to a whole number (1.8 ml/hr = 2 ml/hr). When calculating concentration per minute and hour and volume per minute, carry out the problem to three decimal places, if necessary, before rounding off. The volume per hour, if fractional, can then be rounded off, making the volume per hour as accurate as possible. There are two exceptions to rounding off fractional infusion rates:

1. If the client's condition is labile, the difference between 1 or 2 ml could be important.
2. Because physicians order the medication, they must be consulted if rounding off would significantly change the drug dosage.

Micrograms per Kilogram Body Weight

EXAMPLES

PROBLEM: Infuse dobutamine 250 mg in 500 ml D$_5$W at 10 mcg/kg/min. Patient weighs 143 lb. Concentration of solution is 500 mcg/ml. How many micrograms of dobutamine would be infused per minute? Per hour?

Convert pounds to kilograms:

Divide pounds by 2.2.	$\dfrac{143 \text{ lb}}{2.2 \text{ lb/kg}} = \text{kg}$

Find concentration per minute:

Method: mcg/min

Multiply client's weight by the desired dose of mcg/kg/min.	65 kg × 10 mcg/kg/min = 650 mcg/min

Find concentration per hour:

Method: mcg/hr

Multiply concentration/min by 60 min/hr.	650 mcg/min × 60 min/hr = 39,000 mcg/hr

Answer: The concentration of dobutamine infused per minute and per hour is 650 mcg/min and 39,000 mcg/hr for the patient's body weight.

How many milliliters of dobutamine will be infused per minute? Per hour? Find volume per minute:

Method: ml/min

Divide the concentration/minute by the concentration of the solution.	$\dfrac{650 \text{ mcg/min}}{500 \text{ mcg/ml}} = 1.241 \text{ ml/min}$

Find volume per hour:

Method: ml/hr

Multiply volume/minute by 60 min/hr.	1.241 ml/min $\times$ 60 min/hr = 74.46 or 74 ml/hr

Answer: The volume of dobutamine infused per minute is 1.241 ml/min, and the infusion rate is 74 ml/hr.

BASIC FRACTIONAL FORMULA

A fractional equation can create a basic formula that can be used as another quick method to determine any one of the following quantities: concentration of solution, volume per hour, and desired concentration per minute ($\times$ kilogram of body weight, if required). The equation has one constant, the drop rate of the IV set, 60 gtt/ml. The unknown quantity can be represented by X. (See Chapter 3 for fractional equations.) The basic formula is not accurate to the nearest hundredth, as are the other methods in this section:

$$\frac{\text{Concentration of solution (U, mg, mcg/ml)}}{\text{Drop rate of set (60 gtt/ml)}} = $$

$$\frac{\text{Desired concentration/min} \times \text{kg body weight}}{\text{Volume/hr (ml/hr or gtt/min)}}$$

Using Basic Formula to Find Volume per Hour or Drops per Minute

EXAMPLE   PROBLEM: Infuse heparin 5000 U in 250 ml D$_5$W at 0.15 U/kg/min.

Client weighs 70 kg. The concentration of solution is 20 U/ml.

Desired concentration/minute: 0.15 U/kg/min $\times$ 70 kg = 10.5 U/min

$$\frac{20 \text{ U/ml}}{60 \text{ gtt/ml}} = \frac{10.5 \text{ U/min}}{\text{X (ml/hr or gtt/min)}}$$
$$20 \text{ X} = 630$$
$$\text{X} = 31 \text{ ml/hr or 31 gtt/min}$$

Using Basic Formula to Find Desired Concentration per Minute

EXAMPLE   PROBLEM: Infuse lidocaine 2 g in 500 ml D$_5$W at 30 ml/hr. The concentration of the solution is 4 mg/ml.

$$\frac{4 \text{ mg/ml}}{60 \text{ gtt/ml}} = \frac{\text{X}}{30 \text{ ml/hr}}$$
$$60 \text{ X} = 120$$
$$\text{X} = 2 \text{ mg/min}$$

Using Basic Formula to Find Concentration of Solution

EXAMPLE

PROBLEM: Infuse dobutamine 250 mg in D_5W 500 ml at 10 mcg/kg/min with rate of 74 ml/hr. Client weights 65 kg.

$$\text{Desired concentration per minute} = 10 \text{ mcg/kg/min} \times 65 \text{ kg}$$
$$= 650 \text{ mcg/min}$$
$$\frac{X}{60 \text{ gtt/ml}} = \frac{650 \text{ mcg/min}}{74 \text{ ml/hr}}$$
$$74 X = 39,000$$
$$X = 527 \text{ mcg/ml}$$

PRACTICE
PROBLEMS III **Calculating Infusion Rate for Specific Body Weight**

Answers can be found on page 286.

Determine the infusion rates for specific body weight by calculating the following:

- Concentration of the solution

- Weight in kilograms

- Infusion rates:

  a. Concentration per minute

  b. Concentration per hour (not always measured)

  c. Volume per minute

  d. Volume per hour

  You can use the basic fractional formula and compare answers.

1. Infuse dobutamine 500 mg in 250 ml D_5W at 5 mcg/kg/min. Client weighs 182 lb.

_____

2. Infuse amrinone 250 mg in 250 ml NSS at 5 mcg/kg/min. Client weighs 165 lb.

_____

3. Infuse dopamine 400 mg in 250 ml D_5W at 10 mcg/kg/min. Client weighs 140 lb.

_____

4. Infuse nitroprusside 100 mg in 500 ml D_5W at 3 mcg/kg/min. Client weighs 55 kg.

_____

5. Infuse dobutamine 1000 mg in 500 ml D_5W at 15 mcg/kg/min. Client weighs 110 lb.

_____

6. Infuse propofol (Diprivan) 500 mg/50 ml infusion bottle at 10 mcg/kg/min. Client weighs 187 lb.

7. Infuse alfentanil (Alfenta) 10,000 mcg in D_5W 250 ml at 0.5 mcg/kg/min. Client weighs 175 lb.

8. Infuse milrinone (Primacor) 20 mg in D_5W 100 ml at 0.375 mcg/kg/min. Client weighs 160 lb.

9. Infuse theophylline 400 mg in D_5W 500 ml at 0.55 mg/kg/hr. Client weighs 70 kg.

10. Infuse esmolol 2.5 g in NSS 250 ml at 150 mcg/kg/min. Client weighs 148 lb.

 Additional practice problems for "Critical Care Medications" are available on the CD-ROM in the "Calculating Dosages" section.

TITRATION OF INFUSION RATE

Titration of drugs administered by infusion is based on (1) *concentration of solution,* (2) *infusion rates,* (3) *specific concentration per kilogram of body weight,* and (4) *titration factor.* The *titration factor* is the concentration of drug per drop in units (U/gtt), milligrams (mg/gtt), or micrograms (mcg/gtt or μg/gtt). For the programmable volumetric infusion pump, the titration factor is the increment of increase or decrease in units, micrograms, or milligrams. If the only IV equipment available has the ml/hr feature, the titration factor of concentration per drop can be used. Advanced volumetric infusion pumps can infuse medication volume in increments of 0.1 ml/hr. Other pump features include a drug-specific dose calculator that allows the nurse to select a drug name, input the dosage, the concentration of the drug, and the weight of the patient (Figure 11-1). These infusion pumps make drug delivery and titration safer and easier. Any dose changes can be easily reprogrammed by the drug-specific dose calculator. The safety features of the advanced infusion pumps decrease medication errors. Many drug manufacturers are recommending infusion pumps for the delivery of all vasoactive medications used in critical care.

Calculating the titration factor is necessary when the technology of the advanced infusion pumps is unavailable. The titration factor can be added to or subtracted from the baseline infusion rate to determine the exact concentration of an infusion. Because the titration method of drug administration is primarily used when a cient's condition is labile, calculating the titration factor gives the nurse the means of determining the exact amount of drug to be infused.

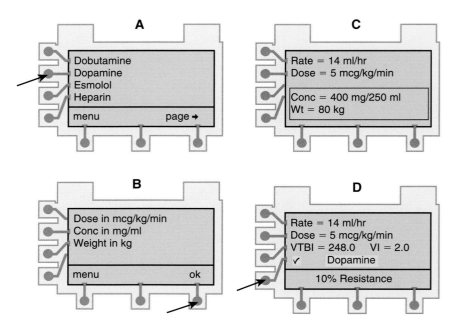

FIGURE 11-1 Example of a display screen of a dose rate calculator on an advanced infusion pump. Screen A selects drug. Screen B shows parameters. Screen C displays data input, and Screen D shows active data. (Modified from *Volumetric Infusion Pump Manual,* 1999, Alaris Medical Systems, San Diego, CA.)

Charts for drug infusion, developed by drug manufacturers, can be used to adjust infusion rates for drug titrations. Often, the amount of drug being infused falls between calibrations on the charts. When this occurs, the titration factor can be used to determine the exact concentration of drug being administered. The titration factor can also be used to verify the correct selection from the chart.

EXAMPLES

PROBLEM: Infuse Isuprel 2 mg in 250 ml D₅W. Titrate 1-3 mcg/min to maintain heart rate >50 beats/min and <130 beats/min and blood pressure >90 mm Hg systolic.

a. Find concentration of solution:

Convert mg to mcg. Set up ratio and proportion.

$$2 \text{ mg} = 2000 \text{ mcg}$$
$$2000 \text{ mcg} : 250 \text{ ml} :: X \text{ mcg} : \text{ml}$$
$$250 \text{ X} = 2000$$
$$X = 8 \text{ mcg}$$
$$8 \text{ mcg/ml}$$

b. Infusion rate by volume per unit time:
Desired infusion rate by concentration is stated in the problem.
Note that the upper dosage and lower dosage must be determined.

REMEMBER   Hourly rate and the number of drops per minute are the same with a microdrip administration set.

Find volume rate per minute: ml/min:

Divide concentration/ minute by concentration of solution.	Lower	Upper
	$\dfrac{1 \text{ mcg/min}}{8 \text{ mcg/ml}}$	$\dfrac{3 \text{ mcg/min}}{8 \text{ mcg/ml}}$
	= 0.125 ml/min	= 0.375 ml/min

Find volume rate per hour: ml/hr (equivalent to gtt/min):

Multiply volume rate/minute by 60 min.	*Lower*
	0.125 ml/min × 60 min/hr
	= 7.5 ml/hr (7.5 gtt/min)
	Upper
	0.375 ml/hr × 60 min/hr
	= 22.5 ml/hr (22.5 gtt/min)

c. Determine the titration factor:

Find rate in gtt/min. Divide concentration/minute by gtt/min.	7.5 gtt/min
	$\dfrac{1 \text{ mcg/min}}{7.5 \text{ gtt/min}} = 0.133 \text{ mcg/gtt}$

The *titration factor* is 0.133 mcg/gtt in a solution of Isuprel 2 mg in 250 ml D₅W. In other words, changing drops per minute results in a corresponding change in milliliters per hour. If the baseline infusion rates are **1 mcg/min** for concentration and **7.5 ml/hr** for volume, increasing the infusion rate by **1 gtt/min** changes the concentration/minute by **0.133 mcg** and increases the hourly volume by **1 ml** to give a rate of **8.5 ml/hr.**

    d. Increasing or decreasing infusion rates.
       To increase the infusion rate by 5 gtt/min from a baseline rate of 1 mcg/min, set up a ratio and proportion or multiply the titration factor (mcg/gtt) by 5 to obtain the increment of increase.

EXAMPLES

Set up a ratio and proportion with rate in gtt/min as the known variable.	7.5 gtt : 1 mcg ∷ 5 gtt : X mcg
	7.5 X = 5
	X = 0.666 mcg
	5 gtt/0.66 mcg

or

Multiply titration factor in mcg/gtt by 5.	0.133 mcg/gtt × 5 gtt = 0.665 mcg

Adding 5 gtt/min increases the volume infusion rate by 5 ml/hr, from 7.5 to 12.5 ml/hr. The concentration of drug delivered is increased by 0.665 mcg/min to 1.665 mcg/min. For example,

$$
\begin{array}{ll}
1.000 \text{ mcg/min} & \text{baseline rate} \\
\underline{+ \ 0.665} \text{ mcg/min} & \text{increment of rate increased} \\
1.665 \text{ mcg/min} & \text{adjusted infusion rate}
\end{array}
$$

Suppose the infusion rate was 3 mcg/min and a decrease was needed. To decrease the infusion rate by 10 gtt, set up another ratio and proportion or multiply the titration factor (mcg/gtt) by 10.

EXAMPLES

| Set up a ratio and proportion with rate in gtt/mcg as the known variable. | 7.5 gtt : 1 mcg :: 10 gtt : X mcg
7.5 X = 10
X = 1.33 mcg
1.33 mcg/10 gtt |

or

| Multiply titration factor in mcg/gtt by 10. | 0.133 mcg/gtt × 10 gtt = 1.33 mcg |

Subtracting 10 gtt/min decreases the infusion rate by 10 ml/hr, from 22.5 to 12.5 ml/hr. The amount of drug delivered is decreased by 1.33 mcg/min to 1.67 mcg/min. For example,

$$
\begin{array}{ll}
3.00 \text{ mcg/min} & \text{baseline infusion rate} \\
\underline{-1.33} \text{ mcg/min} & \text{increment of rate decreased} \\
1.67 \text{ mcg/min} & \text{adjusted infusion rate}
\end{array}
$$

PRACTICE PROBLEMS IV Titration of Infusion Rate

Answers can be found on page 290.

1. What are the units of measure for the following terms?

   a. Concentration of solution per minute for specific body weight

   _____

   b. Concentration of solution

   _____

   c. Volume per hour

   _____

   d. Concentration per minute

   _____

   e. Volume per minute

   _____

   f. Concentration per minute

   _____

2. Order: nitroprusside 50 mg in 250 ml D$_5$W. Titrate 0.5 to 1.5 mcg/kg/min to maintain mean systolic blood pressure at 100 mm Hg. Client weighs 70 kg.

   Find the following:

   a. Concentration of solution

   _____

   b. Concentraton per minute

   _____

   c. Volume per minute and hour

   _____

   d. Titration factor

   _____

   e. Increase the infusion rate of 11 gtt/min by 5 gtt. What is the concentration per minute? What is the volume per hour?

   _____

   f. Increase the infusion rate of 16 gtt/ml by 13 gtt. What is the concentration per minute? What is the volume per hour?

   _____

3. Order: dopamine 400 mg in 250 ml D$_5$W. Titrate beginning at 4 mcg/kg/min to maintain a mean systolic blood pressure of 100 to 120 mm Hg. Client weighs 75 kg.

   Find the following:

   a. Concentration of solution

   _____

   b. Concentration per minute

   _____

   c. Volume per minute and hour

   _____

   d. Titration factor

   _____

   e. Increase the infusion rate of 113 gtt/min by 7 gtt. What is the concentration per minute? What is the volume per hour?

   _____

   f. Decrease the infusion rate of 120 ml/hr (120 gtt/min) by 5 gtt. What is the concentration per minute? What is the volume per hour?

   _____

Additional problems for "Titrating Medications" are available on the CD-ROM in the "Calculating Dosages" section.

TOTAL AMOUNT OF DRUG INFUSED OVER TIME

Determining the total amount of drug infused over time is useful when changes in drug therapy occur. If adverse effects, toxic levels, therapeutic failure, or discontinuance of a drug occurs, knowing the amount that was administered can be important for charting and for determining future therapies.

For this calculation, the concentration of the drug in solution must be known, as must the time that drug therapy began to the nearest minute. Again, with 60-gtt sets, the hourly rate is the same as the drip rate per minute.

EXAMPLES

PROBLEM: Heparin 10,000 U in 250 ml D₅W at 30 ml/hr has been infusing for 3 hours. The drug is discontinued.

How much heparin did the client receive?

Find concentration of solution:

Set up a ratio and proportion. Solve for X.	10,000 U : 250 ml :: X U : ml 250 X = 10,000 X = 40 U 40 U/ml

Find concentration per hour:

Multiply concentration of solution by volume/hour.	40 U/ml × 30 ml/hr = 1200 U/hr

Calculate total amount of drug infused:

Multiply concentration/hour by length of administration.	1200 U/hr × 3 hr = 3600 U/hr

Answer: The total amount of heparin infused over 3 hours was 3600 U.

PRACTICE PROBLEMS ▽ Total Amount of Drug Infused Over Time

Answers can be found on page 291.

Solve for the amount of drug infused over time.

1. In 1 hour, a client received two boluses of lidocaine 100 mg and an IV infusion of 4 mg/ml at 40 ml/hr for 30 minutes. How many milligrams have been infused?

   Note: Do not exceed 300 mg/hr of lidocaine.

2. Heparin 20,000 U in 500 ml D₅W at 50 ml/hr has been infused for 5½ hours. The drug is discontinued. How much heparin has been given?

ANSWERS

I   Calculating Concentration of a Solution

1. 10,000 U:250 ml :: X U:ml

250 X = 10,000

X = 40 U

The concentration of solution is 40 U/ml.

2. 250 mg:500 ml :: X mg: ml

500 X = 250

X = 0.5 mg

The concentration of solution is 0.5 mg/ml.

3. 100 U:500 ml :: X U:ml

500 X = 100

X = 0.2 U

The concentration of solution is 0.2 U/ml.

4.   1 g = 1000 mg

1000 mg:1000 ml :: X mg:ml

1000 X = 1000

X = 1 mg

The concentration of solution is 1 mg/ml.

5.   4 mg = 4000 mcg

4000 mcg:500 ml :: X mcg:ml

500 X = 4000

X = 8 mcg

The concentration of solution is 8 mcg/ml.

6. 500 mg:250 ml :: X mcg:ml

250 X = 500

X = 2 mg

The concentration of solution is 2 mg/ml.

7. 400 mg:250 ml :: X mg:ml

250 X = 400

X = 1.6 mg

The concentration of solution is 1.6 mg/ml.

8.   2 mg = 2000 mcg

2000 mcg:250 ml :: X mcg:ml

250 X = 2000

X = 8 mcg

The concentration of solution is 8 mcg/ml.

9. 750,000 U:50 ml :: X U:ml

50 X = 750,000

X = 15,000 U

The concentration of solution is 15,000 U/ml.

10.   50 mg = 50,000 mcg
      50,000 mcg:500 ml :: X mcg:ml
              500 X = 50,000
              X = 100 mcg
The concentration of solution is 100 mcg/ml.

11.   1 g = 1000 mg
      1000 mg:250 ml :: X mg:ml
              250 X = 1000
              X = 4 mg
The concentration of solution is 4 mg/ml.

12.   2 g = 2000 mg
      2000 mg:250 ml :: X mg:ml
              250 X = 2000
              X = 8 mg
The concentration of solution is 8 mg/ml.

13. 25,000 U:250 ml :: X mg:ml
              250 X = 25,000
              X = 100 U
The concentration of solution is 100 U/ml.

14.   1 g = 1000 mg
      1000 mg:500 ml :: X mg:ml
              500 X = 1000
              X = 2 mg
The concentration of solution is 2 mg/ml.

15.   50 mg = 50,000 mcg
      50,000 mcg:250 ml :: X mcg:ml
              250 X = 50,000 mcg
              X = 200 mcg
The concentration of solution is 200 mcg/ml.

16. 100 mg:100 ml :: X mg:ml
              100 X = 100
              X = 1 mg/ml
The concentration of solution is 1 mg/ml.

17. 800 mg:500 ml :: X mg:ml
              500 X = 800
              X = 1.6 mg/ml
The concentration of solution is 1.6 mg/ml.

18. 20 mg:100 ml :: X mg:ml
              100 X = 20
              X = .2 mg/ml
The concentration of solution is 0.2 mg/ml.

19. 1,500,000 U:100 ml :: X mg:ml
              100 X = 1,500,000
              X = 15,000 U/ml
The concentration of solution is 15,000 U/ml.

20. 150 mg:100 ml :: X mg:ml
$$100 X = 150$$
$$X = 1.5 \text{ mg/ml}$$
The concentration of solution is 1.5 mg/ml.

II Calculating Infusion Rate

1. *Concentration of solution:*
1000 U:500 ml = X U:ml
$$500 X = 1000$$
$$X = 2 \text{ U}$$
The concentration of solution is 2 U/ml.
Infusion rates:
a. Volume/min:
50 ml:60 min :: X ml:min
$$60 X = 50$$
$$X = 0.833 \text{ ml or } 0.83 \text{ ml}$$
$$0.83 \text{ ml/min}$$
b. Volume/hr:
50 ml/hr
c. Concentration/min:
2 U/ml × 0.83 ml/min = 1.66 U/min
d. Concentration/hr:
1.66 U/min × 60 min/hr = 99.6 U/hr or 100 U/hr
2. *Concentration of solution.*
100 mg:500 ml :: X mg:ml
$$500 X = 100$$
$$X = 0.2 \text{ mg}$$
The concentration of solution is 0.2 mg/ml.
Infusion rates:
a. Volume/min:
60 ml:60 min :: X ml:min
$$60 X = 60$$
$$X = 1 \text{ ml}$$
$$1 \text{ ml/min}$$
b. Volume/hr:
60 ml/hr
c. Concentration/min:
0.2 mg/ml × 1 ml/min = 0.2 mg/min
d. Concentration/hr:
0.2 mg/min × 60 min/hr = 12 mg/hr
3. *Concentration of solution:*
25 mg = 25,000 mcg
25,000 mcg:250 ml :: X mcg:ml
$$250 X = 25,000$$
$$X = 100 \text{ mcg}$$
The concentration of solution is 100 mcg/ml.

Infusion rates:

a. Volume/min:
$$\frac{50 \text{ mcg/min}}{100 \text{ mcg/ml}} = 0.5 \text{ ml/min}$$

b. Volume/hr:

0.5 ml/min × 60 min/hr = 30 ml/hr

c. Concentration/min:

50 mcg/min

d. Concentration/hr:

50 mcg/min × 60 min/hr = 3000 mcg/hr

4. *Concentration of solution:*

800 mg = 800,000 mcg

800,000 mcg : 500 ml :: X mcg : ml

500 X = 800,000

X = 1600 mcg

The concentration of solution is 1600 mcg/ml.

Infusion rates:

a. Volume/min:
$$\frac{400 \text{ mcg/min}}{1600 \text{ mcg/ml}} = 0.25 \text{ ml/min}$$

b. Volume/hr:

0.25 ml/min × 60 min/hr = 15 ml/hr

c. Concentration/min:

400 mcg/min

d. Concentration/hr:

400 mcg/min × 60 min/hr = 24,000 mcg/hr

5. *Concentration of solution:*

2 mg = 2000 mcg

2000 mcg : 250 ml :: X mcg : ml

250 X = 2000

X = 8 mcg

The concentration of solution is 8 mcg/ml.

Infusion rates:

a. Volume/min:

45 ml : 60 min :: X ml : min

60 X = 45

X = 0.75 ml/min

b. Volume/hr:

45 ml/hr

c. Concentration/min:

8 mcg/ml × 0.75 ml/min = 6 mcg/min

d. Concentration/hr:

6 mcg/min × 60 min/hr = 360 mcg/hr

6. *Concentration of solution:*

$$1000 \text{ mg} = 1{,}000{,}000 \text{ mcg}$$
$$1{,}000{,}000 \text{ mcg} : 500 \text{ ml} :: X \text{ mcg} : \text{ml}$$
$$500 \text{ X} = 1{,}000{,}000$$
$$X = 2000 \text{ mcg}$$

The concentration of solution is 2000 mcg/ml.

Infusion rates:

a. Volume/min:

$$12 \text{ ml} : 60 \text{ min} :: X \text{ ml} : \text{min}$$
$$60 \text{ X} = 12$$
$$X = 0.2 \text{ ml}$$
$$0.2 \text{ ml/min}$$

b. Volume/hr:

12 ml/hr

c. Concentration/min:

$$2000 \text{ mcg/ml} \times 0.2 \text{ ml/min} = 400 \text{ mcg/min}$$

d. Concentration/hr:

$$400 \text{ mcg/min} \times 60 \text{ min/hr} = 24{,}000 \text{ mcg/hr}$$

7. *Concentration of solution:*

$$250 \text{ mg} = 250{,}000 \text{ mcg}$$
$$250{,}000 \text{ mcg} : 250 \text{ ml} :: X \text{ mcg} : \text{ml}$$
$$250 \text{ X} = 250{,}000$$
$$X = 1000 \text{ mcg}$$

The concentration of solution is 1000 mcg/ml.

Infusion rates:

a. Volume/min:

$$60 \text{ ml} : 60 \text{ min} :: X \text{ ml} : 1 \text{ min}$$
$$60 \text{ X} = 10 \text{ ml}$$
$$X = 0.1666 \text{ ml or } 0.167 \text{ ml}$$
$$0.167 \text{ ml/min}$$

b. Volume/hr:

10 ml/hr

c. Concentration/min:

$$1000 \text{ mcg/ml} \times 0.167 \text{ ml/min} = 167 \text{ mcg/min}$$

d. Concentration/hr:

$$167 \text{ mcg/min} \times 60 \text{ min/hr} = 10{,}020 \text{ mcg/hr or } 10{,}000 \text{ mcg/hr}$$

8. *Concentration of solution:*

$$2 \text{ g} = 2000 \text{ mg}$$
$$2000 \text{ mg} : 500 \text{ ml} :: X \text{ mg} : \text{ml}$$
$$500 \text{ X} = 2000$$
$$X = 4 \text{ mg}$$

The concentration of solution is 4 mg/ml.

Infusion rates:
a. Volume/min:

$$\frac{4 \text{ mg/ml}}{4 \text{ mg/min}} = 1 \text{ ml/min}$$

b. Volume/hr:
1 ml/min × 60 min/hr = 60 ml/hr
c. Concentration/min:
4 mg/min
d. Concentration/hr:
4 mg/min × 60 min/hr = 240 mg/hr

9. *Concentration of solution:*

400 mg : 250 ml :: X mg : ml
$$250 \text{ X} = 400$$
$$\text{X} = 1.6 \text{ mg}$$

The concentration of solution is 1.6 mg/ml.
Infusion rates:
a. Volume/min:

60 ml : 60 min :: X ml : min
$$60 \text{ X} = 60$$
$$\text{X} = 1 \text{ ml}$$
1 ml/min

b. Volume/hr:
60 ml/hr
c. Concentration/min:
1.6 mg/ml × 1 ml/min = 1.6 mg/min
d. Concentration/hr:
1.6 mg/min × 60 min/hr = 96 mg/hr

10. *Concentration of solution:*

4 mg = 4000 mcg
4000 mcg : 500 ml :: X mcg : ml
$$500 \text{ X} = 4000$$
$$\text{X} = 8 \text{ mcg}$$

The concentration of solution is 8 mcg/ml.
Infusion rates:
a. Volume/min:

65 ml : 60 min :: X ml : min
$$60 \text{ X} = 65$$
$$\text{X} = 1.083 \text{ ml}$$
1.08 ml/min

b. Volume/hr:
65 ml/hr
c. Concentration/min:
8 mcg/ml × 1.08 ml/min = 8.64 mcg/min
d. Concentration/hr:
8.64 mcg/min × 60 min/hr = 518.4 mcg/hr

11. *Concentration of solution:*

50 mg : 150 ml :: X mg : ml

150 X = 50

X = 0.33 mg

The concentration of solution is 0.33 mg/ml.

Infusion rates:

a. Concentration/min:

3 mg : 60 min :: X mg : min

60 X = 3

X = 0.05 mg/min

b. Concentration/hr:

3 mg/hr

c. Volume/min:

$$\frac{0.05 \text{ mg/min}}{0.33 \text{ mg/ml}} = 0.15 \text{ ml/min}$$

d. Volume/hr:

$$\frac{3 \text{ mg/hr}}{0.33 \text{ mg/ml}} = 9.09 \text{ or } 9 \text{ ml/hr}$$

12. *Concentration of solution:*

50 U : 250 ml :: X mg : ml

250 X = 50

X = 0.2 U

The concentration of solution is 0.2 U/ml.

Infusion rates:

a. Concentration/min:

4 U : 60 min :: X U : min

60 X = 4

X = 0.066 U/min

b. Concentration/hr:

4 U/hr

c. Volume/min:

$$\frac{0.66 \text{ U/min}}{0.2 \text{ U/ml}} = 0.33 \text{ ml/min}$$

d. Volume/hr:

$$\frac{4 \text{ U/hr}}{0.2 \text{ U/ml}} = 20 \text{ ml/hr}$$

13. *Concentration of solution:*

2 g = 2000 mg

2000 mg : 250 ml :: X mg : ml

250 X = 2000

X = 8 mg

The concentration of solution is 8 mg/ml.

Infusion rates:

a. Volume/hr = 20 ml/hr

b. Volume/min:

20 ml:60 min/hr :: X ml:min

60 X = 20

X = 0.3 ml/min

c. Concentration/min:

8 mg/ml × 0.3 ml/min = 2.4 mg/min

d. Concentration/hr:

2.4 mg/min × 60 min/hr = 360 mg/hr

14. *Concentration of solution:*

50 mg = 50,000 mcg

50,000 mcg:250 ml :: X mg:ml

250 X = 50,000

X = 200 mcg

The concentration of solution is 200 mcg/ml.

Infusion rates:

a. Volume/hr = 24 ml/hr

b. Volume/min:

24 ml/hr:60 min/hr :: X ml:min

60 X = 24

X = 0.4 ml/min

c. Concentration/min:

200 mcg/ml × 0.4 ml/min = 80 mcg/min

d. Concentration/hr:

80 mcg/min × 60 min = 4800 mcg/hr

15. *Concentration of solution:*

25,000 U:500 ml :: X U:ml

500 X = 25,000

X = 50 U

The concentration of solution is 50 U/ml.

Infusion rates:

a. Volume/hr:

10 ml/hr

b. Volume/min:

10 ml:60 min/hr :: X ml:min

60 X = 10

X = 0.165 ml/min

c. Concentration/hr:

50 U/ml × 10 ml/hr = 500 U/hr

d. Concentration/min:

50 U/ml × 0.165 ml/min = 8.25 U/min

16. *Concentration of solution:*

900 mg:500 ml :: X mg:ml

500 X = 900

X = 1.8 mg/ml

The concentration of solution is 1.8 mg/ml.

Infusion rates:
  a. Volume/hr:
     33.3 ml/hr
  b. Volume/min:
     33.3 ml:60 min ∷ X ml:min
            60 X = 33.3
                X = 0.55 ml/min
  c. Concentration/hr:
     1.8 mg/ml × 60 min/hr = 108 mg/hr
  d. Concentration/min:
     1.8 mg/ml × 0.55 ml/min = 0.99 mg/ml
17. *Concentration of solution:*
            1 g = 1000 mg
     1000 mg:250 ml ∷ X mg:ml
            250 X = 1000
                X = 4 mg/ml
The concentration of solution is 4 mg/ml.
Infusion rates:
  a. Volume/min:
     $\dfrac{4 \text{ mg/min}}{4 \text{ mg/ml}}$ = 1 ml/min
  b. Volume/hr:
     1 ml/min × 60 min/hr = 60 ml/hr
  c. Concentration/hr:
     4 mg/min × 60 min/hr = 240 mg/hr
  d. Concentration/min:
     4 mg/min
18. *Concentration of solution:*
     100 mg:100 ml ∷ X mg:ml
            100 X = 100
                X = 1 mg/ml
The concentration of solution is 1 mg/ml.
Infusion rates:
  a. Volume/hr:
     $\dfrac{10 \text{ mg/hr}}{1 \text{ mg/ml}}$ = 10 ml/hr
  b. Volume/min:
     $\dfrac{10 \text{ ml/hr}}{60 \text{ min/hr}}$ = 0.166 ml/min
  c. Concentration/hr:
     10 mg/hr
  d. Concentration/min:
     1 mg/ml × 0.166 ml/min = 0.166 mg/min

19. *Concentration of solution:*

750,000 U:250 ml :: X U:ml

250 X = 750,000

X = 3000 U/ml

The concentration of solution is 3000 U/ml.

Infusion rates:

a. Volume/hr:

$$\frac{100,000 \text{ U/hr}}{3000 \text{ U/ml}} = 33.3 \text{ ml/hr}$$

b. Volume/min:

$$\frac{33.3 \text{ ml/hr}}{60 \text{ min/hr}} = 0.55 \text{ ml/min}$$

c. Concentration/hr:

100,000 U/hr

d. Concentration/min:

$$\frac{100,000 \text{ U/hr}}{60 \text{ min/hr}} = 166.6 \text{ U/min}$$

20. *Concentration of solution:*

1 g = 1000 mg

1000 mg:250 ml :: X mg:ml

250 X = 1000

X = 4 mg/ml

The concentration of solution is 4 mg/ml.

Infusion rates:

a. Volume/min:

$$\frac{1 \text{ mg/min}}{4 \text{ mg/ml}} = 0.25 \text{ ml/min}$$

b. Volume/hr:

0.25 ml/min × 60 min/hr = 15 ml/hr

c. Concentration/hr:

4 mg/ml × 15 ml/hr = 60 mg/hr

d. Concentration/min:

1 mg/min

III Calculating Infusion Rate for Specific Body Weight

1. *Concentration of solution:*

lb to kg

500 mg = 500,000 mcg $\quad \dfrac{182}{2.2} = 82.7$ kg

500,000:250 ml :: X mcg:ml

250 X = 500,000

X = 2000 mcg

The concentration of solution is 2000 mcg/ml.

Infusion rates:

a. Concentration/min:

Body weight × Desired dose/kg/min

82.7 kg × 5 mcg/kg/min

= 413.4 mcg/min

b. Concentration/hr:

413.5 mcg/min × 60 min/hr = 24,810 mcg/hr

c. Volume/min:

$$\frac{413.5 \text{ mcg/min}}{2000 \text{ mcg/ml}} = 0.206 \text{ ml/min}$$

d. Volume/hr:

0.206 ml/min × 60 min/hr = 12.36 or 12 ml/hr

2. *Concentration of solution:*

lb to kg

250 mg = 250,000 mcg $\dfrac{165}{2.2} = 75$ kg

250,000 mcg:250 ml :: X mcg:ml

250 X = 250,000

X = 1000 mcg

The concentration of solution is 1000 mcg/ml.

Infusion rates:

a. Concentration/min:

Body weight × Desired dose/kg/min

75 kg × 5 mcg/kg/min = 375 mcg/min

b. Concentration/hr:

375 mcg/min × 60 min/hr = 22,500 mcg/hr

c. Volume/min:

$$\frac{375 \text{ mcg/min}}{1000 \text{ mcg/ml}} = 0.375 \text{ ml/min}$$

d. Volume/hr:

0.375 ml/min × 60 min/hr = 22.5 ml/hr or 23 ml/hr

3. *Concentration of solution:*

lb to kg

400 mg = 400,000 mcg $\dfrac{140}{2.2} = 63.6$ kg

400,000 mg:250 ml :: X mg:ml

250 X = 400,000

X = 1600 mcg

The concentration of solution is 1600 mcg/ml.

Infusion rates:

a. Concentration/min:

Body weight × Desired dose/kg/min

63.6 kg × 10 mcg/kg/min

= 636 mcg/min

b. Concentration/hr:

636 mcg/min × 60 min/hr = 38,160 mcg/hr

c. Volume/min:

$$\frac{636 \text{ mcg/min}}{1600 \text{ mcg/ml}} = 0.39 \text{ ml/min}$$

d. Volume/hr:

0.39 ml/min × 60 min/hr = 23.4 ml/hr or 23 ml/hr

4. *Concentration of solution:*

Patient weight

$$100 \text{ mg} = 100,000 \text{ mcg} \quad 55 \text{ kg}$$
$$100,000 \text{ mcg} : 500 \text{ ml} :: X \text{ mg} : \text{ml}$$
$$500 X = 100,000$$
$$X = 200 \text{ mcg}$$

The concentration of solution is 200 mcg/ml.

Infusion rates:

a. Concentration/min:

3 mcg/kg/min $\times$ 55 kg = 165 mcg/min

b. Concentration/hr:

165 mcg/min $\times$ 60 min/hr = 9900 mcg/hr

c. Volume/min:

$$\frac{165 \text{ mcg/min}}{200 \text{ mcg/ml}} = 0.825 \text{ ml/min}$$

d. Volume/hr:

0.825 ml/min $\times$ 60 min/hr = 49.5 ml/hr or 50 ml/hr

5. *Concentration of solution:*

lb to kg

$$1000 \text{ mg} = 1,000,000 \text{ mcg} \quad \frac{110}{2.2} = 50 \text{ kg}$$
$$1,000,000 \text{ mcg} : 500 \text{ ml} :: X \text{ mcg} : \text{ml}$$
$$500 X = 1,000,000$$
$$X = 2000 \text{ mcg}$$

The concentration of solution is 2000 mcg/ml.

Infusion rates:

a. Concentration/min:

Body weight $\times$ Desired dose/kg/min

50 kg $\times$ 15 mcg/kg/min

= 750 mcg/min

b. Concentration/hr:

750 mcg/min $\times$ 60 min/hr = 45,000 mcg/hr

c. Volume/min:

$$\frac{750 \text{ mcg/min}}{2000 \text{ mcg/ml}} = 0.375 \text{ ml/min}$$

d. Volume/hr:

0.375 ml/min $\times$ 60 min/hr = 22.5 ml/hr or 23 ml/hr

6. *Concentration of solution:*

lb to kg

$$500 \text{ mg} : 50 \text{ ml} :: X \text{ mg} : \text{ml} \quad \frac{187}{2.2} = 85 \text{ kg}$$
$$50 X = 500$$
$$X = 10 \text{ mg/ml}$$

The concentration of solution is 10 mg/ml or 10,000 mcg/ml.

Infusion rates:

a. Concentration/min:

Body weight $\times$ Desired dose/kg/min

85 kg $\times$ 10 mcg/kg/min

= 850 mcg/min

b. Concentration/hr:

850 mcg/min × 60 min/hr = 51,000 mcg/hr or 51 mg/hr

c. Volume/min:

$$\frac{850 \text{ mcg/min}}{10,000 \text{ mcg/ml}} = 0.085 \text{ ml/min}$$

d. Volume/hr:

0.085 ml/min × 60 min/hr = 5.1 ml/hr

7. *Concentration of solution:*

lb to kg

10,000 mcg:250 ml :: X mcg:ml $\frac{175}{2.2} = 79.5$ kg

250 X = 10,000

X = 40 mcg/ml

Infusion rates:

a. Concentration/min:

Body weight × Desired dose/kg/min

79.5 kg × 0.5 mcg/kg/min

= 39.75 mcg/min

b. Concentration/hr:

39.75 mcg/min × 60 min/hr = 2385 mcg/hr or 2.4 mg/hr

c. Volume/min:

$$\frac{39.75 \text{ mcg/min}}{40 \text{ mcg/ml}} = 0.99 \text{ ml/min or 1 ml/min}$$

d. Volume/hr:

0.99 ml/min × 60 min/hr = 59.6 ml/hr

8. *Concentration of solution:*

lb to kg

20 mg:100 ml :: X mg:ml $\frac{160}{2.2} = 72.70$ kg

100 X = 20

X = 0.2 mg/ml

or 200 mcg/ml

Infusion rates:

a. Concentration/min:

Body weight × Desired dose/kg/min

72.7 kg × 0.375 mcg/kg/min

= 27.2 mcg/min

b. Concentration/hr:

27.2 mcg/min × 60 min/hr = 1635 mcg/hr or 1.6 mg/hr

c. Volume/min:

$$\frac{27.2 \text{ mcg/min}}{200 \text{ mcg/ml}} = 0.136 \text{ ml/min}$$

d. Volume/hr:

0.136 ml/min × 60 min/hr = 8.16 ml/hr

9. *Concentration of solution:*

Client weight

400 mg:500 ml :: X mg:ml   70 kg

500 X = 400

X = 0.8 mg/ml

Infusion rates:

a. Concentration/hr:

Body weight × Desired dose/kg/min

70 kg × 0.55 mg/kg/min

= 38.5 mg/hr

b. Volume/hr:

$$\frac{38.5 \text{ mg/hr}}{0.8 \text{ mg/ml}} = 48.125 \text{ ml/hr}$$

10. *Concentration of solution:*

2500 mg : 250 ml :: X mg : ml

250 X = 2500

X = 10 mg/ml

lb to kg

$$\frac{148}{2.2} = 67.2 \text{ kg}$$

Infusion rates:

a. Concentration/min:

Body weight × Desired dose/kg/min

67.2 × 150 mcg/kg/min

= 10,080 mcg/min or 10 mg/min

b. Concentration/hr:

10 mg/min × 60 min/hr = 600 mg/hr

c. Volume/min:

$$\frac{10 \text{ mg/min}}{10 \text{ mg/ml}} = 1 \text{ ml/min}$$

d. Volume/hr:

1 ml/min × 60 min/hr = 60 ml

IV Titration of Infusion Rate

1. a. (U, mg, mcg)/kg/min

   b. (U, mg, mcg)/ml

   c. ml/hr

   d. (U, mg, mcg)/min

   e. ml/min

   f. (U, mg, mcg)/min

2. a. Concentration of solution:

50 mg = 50,000 mcg

50,000 mcg : 250 ml :: X mcg : 1 ml

250 X = 50,000

X = 200 mcg

The concentration of solution is 200 mcg/ml.

   b. Concentration/min:

Lower: 0.5 mcg/kg/min × 70 kg = 35 mcg/min

Upper: 1.5 mcg/kg/min × 70 kg = 105 mcg/min

   c. Volume/min and volume/hr:

Lower

$$\frac{35 \text{ mcg/min}}{200 \text{ mcg/ml}} = 0.175 \text{ ml/min} \times 60 \text{ min/hr} = 10.5 \text{ or } 11 \text{ ml/hr}$$

Upper

$$\frac{105 \text{ mcg/min}}{200 \text{ mcg/ml}} = 0.525 \text{ ml/min} \times 60 \text{ min/hr} = 31.5 \text{ or } 32 \text{ ml/hr}$$

  d. Titration factor:

11 ml/hr = 11 gtt/min $\dfrac{35 \text{ mcg/min}}{11 \text{ gtt/min}} = 3.18$ or 3 mcg/gtt

  e. Concentration/min and volume/hr:

5 gtt × 3 mcg/gtt = 15 mcg

15 mcg + 35 mcg/min = 50 mcg/min

5 gtt + 11 gtt/min = 16 gtt/min or 16 ml/hr

  f. Concentration/min and volume/hr:

13 gtt × 3 mcg/gtt = 39 mcg

39 mcg + 50 mcg = 89 mcg/min

13 gtt + 16 gtt = 29 gtt/ml or 29 ml/hr

3. a. Concentration of solution:

400 mg = 40,000 mcg

40,000 mcg:250 ml ∷ X mcg:1 ml

250 X = 40,000 mcg

X = 160 mcg

The concentration of solution is 160 mcg/ml.

  b. Concentration/min:

4 mcg/kg/min × 75 kg = 300 mcg/min

  c. Volume/min and volume/hr:

$$\frac{300 \text{ mcg/min}}{160 \text{ mcg/ml}} = 1.875 \text{ ml/min} \times 60 \text{ min/hr} = 112.5 \text{ or } 113 \text{ ml/hr}$$

  d. Titration factor:

113 ml/hr = 113 gtt/min

$$\frac{300 \text{ mcg/min}}{113 \text{ gtt/min}} = 2.65 \text{ or } 3 \text{ mcg/gtt}$$

  e. Concentration/min and volume/hr:

7 gtt × 3 mcg/gtt = 21 mcg

21 mcg + 300 mcg/min = 321 mcg/min

7 gtt + 113 gtt/min = 120 gtt/min or 120 ml/hr

  f. Concentration/min and volume/hr:

5 gtt × 3 mcg/gtt = 15 mcg

321 mcg/min − 15 mcg = 306 mcg/min

120 gtt/min − 5 gtt = 115 gtt/min or 115 ml/hr

V Total Amount of Drug Infused Over Time

1. Lidocaine bolus:

    100 mg

  +100 mg

    200 mg

Lidocaine IV infusion:

  a. Concentration of solution: given as 4 mg/ml in problem.

  b. Concentration/hr:
      4 mg/ml × 40 ml/hr = 160 mg/hr
  c. Concentration over ½ hour:

$$160 \text{ mg/hr} \times \frac{30 \text{ min}}{60 \text{ min/hr}} = 80 \text{ mg over 30 min}$$

  d. Amount of IV drug infused:
      Lidocaine per two boluses: 200 mg
      Lidocaine per IV infusion: +80 mg
      _____
                                   280 mg total amount infused over 1 hr

  Note: The infusion rate is close to exceeding the maximum therapeutic range, which is 200 to 300 mg/hr.

2. Concentration of solution:
   20,000 U : 500 ml :: X U : 1 ml
                 500 X = 20,000
                     X = 40 U

  a. The concentration of solution is 40 U/ml.
  b. Concentration/hr:
      40 U/ml × 50 ml/hr = 2000 U/hr
  c. Amount of IV drug infused over 5½ hours:

$$2000 \text{ U} \times \frac{30 \text{ min}}{60 \text{ min/hr}} = 1000 \text{ U over } \tfrac{1}{2} \text{ hr}$$

$$200 \text{ U} \times 5 \text{ hr} = 10,000 \text{ U/5 hr}$$

          10,000 U
         +1,000 U
         _____
          11,000 U over 5½ hr

Pediatric Critical Care

OBJECTIVES

- Recognize factors that contribute to errors in drug and fluid administration.
- Identify the steps in calculating dilution parameters.
- Determine the accuracy of the dilution parameters in a drug order.

OUTLINE

FACTORS INFLUENCING INTRAVENOUS ADMINISTRATION
CALCULATING ACCURACY OF DILUTION PARAMETERS

In delivery of emergency drugs with complex dilution calculations, it is important for the nurse to evaluate the accuracy of the physician's order and to ensure that a child does not receive excessive fluids. Many institutions are attempting to standardize the concentration of the solution for various pediatric intravenous (IV) dosages to decrease the occurrence of miscalculations.

As noted in Chapter 11, the concepts of concentration of the solution, infusion rates for concentration and volume, and concentration of a drug for specific body weight per unit time that are employed in adult critical care are also used to prepare pediatric doses.

FACTORS INFLUENCING INTRAVENOUS ADMINISTRATION

Excess fluid can be given when the fluid volume of the emergency drug is not considered in the 24-hour fluid intake. Long IV tubing can be another source of fluid excess and can cause errors in drug delivery. When the priming or filling volume of the IV tubing is not considered, the child may receive extra fluid, especially if medication is added to the primary IV set via a secondary IV set. IV medication may not reach the child if the IV infusion rate is low, such as 1 ml/hr, or if the IV tubing has not been primed or filled with the medication before infusion. Most pediatric departments are developing protocols for safe and consistent IV drug delivery.

CALCULATING ACCURACY OF DILUTION PARAMETERS

The nurse may find it necessary to calculate the dilution parameters of a drug order that specifies the concentration per kilogram per minute and the volume per hour infusion rate. The physician should determine all drug dose parameters, including concentration per kilogram per minute, volume per hour, and dilution parameters. The nurse should check the accuracy of the dilution parameters to ensure that the correct drug dosage is given. These methods are also used to prepare the pediatric dose. In many pediatric critical care areas, IV fluids for drug administration are limited to prevent fluid overload. If the physician changes the drug dosage, rather than increasing the volume (ml), the concentration of the solution will be changed.

EXAMPLES

PROBLEM 1: A 6-day-old infant, weight 3.5 kg, is in septic shock.
Order: dopamine 5 mcg/kg/min at 1 ml/hr and dilute as follows:
100 mg in 100 ml D$_5$½ NSS.
Dosage: 2-5 mcg/kg/min.
Drug available: dopamine 40 mg/ml.

The following steps are needed to determine whether dilution orders will result in the correct concentration of solution to deliver 5 mcg/kg/min at 1 ml/hr:

Step 1: Determine infusion rates for concentration per unit time.

1. Find the concentration per minute.

Infant weight × Concentration/kg/min =
3.5 kg × 5 mcg/kg/min = 17.5 mcg/min

2. Calculate the concentration per hour.

17.5 mcg/min × 60 min/hr = 1050 mcg/hr

Step 2: Determine concentration of solution.
Divide the concentration per hour by volume per hour.

$$\frac{1050\ mcg/hr}{1\ ml/hr} = 1050\ mcg/ml\ or\ 1\ mg/ml$$

Step 3: Determine the accuracy of the dilution order.
Find how much dopamine must be added to 100 ml.
Set up a ratio and proportion.

1 mg : 1 ml :: X : 100 ml
X = 100 mg

Dilution order is correct.

Preparation of Drug Dosage

$$\frac{D}{H} \times V = \frac{100}{40} \times 1 = 2.5\ ml \quad \textbf{or} \quad H : V :: D : V$$
$$40\ mg : 1\ ml :: 100\ mg : X\ ml$$
$$40\ X = 100$$
$$X = 2.5\ ml$$

Answer: Add 2.5 ml of dopamine 40 mg/ml to 100 ml D$_5$½ NSS.

PROBLEM 2: A 3-week-old infant, weight 1.6 kg, is in septic shock.
Order: dobutamine 2.5 mcg/kg/min by a syringe pump with a 35-ml syringe at 1 ml/hr.
Dilution: dobutamine 8.4 mg with D$_5$¼ NSS to equal 35 ml.
Dosage: 2.5-40 mcg/kg/min.
Drug available: dobutamine 250 mg/20 ml.
Determine accuracy of dilution order to deliver 2.5 mcg/kg/min at 1 ml/hr.

Step 1: Find the infusion rates for concentration per unit time.

1. Determine the concentration per minute.

Infant weight × Concentration/kg/min =
1.6 kg × 2.5 mcg/kg/min = 4 mcg/min

2. Determine the concentration per hour.

4 mcg/min × 60 min/hr = 240 mcg/hr

Step 2: Determine the concentration of solution.
Divide the concentration per hour by volume per hour.

$$\frac{240\ mcg/hr}{1\ ml/hr} = 240\ mcg/ml$$

Step 3: Determine the accuracy of the dilution order.
Find how much dobutamine must be added to make 35 ml

$$240 \text{ mcg} : 1 \text{ ml} :: X \text{ mcg} : 35 \text{ ml}$$
$$X = 8400 \text{ mcg or } 8.4 \text{ mg}$$

Dilution order is correct.

Preparation of Drug Dosage

$$\frac{D}{H} \times V = \frac{8.4 \text{ mg}}{250 \text{ mg}} \times 20 \text{ ml} = 0.672 \text{ ml}$$

or

$$
\begin{array}{cccc}
H & : & V & D & : & V \\
\end{array}
$$
$$250 \text{ mg} : 20 \text{ ml} :: 8.4 \text{ mg} : X \text{ ml}$$
$$250 \text{ X} = 168$$
$$X = 0.67 \text{ ml}$$

Answer: Add 0.67 ml of dobutamine 250 mg/20 ml to 34.33 ml D$_5$¼ NSS.

PROBLEM 3: For the same infant, the physician increases the dose of dobutamine. Again, fluids must be limited, and another concentration must be prepared.
Order: dobutamine 15 mcg/kg/min by a syringe pump. Dilute 40.5 mg in 35 ml D$_5$¼ NSS and administer 1 ml/hr.
Determine the accuracy of dilution order to deliver 15 mcg/kg/min at 1 ml/hr.

Step 1: Determine the infusion rates for concentration per unit time.
    1. Find the concentration per minute.

$$
\begin{array}{cc}
\text{Infant weight} \times \text{Concentration/kg/min} = \\
1.6 \text{ kg} \quad \times \quad 15 \text{ mcg/kg/min} \quad = 24 \text{ mcg/min}
\end{array}
$$

    2. Find the concentration per hour.

$$24 \text{ mcg/min} \times 60 \text{ min/hr} = 1440 \text{ mcg/hr}$$

Step 2: Calculate the concentration of solution.
Divide the concentration per hour by volume per hour.

$$\frac{1440 \text{ mcg/hr}}{1 \text{ ml/hr}} = 1440 \text{ mcg/ml}$$

Step 3: Determine the accuracy of the dilution order.

$$1440 \text{ mcg} : 1 \text{ ml} :: X \text{ mcg} : 35 \text{ ml}$$
$$X = 50,400 \text{ mcg}$$
$$50,400 \text{ mcg} = 50.4 \text{ mg} \quad \text{or} \quad 50 \text{ mg}$$

Answer: The dilution order is *incorrect:* 50 mg of dobutamine is needed to deliver 15 mcg/kg/min.

SUMMARY PRACTICE PROBLEMS

Determine whether dilution orders will yield the correct concentration of solution. Answers are on page 298.

1. A 2-year-old child with acute status asthmaticus.
   Child weighs 10.5 kg.
   Order: aminophylline 110 mg in 500 ml of D₅W at 40 ml/hr.
   Pediatric dose: 0.85 mg/kg/hr.
   Drug available: aminophylline 250 mg/10 ml.

2. A 9-year-old child with supraventricular tachycardia.
   Child weighs 30 kg.
   Order: lidocaine 20 mcg/kg/min.
   Dilute: 300 mg in 250 ml of D₅W at 30 ml/hr.
   Pediatric dose: 20-40 mcg/kg/min.
   Drug available: lidocaine 1 g/25 ml.

3. A 1-year-old child with septic shock.
   Child weighs 9 kg.
   Order: dopamine 5 mcg/kg/min.
   Dilute: 100 mg in 200 ml of D₅¼ NSS at 6.75 ml/hr.
   Pediatric dose: 2-5 mcg/kg/min.
   Drug available: dopamine 400 mg/5 ml.

4. A 3-year-old child in shock.
   Child weighs 16 kg.
   Order: sodium nitroprusside 2 mcg/kg/min.
   Dilute: 25.25 mg in 250 ml of D₅W at 19 ml/hr.
   Pediatric dose: 200-500 mcg/kg/hr.
   Drug available: sodium nitroprusside 50 mg/5 ml.

5. A 10-year-old child with diabetic ketoacidosis.
   Child weighs 32 kg.
   Order: regular Humulin insulin 50 U in 500 ml of normal saline at 32 ml/hr.
   Pediatric dose: 0.1 U/kg/hr.
   Drug available: 100 U/ml.

6. A 2-day-old infant with patent ductus arteriosus.
   Child weighs 3.4 kg.
   Order: alprostadil 0.1 mcg/kg/min.
   Dilute: 1000 mcg in 50 ml D₅W by syringe pump at 1 ml/hr.
   Pediatric dosage: 0.05-0.1 mcg/kg/min.
   Drug available: alprostadil 500 mcg/ml.

7. A 7-year-old child with pulmonary embolism.
   Child weighs 20 kg.
   Order: Heparin 25 U/kg/hr.
   Dilute: 10,000 U heparin in 50 ml D₅W at 5 ml/hr.
   Pediatric dosage: 25-50 U/kg.
   Drug available: Heparin 10,000 U/ml.

ANSWERS SUMMARY PRACTICE PROBLEMS

1. *Step 1:* Infusion rates for concentration.
    Concentration per hour.

$$10.5 \text{ kg} \times 0.85 \text{ mg/kg/hr} = 8.9 \text{ mg/hr}$$

Step 2: Concentration of solution.

$$\frac{8.9 \text{ mg/hr}}{40 \text{ ml/hr}} = 0.22 \text{ mg/ml}$$

Step 3: Accuracy of dilution order.

$$\text{mg : ml :: mg : ml}$$
$$0.22 : 1 :: X : 500$$
$$X = 110 \text{ mg}$$

Dilution order is correct.

Preparation of drug dosage:

$$\frac{D}{H} \times V = \frac{110}{250} \times 10 = \frac{1100}{250} = 4.4 \text{ ml}$$

or

$$250 \text{ mg} : 10 \text{ ml} :: 110 \text{ mg } X \text{ ml}$$
$$250 X = 1100$$
$$X = 4.4 \text{ ml}$$

2. *Step 1:* Infusion rates for concentration/unit time.
    a. Concentration per minute.

$$30 \text{ kg} \times 20 \text{ mcg/kg/min} = 600 \text{ mcg/min}$$

   b. Concentration per hour.

$$600 \text{ mcg/min} \times 60 \text{ min/hr} = 36,000 \text{ mcg/hr}$$

Step 2: Concentration of solution.

$$\frac{36,000 \text{ mcg/hr}}{30 \text{ ml/hr}} = 1200 \text{ mcg/ml or } 1.2 \text{ mg/ml}$$

Step 3: Accuracy of dilution order.

$$1.2 \text{ mg} : 1 \text{ ml} :: X \text{ mg} : 250 \text{ ml}$$
$$X = 300 \text{ mg}$$

Dilution order is correct.

Preparation of drug dosage:

$$\frac{D}{H} \times V = \frac{300}{1000} \times 25 = \frac{7500}{1000} = 7.5 \text{ ml}$$

or

$$1000 \text{ mg} : 25 \text{ ml} :: 300 \text{ mg} : X \text{ ml}$$
$$1000 X = 7500$$
$$X = 7.5 \text{ ml}$$

Answer: 7.5 ml of lidocaine added to 250 ml.

3. *Step 1:* Infusion rate for concentration.

  a. Concentration per minute.

  $$9 \text{ kg} \times 5 \text{ mcg/kg/min} = 45 \text{ mcg/min}$$

  b. Concentration per hour.

  $$45 \text{ mcg/min} \times 60 \text{ min/hr} = 2700 \text{ mcg/hr}$$

Step 2: Concentration of solution.

$$\frac{2700 \text{ mcg/hr}}{6.75 \text{ ml/hr}} = 400 \text{ mcg/ml}$$

Step 3: Accuracy of dilution order.

$$400 \text{ mcg}:1 \text{ ml} :: X \text{ mcg}:200 \text{ ml}$$
$$X = 80,000 \text{ mcg or 80 mg in 200 ml}$$

Dilution order is incorrect.

4. *Step 1:* Infusion rates for concentration.

  a. Concentration per minute.

  $$16 \text{ kg} \times 2 \text{ mcg/kg/min} = 32 \text{ mcg/min}$$

  b. Concentration per hour.

  $$32 \text{ mcg/min} \times 60 \text{ min/hr} = 1920 \text{ mcg/hr}$$

Step 2: Concentration of solution.

$$\frac{1920 \text{ mcg/hr}}{19 \text{ ml/hr}} = 101 \text{ mcg/ml}$$

Step 3: Accuracy of order.

$$101 \text{ mcg}:1 \text{ ml} :: X \text{ mcg}:250 \text{ ml}$$
$$X = 25,250 \text{ mcg or 25.25 mg}$$

Dilution order is correct.

Preparation of drug dosage:

$$\frac{D}{H} \times V = \frac{25.25}{50} \times 5 = 2.52 \text{ ml}$$

or

$$50 \text{ mg}:5 \text{ ml} :: 25.25 \text{ mg}:X \text{ ml}$$
$$50 \text{ X} = 126.25$$
$$X = 2.52 \text{ ml}$$

Answer: 2.52 ml of sodium nitroprusside added to 250 ml.

5. *Step 1:* Infusion rate for concentration.

  Concentration per hour.

  $$32 \text{ kg} \times 0.1 \text{ U/kg/hr} = 3.2 \text{ U/hr}$$

Step 2: Concentration of solution.

$$\frac{3.2 \text{ U/hr}}{32 \text{ ml/hr}} = 0.10 \text{ U/ml}$$

Step 3: Accuracy of dilution order.

$$0.1 \text{ U}:1 \text{ ml} :: X \text{ U}:500 \text{ ml}$$
$$X = 50 \text{ U}$$

Dilution order is correct.

Preparation of drug dose:

$$\frac{D}{H} \times V = \frac{50 \text{ U}}{100 \text{ U}} \times 1 = 0.5 \text{ ml}$$

Answer: 50 U/0.5 ml—use a U 100 insulin syringe.

6. *Step 1:* Infusion rates for concentration.
     a. Concentration per minute.

$$3.4 \text{ kg} \times 0.1 \text{ mcg/kg/min} = 0.34 \text{ mcg/min}$$

     b. Concentration per hour.

$$0.34 \text{ mcg/min} \times 60 \text{ min/hr} = 20.4 \text{ mcg/hr}$$

Step 2: Concentration of solution.

$$\frac{20.4 \text{ mcg/hr}}{1 \text{ ml/hr}} = 20.4 \text{ mcg/ml or 20 mcg/ml}$$

Step 3: Accuracy of dilution order.

$$20 \text{ mcg} : 1 \text{ ml} :: X \text{ mcg} : 50 \text{ ml}$$
$$X = 1000 \text{ mcg}$$

Dilution order is correct.

7. *Step 1:* Infusion rates for concentration.
     Concentration per hour.

$$20 \text{ kg} \times 25 \text{ U/kg/hr} = 500 \text{ U/hr}$$

Step 2: Concentration of solution.

$$\frac{500 \text{ U/hr}}{5 \text{ ml/hr}} = 100 \text{ U/ml}$$

Step 3: Determine the accuracy of dilution order.

$$100 \text{ U} : 1 \text{ ml} :: X \text{ U} : 5 \text{ ml}$$
$$1X = 500$$
$$X = 500 \text{ U}$$

Accuracy of dilution order.

$$500 \text{ U} : \text{ml} :: X : 50 \text{ ml}$$
$$X = 25,000 \text{ U/ml}$$

Answer: The dilution order is incorrect. Heparin 10,000 U/ml must be diluted in 100 ml D_5W to deliver 25 U/kg/min.

Labor and Delivery

OBJECTIVES

- State the complication related to intravenous fluid administration in the high-risk mother.
- Recognize the different types of fluid administration used in cases of high-risk labor.
- Determine the infusion rates of a drug in solution when the drug is prescribed by concentration or volume.

OUTLINE

FACTORS INFLUENCING INTRAVENOUS FLUID AND DRUG MANAGEMENT

TITRATION OF MEDICATIONS WITH MAINTENANCE INTRAVENOUS FLUIDS
Administration by Concentration
Administration by Volume

INTRAVENOUS LOADING DOSE

INTRAVENOUS FLUID BOLUS

Drug calculations for labor and delivery are the same as those used in critical care. Determinations of the concentration of the solution, infusion rates, and titration factors are the primary calculation skills used. Accurate calculations are essential, as is the monitoring of intravenous (IV) fluid intake for medications and anesthetic procedures. Impaired renal filtration in patients with preeclampsia and the antidiuretic effect of tocolytic drugs make the monitoring of fluid intake vital. Accurate measurement of IV fluid intake along with pulmonary assessment can decrease the risk of fluid overload and the sequelae of acute pulmonary edema in women at high risk for complications.

Physicians' orders and hospital protocols give specific guidelines for administering IV drugs. The nurse is responsible for managing the IV drug therapy, monitoring the patient's fluid balance, and assessing the patient's response to drug therapy.

FACTORS INFLUENCING INTRAVENOUS FLUID AND DRUG MANAGEMENT

The most important concept in labor and delivery is that the drugs given to the mother also affect the unborn baby. Therefore the responses of both the mother and the unborn baby must be closely monitored. Vital signs, urine output, reflexes, and contraction patterns are the main indicators of the mother's status. For the fetus, fetal heart rate is the primary guide.

TITRATION OF MEDICATIONS WITH MAINTENANCE INTRAVENOUS FLUIDS

Women in labor receive IV fluids to prevent dehydration when oral intake is contraindicated. IV drugs are given to stimulate labor, treat preeclampsia, or inhibit preterm labor. Normally, 200 to 500 ml of IV fluids may be given to initially hydrate the mother, especially in preterm labor or before administration of regional anesthesia. Any IV medications that are given by titration are a part of the hourly IV rate. The client has a primary IV line and a secondary IV line for medications. All IV medications should be delivered by a volumetric pump, which ensures that the specified volume and correct dosage are delivered.

Titration of drugs is frequently done for women with preeclampsia and women experiencing preterm labor. The most common use of titration is in the induction or stimulation of labor. In the following example, an oxytocic drug is given, and the primary IV rate is adjusted with the secondary IV drug line to achieve a therapeutic effect and maintain adequate maternal hydration. Note that the drug is ordered to be given by concentration and that the infusion rates for volume per minute and hour must be determined.

Administration by Concentration

EXAMPLES
1. Give IV fluids at 100 ml/hr with D$_5$ $^1/_2$ NSS.
2. Mix 10 U of oxytocin in 1000 NSS. Start at 5 mU/min, increase by 1 or 2 mU/min, q10min, until uterine contractions are 2 to 3 minutes apart. Do not exceed 40 mU/min.

Note: *1 Unit (U) = 1000 milliunits (mU)*

Available: Secondary set:
        oxytocin 10 U/ml
        1000 ml NSS
        microdrop IV set 60 gtt/ml
        infusion pump
    Primary set:
        1000 ml D$_5$ $^1/_2$ NSS
        IV set drop factor 60 gtt/ml

For the *secondary* IV set, the following calculations must be made:
1. Concentration of solution.
2. Infusion rates: volume per minute and volume per hour.
3. Titration factor in concentration per minute (mU/min).

For the *primary* IV set, the following calculations must be made:
1. Drop rate per minute. If a pump is used, set the rate at ml/hr.
2. Balance primary IV flow with secondary IV rate to achieve 100 ml/hr.

Secondary IV (see Chapter 7 for formulas)
1. Concentration of solution:

$$10 \text{ U}:100 \text{ ml} :: \text{X}:1 \text{ ml}$$
$$1000 \text{ X} = 10$$
$$\text{X} = 0.01 \text{ U or } 10 \text{ mU}$$

The concentration of solution is 10 mU/ml.

2. Infusion rates for volume:

$$\frac{\text{Concentration/minute}}{\text{Concentration of solution}} = \text{Volume/min} \times 60 \text{ min} = \text{Volume/hr}$$

Volume per minute	*Volume per hour*

$$\frac{1 \text{ mU/min}}{10 \text{ mU/ml}} = 0.1 \text{ ml/min} \times 60 \text{ min} = 6 \text{ ml/hr}$$

$$\frac{2 \text{ mU/min}}{10 \text{ mU/ml}} = 0.2 \text{ ml/min} \times 60 \text{ min} = 12 \text{ ml/hr}$$

$$\frac{5 \text{ mU/min}}{10 \text{ mU/ml}} = 0.5 \text{ ml/min} \times 60 \text{ min} = 30 \text{ ml/hr}$$

3. Titration factor (see Chapter 11): to increase the concentration by increments of 1 mU/min, the hourly rate on the pump must be increased by 6 ml/hr. The titration factor for this problem is 6 ml/hr. To increase the concentration to a higher rate, multiply the rate of increase times 6 ml/hr. (Example: to increase infusion to 5 mU/min, multiply 5 by 6 ml = 30 ml/hr.)

For the secondary IV line, the concentration of the solution is 10 mU/ml of oxytocin, with the infusion rate of 30 ml/hr to be increased in increments of 6 to 12 ml every 10 minutes until contractions are 2 to 3 minutes apart.

Primary IV

The secondary IV rate will start at 30 ml/hr; therefore the primary rate will be 70 ml/hr. (A balance is needed to achieve 100 ml/hr.)

Drop rate with a 60 gtt/ml set will be the ml/hr rate on a pump.

$$\frac{70 \text{ ml/hr} \times 60 \text{ gtt/ml}}{60 \text{ min}} = 70 \text{ gtt/min}$$

For every increase in rate from the secondary line, a corresponding decrease must be made with the primary IV line. If the rate of the secondary line exceeds the ordered hourly rate, the primary IV line may be shut off completely. The concentration of the solution may be changed by the physician if the mother is receiving too much fluid.

Administration by Volume

In the previous example, the oxytocin was ordered to be infused by concentration (mU/min), which is the recommended method for patient safety. Sometimes in clinical practice, the infusion rate may be ordered by volume (ml/hr).

EXAMPLES

Mix 10 U of oxytocin in 1000 ml NSS. Start at 30 ml/hr and increase by 6 to 12 ml q10min until uterine contractions are 2 to 3 minutes apart. Do not exceed 40 mU/min.

To determine the concentration per hour of infusion, multiply concentration of the solution by volume/hr = concentration/hr:

$$10 \text{ mU/ml} \times 30 \text{ ml/hr} = 300 \text{ mU/hr}$$

To determine the concentration of the infusion per minute, divide:

$$\frac{\text{Concentration/hr}}{60 \text{ min/hr}} = \text{Concentration/min}$$

$$\frac{300 \text{ mU/hr}}{60 \text{ min/hr}} = 5 \text{ mU/min}$$

Therefore an oxytocin solution with a concentration of 10 mU/ml infused at 30 ml/hr will administer 5 mU of the drug per minute.

INTRAVENOUS LOADING DOSE

Some situations require IV medications to be infused over a short period to obtain a serum level for a therapeutic effect. This type of IV drug administration is called a *loading dose*.

In the following example, a patient with preeclampsia receives a loading dose of magnesium sulfate, followed by a maintenance dose of magnesium sulfate via the secondary IV line. A primary IV line is also maintained after the loading dose is given. At the end of this example, the total IV intake is determined for an 8-hour period.

EXAMPLES

1. Mix magnesium sulfate 20 g in 1000 ml of D_5W.
2. Infuse 4 g over 20 minutes, then maintain at 1 g/hr.
3. Start D_5 LRS at 75 ml/hr after magnesium sulfate loading dose.

Available: Secondary set:
        magnesium sulfate 50% (5 g in 10-ml ampules)
        1000 ml D_5W
        microdrip IV set 60 gtt/ml
        infusion pump
     Primary set:
        1000 ml D_2 LRS
        IV set drop factor 10 gtt/ml

For the *secondary* IV line, the following calculations must be made:

1. Dose of magnesium sulfate in IV.
2. Concentration of solution.
3. Volume of loading dose and flow rate for infusion pump (see Chapter 9).
4. Infusion rate: volume per hour of magnesium sulfate infusion.

For the *primary* IV line, the following calculation must be made:

1. Drop rate per minute.

For the total IV intake, the following solutions must be added:

1. Volume of loading dose.
2. Volume of secondary IV for 8 hours.
3. Volume of primary IV for 8 hours.

Secondary IV

1. $\dfrac{D}{H} \times V = \dfrac{20\ g}{5\ g} \times 10\ ml = 40\ ml$ of magnesium sulfate or 4 ampules

2. Concentration of solution:
$$20\ g = 20{,}000\ mg$$
$$20{,}000\ mg : 1000\ ml :: X : 1\ ml$$
$$1000\ X = 20{,}000$$
$$X = 20\ mg$$
The concentration of solution is 20 mg/ml.

3. Volume of loading dose:
$$4\ g = 4000\ mg$$
$$20\ mg : 1\ ml :: 4000\ mg : X\ ml$$
$$20\ X = 4000$$
$$X = 200\ ml$$

Flow rate for the pump:

$$200\ ml \div \dfrac{20\ min}{60\ min/hr} = 200 \times \dfrac{\overset{3}{\cancel{60}}}{\underset{1}{\cancel{20}}} = 600\ ml/hr$$

The rate on the infusion pump for the 4-g infusion of magnesium sulfate over 20 minutes is 600 ml/hr. If the pump cannot be adjusted to that rate, then the infusion rate must be monitored closely, and the patient must be observed for response to drug therapy.

4. Infusion rate: volume per hour:

$$1 \text{ g} = 1000 \text{ mg}$$

$$\frac{\text{Concentration/hr}}{\text{Concentration of solution}} = \text{Volume/hr} \qquad \frac{100 \text{ mg/hr}}{20 \text{ mg/ml}} = 50 \text{ ml/hr}$$

The rate on the pump for the 1 g/hr infusion is 50 ml/hr.

Primary IV

After the loading dose of magnesium sulfate, the primary IV will run at 75 ml/hr. Drop rate with a 10 gtt/ml set is:

$$\frac{75 \text{ ml/hr} \times 10 \text{ gtt/min}}{60 \text{ min}} = 12.5 \text{ or } 13 \text{ gtt/min}$$

Total IV Intake Over 8 Hours

Volume of loading dose		200 ml
Volume of secondary IV	50 ml × 8 =	400 ml
Volume of primary IV	75 ml × 8 =	+ 600 ml
		1200 ml

Because fluid overload is a potential problem for patients with preeclampsia, all IV fluids must be calculated accurately. The use of infusion pumps, if available, when high volumes of fluid need to be infused, will provide accuracy when drops are too fast to count.

INTRAVENOUS FLUID BOLUS

An IV fluid *bolus* is a large volume, 200 to 500 ml, of IV fluid infused over a short time (1 hour or less). A bolus may be given before administration of regional anesthesia or to a patient experiencing preterm labor.

In the next example, calculate the flow rate of an IV bolus from the primary IV followed by an infusion of a tocolytic drug given by titration. At the end of this example, calculate the patient's fluid intake for 8 hours.

EXAMPLES

1. Start 1000 D$_5$ LRS at 300 ml/10 min, then reduce to 125 ml/hr.
2. Mix terbutaline 5 mg in 1000 ml of NSS; start at 10 mcg/min; increase 5 mcg/min q10min until contractions subside.

Available: Primary set:
    1000 ml D$_5$ LRS
    IV set drop factor 10 gtt/ml
  Secondary set:
    terbutaline 1 mg/ml
    500 ml NSS
    microdrip IV set 60 gtt/ml
    infusion pump

For the *secondary* IV line, the following calculations must be made:

1. The dose of terbutaline in IV.
2. Concentration of solution.
3. Infusion rates: volume per minute and hour.
4. Titration factor for 5 mcg/ml.

For the *primary* IV line, determine the following:

1. Drop rate per minute for 300 ml over 10 minutes and 125 ml/hr.
2. Balance the primary IV with the secondary IV to achieve a rate of 125 ml/hr. Total the IV fluids for 8 hours.

Secondary IV

1. $\dfrac{D}{H} \times V = \dfrac{5 \text{ mg}}{1 \text{ mg}} \times 1 \text{ ml} = 5 \text{ ml of terbutaline}$

2. Concentration of solution:

$$5 \text{ mg} = 5000 \text{ mcg}$$
$$5000 \text{ mcg} : 1000 \text{ ml} :: X \text{ mcg} : 1 \text{ ml}$$
$$1000 \text{ X} = 5000$$
$$X = 5 \text{ mcg}$$

The concentration of solution is 5 mcg/ml.

3. Infusion rates: volume per minute and volume per hour.

$$\frac{10 \text{ mcg/min}}{5 \text{ mcg/ml}} = 2 \text{ ml/min} \times 60 \text{ min/hr} = 120 \text{ ml/hr}$$

4. Titration factor: to increase the concentration by increments of 5 mcg/min, the volume of the increment of change must be calculated per minute and per hour:

$$\frac{\text{Concentration/minute}}{\text{Concentration of solution}} = \text{ml/min} \qquad \frac{5 \text{ mcg/min}}{5 \text{ mcg/ml}} = 1 \text{ ml/min}$$

$$\text{Volume/min} \times 60 \text{ min/hr} = \text{Volume/hr}$$
$$1 \text{ ml/min} \times 60 \text{ min/hr} = 60 \text{ ml/hr}$$

The titration factor is 1 ml/min or 60 ml/hr. Increasing or decreasing the infusion rate by 5 mcg/min will correspond to an increase or decrease in volume by 1 ml/min or 60 ml/hr.

Primary IV

1. Drop rate for 300 ml over 10 minutes:

$$\frac{300 \text{ ml} \times \overset{1}{\cancel{10}} \text{ gtt/ml}}{\underset{1}{\cancel{10}} \text{ min}} = 300 \text{ gtt/min}$$

Because this rate is too fast to count, the flow must be monitored closely. Drop rate for 125 ml/hr:

$$\frac{125 \text{ ml} \times \overset{1}{\cancel{10}} \text{ gtt/ml}}{\underset{6}{\cancel{60}} \text{ min}} = 20.8 \text{ or } 21 \text{ gtt/min}$$

Total IV Intake Over 8 Hours

Volume of loading dose		300 ml
Volume of primary set	125 ml × 8 =	1000 ml
Volume of secondary set	180 ml × 8 =	+ 1440 ml
		2740 ml

Assume that an average of 180 ml/hr was given.

SUMMARY PRACTICE PROBLEMS

Answers are on page 309.

1. Preterm labor.

   a. Give NSS 500 ml over 15 minutes, then infuse at 100 ml/hr

   b. If contractions are still regular, mix ritodrine 150 mg in 500 ml NSS. Infuse at 50 mcg/min and increase by 50 mcg q10min until contractions cease. Do not infuse more than 350 mcg/min.

   Available: Primary set:
       1000 ml NSS
       IV set with drop factor of 10 gtt/ml
      Secondary set:
       ritodrine 50 mg in 5-ml ampules
       500 ml NSS
       microdrip set 60 gtt/ml
       infusion pump

   Determine the following:

   a. Secondary IV:
    (1) Ritodrine dosage.
    (2) Concentration of solution.
    (3) Infusion rate for volume per minute and hour.
    (4) Titration factor.

   b. Primary IV: drop rate for 500 ml over 15 minutes and 100 ml/hr.

   c. Total fluid intake for 8 hours.

2. Preeclamptic labor.

   a. Mix magnesium sulfate 20 g in 1000 ml D$_5$W.

   b. Infuse 4 g over 30 minutes, then maintain at 2 g/hr.

   c. Start LRS 1000 ml at 50 ml/hr after loading dose of magnesium sulfate.

   Available: Secondary set:
       magnesium sulfate 50% (5 g in 10 ml)
       1000 ml D$_5$W
       microdrip IV set 60 gtt/ml
       infusion pump

Primary set:
1000 ml LRS
IV set 10 gtt/ml

Determine the following:

a. Secondary IV:
   (1) Magnesium sulfate dosage.
   (2) Concentration of solution.
   (3) Volume of loading dose and infusion rate for pump.
   (4) Infusion rate per hour of magnesium sulfate.

b. Primary IV: drop rate for 50 ml/hr.

c. Total fluid intake for 8 hours.

ANSWERS SUMMARY PRACTICE PROBLEMS

1. a. Secondary IV:
   (1) Ritodrine dosage:

   $$\frac{D}{H} \times V = \frac{150 \text{ mg}}{50 \text{ mg}} \times 5 \text{ ml} = 15 \text{ ml}$$

   Add 15 ml or 3 ampules of ritodrine to 500 ml NSS.
   (2) Concentration of solution:

   $$150 \text{ mg} : 500 \text{ ml} :: X \text{ mg} : 1 \text{ ml}$$
   $$500 \text{ X} = 150$$
   $$X = 0.3 \text{ mg/ml}$$
   or
   $$300 \text{ mcg/ml}$$

   (3) Infusion rates: volume per minute and per hour:

   $$\frac{50 \text{ mcg/min}}{300 \text{ mcg/ml}} = 0.16 \text{ ml/min} \times 60 \text{ min/hr} = 9.6 \text{ or } 10 \text{ ml/hr}$$

   (4) Titration factor: because the increment of increase is 50 mcg/min, the volume per hour, 10 ml/hr, is the titration factor, which increases the concentration by 50 mcg.

   b. Primary IV:
   (1) Drop rate for 500 ml over 15 minutes:

   $$\frac{500 \text{ ml} \times 10 \text{ gtt/ml}}{15 \text{ min}} = 333 \text{ gtt/min}$$

   This rate is impossible to count. Therefore the infusion must be monitored closely during infusion time.
   (2) Drop rate for 100 ml/hr:

   $$\frac{100 \text{ ml} \times 10 \text{ gtt/ml}}{60 \text{ min}} = 16.6 \text{ or } 17 \text{ gtt ml}$$

c. Total IV intake for 8 hours:

IV fluid bolus	500 ml
Primary IV 100 ml × 8 hr	800 ml
Secondary IV 50 ml × 8 hr	+ 400 ml
	1700 ml

Assume that an average of 50 ml/hr was given.

2. a. Secondary IV:

(1) Magnesium sulfate dosage:

$$\frac{D}{H} \times V = \frac{20\text{ g}}{5\text{ g}} \times 10\text{ ml} = 40\text{ ml or 4 ampules of magnesium sulfate}$$

(2) Concentration of solution:

$$20\text{ g} = 200{,}000\text{ mg}$$
$$20{,}000\text{ mg}:1000\text{ ml} :: X\text{ mg}:1\text{ ml}$$
$$1000\text{ X} = 20{,}000$$
$$X = 20\text{ mg}$$

The concentration of solution is 20 mg/ml.

(3) Volume of loading dose:

$$4\text{ g} = 4000\text{ mg}$$
$$20\text{ mg}:1\text{ ml} :: 4000\text{ mg}:X\text{ ml}$$
$$20\text{ X} = 4000$$
$$X = 200\text{ ml}$$

Infusion rate for 30 minutes:

$$200\text{ ml} \div \frac{30\text{ min}}{60\text{ min/hr}} = 200 \times \frac{\overset{2}{\cancel{60}}}{\underset{1}{\cancel{30}}} = 400\text{ ml/hr}$$

(4) Infusion rate: volume per hour:

$$2\text{ g} = 2000\text{ mg}$$

$$\frac{2000\text{ mg/hr}}{20\text{ mg/ml}} = 100\text{ ml/hr}$$

b. Primary IV:

After the loading dose:

$$\frac{50\text{ ml/hr} \times 10\text{ gtt/min}}{60\text{ min}} = 8.3\text{ or 8 gtt/min}$$

c. Total IV intake over 8 hours:

Volume of loading dose		200 ml
Volume of secondary IV	100 ml × 8 =	800 ml
Volume of primary IV	50 ml × 8 =	+ 400 ml
		1400 ml

Community

OBJECTIVES

- Identify the problems with conversion of metric to household measure.
- Name the components of a solution.
- List three methods for preparing a solution.
- Describe three ways solutions are labeled.
- State the formula used for calculating a solution of a desired concentration.
- State the formula used for calculating a weaker solution from a stronger solution.
- Identify the types of devices used for home infusion therapy.

OUTLINE

METRIC TO HOUSEHOLD CONVERSION
PREPARING A SOLUTION OF A DESIRED CONCENTRATION
    Changing a Ratio to Fractions and Percentages
    Calculating a Solution from a Ratio
    Calculating a Solution from a Percentage
PREPARING A WEAKER SOLUTION FROM A STRONGER SOLUTION
    Guidelines for Home Solutions
HOME INFUSION THERAPY
    Home Infusion Devices

Although the metric system has become widespread in the clinical area, the home setting generally does not have the devices of metric measure. This becomes a problem when liquid medication is prescribed in metric measure for the home patient. The community nurse should be able to assist the patient in converting metric to household measure when necessary.

Preparation of solutions in the home setting may involve conversion between the metric and household systems. Solutions used in the home setting can be used for oral fluid replacement, topical application, irrigation, or disinfection. Although the majority of the solutions are commercially available, solutions that can be prepared in the home can be effective and less costly than the premixed items.

When commercially prepared drugs are too concentrated for the patient's use and must be diluted, it is necessary to calculate the strength of the solution to meet the therapeutic need as prescribed by the physician. Knowledge of solution preparation and metric–household conversion can be a useful skill for the community nurse.

METRIC TO HOUSEHOLD CONVERSION

When changing from metric to household measure, use the ounce from the apothecary system as an intermediary, because there is no clear conversion between the two systems.

The conversion factors for volume are:

Ounces to milliliters: multiply ounces × 29.57

Milliliters to ounces: multiply milliliters × 0.034

The conversion factors for weight are:

Ounces to grams: multiply ounces × 28.35

Grams to ounces: multiply grams × 0.035

Note that weight and volume measures differ in the metric system. The properties of crystals, powders, and other solids account for the differences more so than the liquids. Also, as liquid measures increase in volume, there are greater discrepancies between metric and standard household measure. Table 14-1 shows the current approximate equivalents. Deciliters and liters are also included with the volume measurements. These terms will be seen more commonly as the use of the metric system increases. Although conversion charts are helpful guides, a metric measuring device would be optimal for drug administration. Standard household measuring devices should be used instead of tableware if a metric device is not available.

 PRACTICE PROBLEMS ▌ **Metric to Household Conversion**

Answers can be found on page 322.

Use Table 14-1 to convert metric to household measure.

Table 14-1

Household to Metric Conversions (Approximate)

Standard Household Measure	Apothecary	Metric Volume	Metric Weight
$^1/_8$ teaspoon	7-8 gtt/$^1/_{48}$ oz	0.6 ml	0.6 g
$^1/_4$ teaspoon	15 gtt/$^1/_{24}$ oz	1.25 ml	1.25 g
$^1/_2$ teaspoon	30 gtt/$^1/_{12}$ oz	2.5 ml	2.5 g
1 teaspoon	60 gtt/$^1/_6$ oz	5 ml	5 g
1 tablespoon/3 teaspoons	$^1/_2$ oz	15 ml	15 g
2 tablespoons/6 teaspoons	1 oz	$^1/_4$ dl/30 ml	30 g
$^1/_4$ cup/4 tablespoons	2 oz	$^1/_2$ dl/60 ml	60 g
$^1/_3$ cup/5 tablespoons	$2^1/_2$ oz	$^3/_4$ dl/75 ml	75 g
$^1/_2$ cup	4 oz	1 dl/120 ml	120 g
1 cup	8 oz	$^1/_4$ L/250 ml	230 g
1 pint	16 oz	$^1/_2$ L/480-500 ml	
1 quart	32 oz	1 L/1000 ml	
2 quarts/$^1/_2$ gallon	64 oz	2 L/2000 ml	
1 gallon	128 oz	$3^3/_4$ L/3840-4000 ml	

1. Dimetapp 2.5 ml every 6 hours as necessary.

2. Ceclor 5 ml four times per day.

3. Tylenol elixir 1.25 ml every 6 hours as necessary for temperature greater than 102° F.

4. Maalox 30 ml after meals and at bedtime.

5. Neo-Calglucon 7.5 ml three times per day.

6. Gani-Tuss NR liquid 10 ml, q6h, prn.

7. Castor oil 60 ml at bedtime.

8. Metamucil 5 g in 1 glass of water every morning.

9. Dilantin-30 Pediatric suspension 10 ml twice per day.

10. Homemade pediatric electrolyte solution:

    H_2O 1 L, boiled _____

    Sugar 30 g _____

    Salt 1.5 g _____

    Lite salt 2.5 g _____

    Baking soda 2.5 g _____

11. A nonalcoholic mouthwash:

    H_2O 500 ml boiled _____

    Table salt 5 ml _____

    Baking soda 5 ml _____

12. Magic mouthwash:

    Benadryl 50 mg/10 ml _____

    Maalox 10 ml _____

13. Gastrointestinal cocktail for gastric upset.

    Belladonna/Phenobarbital elixir, 10 ml _____

    Maalox, 30 ml _____

    Viscous lidocaine, 10 ml _____

PREPARING A SOLUTION OF A DESIRED CONCENTRATION

All solutions contain a solute (drug) and a solvent (liquid). Solutions can be mixed three different ways:

1. *Weight to weight:* Involves mixing the weight of a given solute with the weight of a given liquid.

    Example: 5 g sugar with 100 g H_2O

    This type of preparation is used in the pharmaceutical setting and is the *most accurate.* Scales for weight to weight preparation are not usually found in the home setting.

2. *Weight to volume:* Uses the weight of a given solute with the volume of an appropriate amount of solvent.

    Example: 10 g of salt in 1 L of H_2O

    or

    $\frac{1}{3}$ oz of salt in 1 qt of H_2O

    Again, a scale is needed for this preparation.

3. *Volume to volume:* Means that a given volume of solution is mixed with a given volume of solution.

Example: 10 ml of hydrogen peroxide 3% in 1 dl H_2O

or

2 T of hydrogen peroxide 3% in $^1/_2$ c H_2O

Preparation of solutions volume to volume is commonly used in both clinical and home settings.

After a solution is prepared, the strength can be expressed numerically in three different ways:

1. A ratio—1:20 acetic acid
2. A fraction—5 g/100 ml acetic acid
3. A percentage—5% acetic acid

With a ratio, the first number is the solute and the second number is the solvent. In a fraction, the numerator is the solid and the denominator is the liquid. A solution labeled by percentage indicates the amount of solute in 100 ml of liquid. All pharmaceutically prepared solutions use the metric system, and the ratio, fraction, and percentages are interpreted in *grams per milliliter.*

Changing a Ratio to Fractions and Percentages

Change a ratio to a percentage or a fraction by setting up a proportion using the following variables:

Known drug : Known volume : : Desired drug : Desired volume

A proportion can also be set up like a fraction:

$$\frac{\text{Known drug}}{\text{Known volume}} = \frac{\text{Desired drug}}{\text{Desired volume}}$$

REMEMBER Any variable in this formula can be found if the other three variables are known.

EXAMPLE   PROBLEM 1: Change acetic acid 1:20 to a percentage
1 g:20 ml = X g:100 ml
20 X = 100
X = 5 g
1 g:20 ml = 5 g:100 ml

Note: *In percentage, the volume of liquid is 100 ml.*

The ratio can be expressed as a fraction, 5 g/100 ml, or as a percentage, 5%. Another method of changing a ratio to a percentage involves finding a multiple of 100 for volume (denominator), then multiplying both terms by that multiple.

Preparing a Solution of a Desired Concentration

Answers can be found on page 323.

Change the following ratios to fractions and percentages.

1. 4:1   **6.** 1:10,000

2. 2:1   **7.** 1:4

3. 1:50   **8.** 1:5000

4. 1:3   **9.** 1:200

5. 1:1000   **10.** 1:10

In the previous problems, grams per milliliter is the unit of measure used for preparing solutions. Scales for measuring grams are rarely found in the clinical area or the home environment. Volume (in milliliters) is the common measurement of drugs for administration. Drugs that are powders, crystals, or liquids are measured in graduated measuring cups with metric, apothecary, or household units. The milliliter, although a volume measure, can be substituted for a gram, a measure of mass, because at 4° C, 1 ml of water weighs 1 g. Mass and volume differ with the type of substance; thus grams and milliliters are not exact equivalents in all instances, but they can be accepted as approximate values for preparation of solutions.

Calculating a Solution from a Ratio

To obtain a solution from a ratio, use the proportion or fraction method.

EXAMPLES

PROBLEM 1: Prepare 500 ml of a 1:100 vinegar-water solution for a vaginal douche.

Known drug : Known volume :: Desired drug : Desired volume
     1 ml   :   100 ml   ::   X ml   :   500 ml
                        100 X = 500
                           X = 5 ml

or

$$\frac{\text{Known drug}}{\text{Known volume}} = \frac{\text{Desired drug}}{\text{Desired volume}}$$

$$\frac{1 \text{ mL}}{100 \text{ ml}} = \frac{X}{500 \text{ ml}}$$

$$100 X = 500$$
$$X = 5 \text{ ml}$$

Answer: 5 ml of vinegar added to 500 ml of water is a 1:100 vinegar-water solution.

Note: Five milliliters did not increase the volume of the solution by a large amount. When volume and volume solutions are mixed, the total amount of *desired volume* should not be exceeded. Therefore it is important to determine the volume of desired drug first, then remove that volume from the appropriate amount of solvent (solution). When mixing the solution, begin with the desired drug and add the premeasured solvent. This process ensures that the solution has an accurate concentration.

PROBLEM 2: Prepare 100 ml of a 1:4 hydrogen peroxide 3% and normal saline mouthwash.

Known drug:Known volume :: Desired drug:Desired volume

1 ml   :   4 ml   ::   X ml   :   100 ml

4 X = 100 ml

X = 25 ml

25 ml of hydrogen peroxide 3% is the amount of desired drug. To calculate the amount of normal saline, use the following formula:

Desired volume − Desired drug = Desired solvent

100 ml   −   25 ml   =   75 ml

Answer: *75 ml of saline and 25 ml of hydrogen peroxide 3% make 100 ml of a 1:4 mouthwash.*

Calculating a Solution from a Percentage

To obtain a solution from a percentage, use the same formula with either the proportion or fraction method.

EXAMPLE   PROBLEM 1: Prepare 1000 ml of a 0.9% NaCl solution.

Known drug:Known volume :: Desired drug:Desired volume

0.9 g   :   100 ml   ::   X g   :   1000 ml

100 X = 900

X = 9 g or 9 ml

Answer: *9 g or 9 ml of NaCl in 1000 ml makes a 0.9% NaCl solution.*

PREPARING A WEAKER SOLUTION FROM A STRONGER SOLUTION

When a situation requires the preparation of a weaker solution from a stronger solution, the amount of desired drug must be determined. The known variables are the desired solution, the available or on-hand solution, and the desired volume. The formula can be set up with the strength of the solutions expressed in either ratio or percentage. The proportion method or the fractional method can be used to solve the problem. The first ratio or fraction, the desired solution (weaker solution), is the numerator, and the available or on-hand solution (stronger solution) is the denominator.

Desired solution : Available solution :: Desired drug : Desired volume

or

$$\frac{\text{Desired solution}}{\text{Available solution}} = \frac{\text{Desired drug}}{\text{Desired volume}}$$

EXAMPLES

PROBLEM 1: Prepare 500 ml of a 2.5% aluminum acetate solution from a 5% aluminum acetate solution. Use water as the solvent.

$$2.5\% : 5\% \ :: \ X : 500 \text{ ml}$$
$$2.5 \text{ ml} : 5 \text{ ml} \ :: \ X : 500 \text{ ml}$$
$$5 \text{ X} = 1250$$
$$X = 250 \text{ ml}$$

Answer: Use 250 ml of 5% aluminum acetate to make 500 ml of 2.5% aluminum acetate solution.

Determine the amount of water needed.

Desired volume − Desired drug = Desired solvent
500 ml   −   250 ml   =   250 ml

or

Same problem using the fractional method:

$$\frac{2.5\%}{5\%} \times \frac{X}{500 \text{ ml}} =$$

$$5 \text{ X} = 1250$$
$$X = 250 \text{ ml of 5\% aluminum acetate}$$

or

Same problem but stated as a ratio:

Prepare 500 ml of a 1 : 40 aluminum acetate solution from a 1 : 20 aluminum acetate solution with water as the solvent.

$$\frac{1}{40} : \frac{1}{20} \ :: \ X : 500 \text{ ml}$$

$$\frac{1}{20 \text{ X}} = \frac{500}{40}$$

$$X = \frac{500}{\overset{}{\underset{2}{40}}} \times \frac{\overset{1}{20}}{1} = \frac{500}{2}$$

$$X = 250 \text{ ml of 5\% aluminum acetate solution}$$

Guidelines for Home Solutions

For solutions prepared by clients in the home, directions need to be very specific and in written form, if possible. People often think that more is better. Teach the client that solutions can be dangerous if they are too concentrated. Higher concentrations of solutions can irritate tissues and prevent the desired effect. Recommend that standard measuring spoons and cups be used rather than tableware. Level measures rather than heaping measures of dry solutes should be used. Utensils and containers for solution preparation should be *clean or sterilized by boiling* if used for infants. Mixing acidic solutions in aluminum containers should be avoided, especially if the solution is for oral use. Although there is no evidence of toxicity, a metallic taste is noticeable. Glass, enamel, or plastic containers can be used. Solutions should be made fresh daily or just before use. Oral solutions, especially for infants, require refrigeration; topical solutions do not.

When preparing the solution, start with the desired drug and then add the solvent. This helps to disperse the drug and ensures that the desired volume of solution is not exceeded.

Solution problems are best calculated within the metric system. Fractional and percentage dosages are difficult to determine within the household system.

PRACTICE PROBLEMS ▍▍▍ **Preparing a Weaker Solution from a Stronger One**

Answers can be found on page 324.

Identify the known variables and choose the appropriate formula. Perform calculations needed to obtain the following solutions using the metric system. Use Table 14–1 to obtain the household equivalent.

1. Prepare 250 ml of a 0.6% NaCl and sterile water solution for nose drops.

2. Prepare 250 ml of a 5% glucose and sterile water solution for an infant feeding.

3. Prepare 1000 ml of a 25% Betadine solution with sterile saline for a foot soak.

4. Prepare 2 L of a 2% Lysol solution for cleaning a changing area.

5. Prepare 20 L of a 2% sodium bicarbonate solution for a bath.

6. Prepare 100 ml of a 50% hydrogen peroxide 3% and water mouthwash.

7. Prepare 500 ml of a modified Dakin's solution 0.5% from a 5% sodium hypochlorite solution with sterile water as the solvent.

8. Prepare 1500 ml of a 0.9% NaCl solution for an enema.

_____

9. Prepare 2 L of a 1:1000 Neosporin bladder irrigation with sterile saline. (Omit the household conversion.)

_____

10. Determine how much alcohol is needed for a 3:1 alcohol and white vinegar solution for an external ear irrigation. Vinegar 30 ml is used. Solve using the proportion method.

_____

11. Prepare 1000 ml of a 1:10 sodium hypochlorite and water solution for cleaning.

_____

12. Prepare 1000 ml of a 3% sodium hypochlorite and water solution.

_____

13. Prepare 2000 L of a 1:9 Lysol solution to clean color-fast linens soiled with body fluids. (Omit the household conversion.)

_____

HOME INFUSION THERAPY

Home Infusion Devices

Home infusion therapy is the administration of a wide range of intravenous (IV) products by the nurse or family member to a patient in the home setting. The IV products include total parental nutrition (TPN) antibiotics, potent vasopressors (dobutamine and milrinone), blood products, chemotherapeutic agents, pain medication, and immunoglobulins. The criteria for home infusion therapy are as follows:

- Patent venous access
- Safe home environment
- A responsible care giver
- A medication that is safe to administer at home

Medication and IV fluids for home infusions are generally premixed by a pharmacy working with the infusion agency. Although most fluids are premixed, TPN solutions may require other pharmaceuticals such as multivitamins, histamine$_2$-blocking agents, and insulin to be added before infusion. Home infusion therapy has led to innovative technologies for fluid and medication delivery (Table 14-2). The new devices are pump-types that are small, portable, quiet, and lightweight (Figures 14-1 and 14-2).

Table 14-2

Home Infusion Devices

Mechanical Infusion Devices

Elastometric balloon	Portable, hard outer shell with a balloon inside that inflates with air. A sterile reservoir inside is filled with medication. Positive pressure in balloon pushes medication through a regulator, which controls flow rate. Used for small volumes of antibiotic or chemotherapeutic agents. Single-use and disposable. Comes in various volumes, 50 to 500 ml. Designed for ambulatory care and used in pediatrics.
Spring-coil container	Pocket-sized round disk contains a spring-loaded pressure plate and a sterile reservoir. Spring plate presses against reservoir, and positive pressure forces fluid from reservoir, through the regulator. Used for small volumes of intermittent IV drugs, analgesics, antibiotics, and chemotherapy. Volume sizes are limited. Designed for ambulatory care.

Electronic Infusion Devices

Stationary pump	Usually mounted on a pole. Can be used with any type of fluid or medication. Programmable with tamperproof abilities. Used primarily in hospitals. See Chapter 9.
Ambulatory	Small, battery-powered. Used for small or large volumes. Sets up like a stationary pump. Can be used for continuous or bolus infusions. Versatile, can infuse any type of fluid. Small, lightweight, can be carried in a backpack with IV fluid. Used in ambulatory care. Allows for continuous and bolus infusions. Special tubing needed.
Implantable	Small, light, preprogrammed. Can be surgically implanted into a pocket of subcutaneous fat. Titanium pump can hold 10 to 20 ml of medication. Can be refilled with a needle inserted into the filling port of the pump. Used for control of chronic pain. Can infuse antibiotics or chemotherapeutic agents.

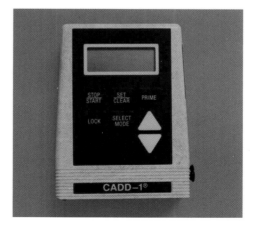

FIGURE 14-1 CADD pump is a small portable pump with a cassette of medication that snaps onto the base. Rate can be adjusted or locked out so no further adjustments can be made. Pump can be reused but medication cassettes must be changed.

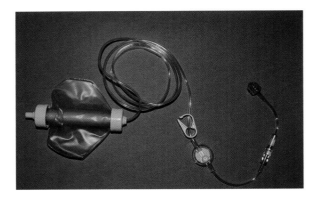

FIGURE 14-2 Elastometric balloon infusion device allows air pressure to squeeze medication cylinder in the center of the balloon to deliver the drug at a set rate. Tubing must be preprimed. It is a one-time-use-only product.

ANSWERS

I Metric to Household Conversion

1. Dimetapp 2.5 ml = $^1/_2$ t
2. Ceclor 5 ml = 1 t
3. Tylenol elixir 1.25 ml = $^1/_4$ t
4. Maalox 30 ml = 2 T
5. Neo-Calglucon 7.5 ml = 1$^1/_2$ t
6. Gani-Tuss NR, 10 ml = 2 t
7. Castor oil 60 ml = 4 T or $^1/_4$ c
8. Metamucil 5 g = 1 t
9. Dilantin-30 Pediatric suspension 10 ml = 2 t
10. H_2O 1 L = 1 qt
 Sugar 30 g = 2 T
 Salt 1.25 g = $^1/_4$ t
 Lite salt 2.5 g = $^1/_2$ t
 Baking soda 2.5 g = $^1/_2$ t
11. H_2O 500 ml = 1 qt
 Table salt 5 ml = 1 t
 Baking soda 5 ml = 1 t
12. Benadryl 50 mg/10 ml = 2 t
 Maalox 10 ml = 2 t
13. Belladonna/Phenobarbital elixir, 10 ml = 2 t
 Maalox 30 ml = 2 T
 Viscous lidocaine 10 ml = 2 t

II Preparing a Solution of a Desired Concentration

1. $4:1 = X:100$

   $X = 400$

   $\dfrac{400}{100}$, 400%

2. $2:1 = X:100$

   $X = 200$

   $\dfrac{200}{100}$, 200%

3. $1:50 = X:100$

   $50\,X = 100$

   $X = 2$

   $\dfrac{2}{100}$, 2%

4. $1:3 = X:100$

   $3\,X = 100$

   $X = 33.3$

   $\dfrac{33.3}{100}$, 33.3%

5. $1:100 = X:100$

   $1000\,X = 100$

   $X = 0.1$

   $\dfrac{0.1}{100}$, 0.1%

6. $1:10,000 = X:100$

   $10,000\,X = 100$

   $X = 0.01$

   $\dfrac{1}{10,000}$, 0.01%

7. $1:4 = X:100$

   $4\,X = 100$

   $X = 25$

   $\dfrac{25}{100}$, 25%

8. $1:5000 = X:100$

   $5000\,X = 100$

   $X = 0.02$

   $\dfrac{0.02}{100}$, 0.02%

9. $1:200 = X:100$

   $200\,X = 100$

   $X = 0.5$

   $\dfrac{0.5}{100}$, 0.5%

10. 1:10 = X:100
$\qquad$ 10X = 100
$\qquad\quad$ X = 10
$\qquad \dfrac{10}{100},$ 10%

III Preparing a Weaker Solution from a Stronger One

1.

Known drug:	0.6% NaCl	0.6:100 :: X:250
Known volume:	100 ml	100 X = 150
Desired drug:	X	X = 1.5 ml
Desired volume:	250 ml	

1.5 ml of NaCl in 250 ml of water yields a 0.6% NaCl solution. Household equivalents are approximately $^1/_4$ teaspoon salt and 1 cup sterile water.

2.

Known drug:	5% glucose (sugar)	5:100 :: X:250
Known volume:	100 ml	100 X = 1250
Desired drug:	X	X = 12.5 ml
Desired volume:	250 ml	

12.5 ml of sugar in 250 ml of water yields a 5% glucose solution. Household equivalents are approximately 1 tablespoon in 1 cup of sterile water.

3.

Known drug:	25% Betadine	25:100 :: X:1000
Known volume:	100 ml	100 X = 25,000
Desired drug:	X	X = 250 ml
Desired volume:	1000 ml	1000 ml − 250 ml = 750 ml

250 ml of Betadine in 750 ml saline yields a 25% Betadine solution. Household equivalents are 1 cup Betadine in 3 cups sterile saline.

4.

Known drug:	2% Lysol	2:100 :: X:2000 ml
Known volume:	100 ml	100 X = 4000
Desired drug:	X	X = 40 ml
Desired volume:	2 L = 2000 ml	

40 ml of Lysol in 2 L of water yields a 2% Lysol solution. Household equivalents are 2 tablespoons and 2 teaspoons (40 ml) of Lysol to 2 quarts or $^1/_2$ gallon of water.

5.

Known drug:	2% sodium bicarbonate	2:100 :: X:20,000 ml
Known volume:	100 ml	X = 40,000
Desired drug:	X	X = 400 ml or 400 g
Desired volume:	20,000 ml	

400 ml or 400 g of sodium bicarbonate (baking soda) in 20,000 ml of water yields a 2% sodium bicarbonate solution. Household equivalents are $1^1/_2$ cups and 2 tablespoons baking soda in 5 gallons of water.

6.

Known drug:	50% hydrogen peroxide	50:100 :: X:100
Known volume:	100 ml	100 X = 5000

Desired drug:	X	X = 50 ml
Desired volume:	100 ml	100 ml − 50 ml = 50 ml

50 ml of hydrogen peroxide 3% in 50 ml water yields a 50% solution. Household equivalents are approximately 3 tablespoons of hydrogen peroxide 3% in 3 tablespoons of water.

7.

Known drug:	0.5%	0.5:5 :: X:500
Available solution:	5%	5 X = 250
Desired drug:	X	X = 50 ml
Desired volume:	500 ml	500 ml − 50 ml = 450 ml

50 ml of sodium hypochlorite in 450 ml sterile water yields a 0.5% modified Dakin's solution. Household equivalents are 3 tablespoons and 1 teaspoon of Dakin's solution in 1 pint minus 3 tablespoons of water.

8.

Known drug:	0.9%	0.9:100 :: X:1500
Known volume:	100 ml	100 X = 1350
Desired drug:	X	X = 13.5 ml
Desired volume:	1500 ml	

13.5 ml of NaCl in 1500 ml water yields a 0.9% NaCl solution. Household equivalents are $2\frac{1}{2}$ teaspoons of salt in $1\frac{1}{2}$ quarts of water.

9.

Known drug:	1 ml	1:100 :: X:2000
Known volume:	1000 ml	1000 X = 2000
Desired drug:	X	X = 2 ml
Desired volume:	2000 ml	

2 ml of Neosporin irrigant in 2000 ml of sterile saline yields a 1:1000 solution for continuous bladder irrigation. This treatment is done primarily in the clinical setting.

10. Use ratio and proportion to solve this problem.
   3:1 :: X:30 ml
     X = 90 ml

Add 90 ml of alcohol to 30 ml of vinegar to yield a 3:1 solution for an external ear wash. Household equivalents are 6 tablespoons of alcohol and 2 tablespoons of vinegar.

11.

Known drug:	1 ml	1:10 :: X:1000
Known volume:	10 ml	10 X = 1000
Desired drug:	X	X = 100 ml
Desired volume:	1000 ml	1000 ml − 100 ml = 900 ml

100 ml of sodium hypochlorite (bleach) in 900 ml water yields a 1:10 sodium hypochlorite solution. Household equivalents are $\frac{1}{3}$ cup and 2 tablespoons sodium hypochlorite in approximately 1 quart minus $\frac{1}{3}$ cup and 2 tablespoons of water.

12.

Known drug:	3 ml	3:100 :: X:1000
Known volume:	100 ml	100 X = 3000
Desired drug:	X	X = 30 ml
Desired volume:	1000 ml	1000 ml − 30 ml = 970 ml

30 ml of sodium hypochlorite (bleach) in 970 ml water yields a 3% sodium hypochlorite solution. Household equivalents are 2 tablespoons in 1 quart minus 2 tablespoons of water.

13. Use ratio and proportion to solve this problem.

$$1:9 :: X:2000 \text{ ml}$$
$$9X = 2000 \text{ ml}$$
$$X = 222 \text{ ml}$$
$$\text{Desired volume} - \text{Desired drug} = \text{Desired solvent}$$
$$2000 \text{ ml} - 222 \text{ ml} = 1778 \text{ ml}$$

222 ml of Lysol in 1778 ml of H_2O yields a 1:9 solution cleansing solution for colorfast linens soiled with body fluids.

PART V

POST-TEST: ORAL PREPARATIONS, INJECTABLES, INTRAVENOUS, AND PEDIATRICS

The post-test is for testing content of Part III, orals, injectables, intravenous, and Chapter 10 pediatrics. The test is divided into four sections. There are 50 drug problems, and the test should take 1 to 1½ hours to complete. You may use a conversion table as needed. Minimum passing score is 44 correct or 88%. If you get more than two drug problems wrong in a section of the test, return to the chapter in the book for that test section and rework the practice problems.

ORAL PREPARATIONS

1. Order: nifedipine (Adalat CC) 60 mg, po, daily for 1 wk; then 90 mg, po, daily.
   Drug available:

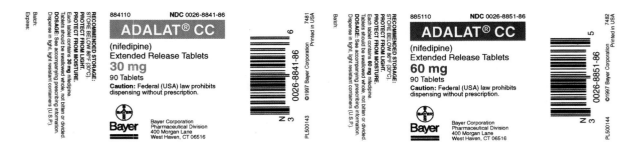

   a. Which Adalat CC container would you use for the first week? _____

   b. Explain how you would give 90 mg. _____

2. Order: rofecoxib (Vioxx) 12.5 mg, po, prn, daily.
   Drug available:

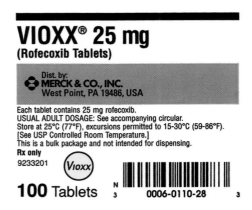

How many tablet(s) of Vioxx would you give? _____

3. Order: pravastatin sodium (Pravachol) 20 mg, po, hs.

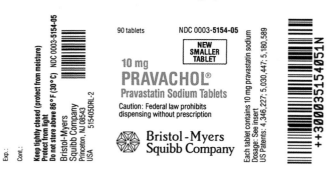

a. What does hs mean? _____

b. How many tablets of Pravachol should the client receive? _____

4. Order: nitroglycerin (Nitrostat) gr 1/200, SL, STAT.
Drug available:

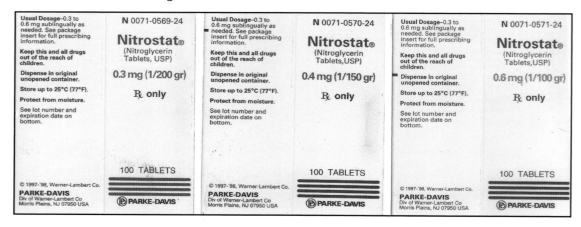

The drug is available in three different strengths. Which drug label would you

select? Why? _____

_____

5. Order: clorazepate sodium (Tranxene) gr 1/4/d, po, hs.
Drug available:

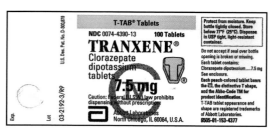

a. Change grain ¼ to milligrams. Use conversion table if needed. How many milligrams (mg) is equivalent to grain ¼? _____

b. How many tablets should the client receive? _____

6. Order: clarithromycin (Biaxin) 0.5 g, bid × 10 d, po.
Drug available:

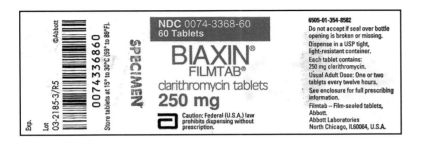

a. 0.5 gram is equivalent to _____ milligram (mg).

b. How many tablets would you give? _____

7. Order: acetaminophen (Tylenol) gr x, po, prn, for headache.
Drug available:

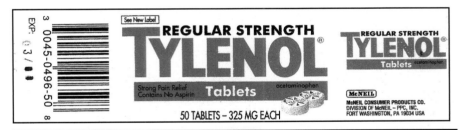

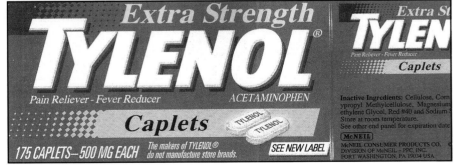

a. Grain x is equivalent to _____ milligrams (mg).

b. Which Tylenol bottle would you select? _____

c. How many tablets or caplets should the client receive? _____

8. Order: allopurinol (Zyloprim) 0.2 g, po, bid.
Drug available:

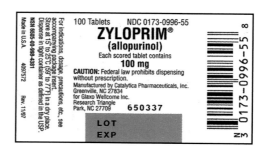

a. 0.2 g is equivalent to _____ milligrams (mg).

b. The client should receive how many tablets of allopurinol per day?

_____

9. Order: prochlorperazine (Compazine) 10 mg, po, tid.
Drug available:

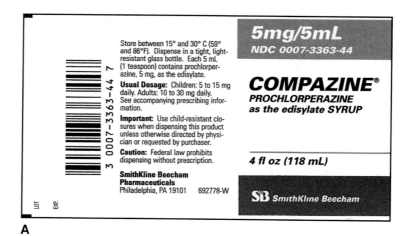

a. Which Compazine bottle would you select? Why? _____

b. How many milliliters would you give? _____

10. Order: cefuroxime axetil (Ceftin) 500 mg, po, q12h.

Drug available:

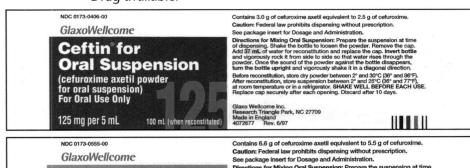

a. Which Ceftin bottle would you select? Explain. _____

b. The client would receive how many grams (g) _____ or

milligrams (mg) _____ of Ceftin per day?

c. How many milliliters should the client receive? _____

11. Order: cefaclor (Ceclor) 250 mg, po, q8h.
Drug available:

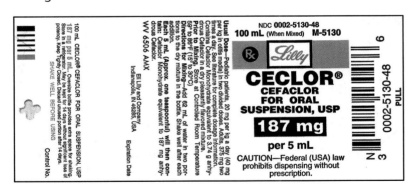

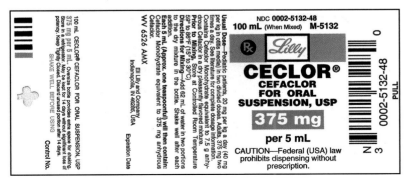

    a. Which Ceclor bottle would you select? _____

    b. How many milliliters should the client receive per dose? _____

    c. Is there another solution to this drug problem? _____

12. Order: simvastatin (Zocor) 40 mg, po, qd.
Drug available:

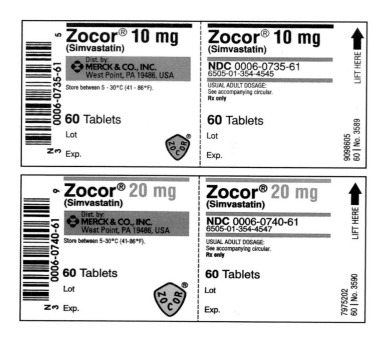

    a. Which Zocor bottle would you select? Why? _____

    b. How many tablets should the client receive? _____

13. Order: etretinate (Tegison) 0.75 mg/kg/day, po, in two divided doses. Client weighs 150 pounds.
Drug available: Tegison 10-mg and 25-mg capsules.

    a. How many kilograms does the client weigh? _____

    b. How many milligrams of Tegison should the client receive per day?

    _____

    c. How many capsules of Tegison per dose? _____

14. Order: theophylline 5 mg/kg/LD (loading dose), po. Client weighs 70 kg.
Drug available: Oral solution 80 mg/15 ml and 150 mg/15 ml.

    a. Which oral solution bottle would you select? _____

    b. How many milliliters of theophylline should the client receive as a loading dose? _____

15. Order: docusate sodium (Colace) 100 mg, po, bid per NG (nasogastric) tube. Drug available: Colace 50 mg/5 ml. Osmolality of docusate sodium is 3900 mOsm. The desired osmolality is 500 mOsm.

   a. How many milliliters of Colace should the client receive? _____

   b. How much water dilution is needed to obtain the desired osmolality?

   _____

INJECTABLES

16. Order: hydroxyzine (Vistaril) 25 mg, deep IM, STAT.
   Drug available:

   How many milliliters of Vistaril would you give? _____

17. Order: digoxin (Lanoxin) 0.25 mg, IM, qd.
   Drug available:

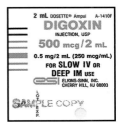

   How many milliliters of digoxin would you give? _____

18. Order: meperidine (Demerol) 40 mg and atropine sulfate 0.5 mg, IM, STAT.
   Drug available:

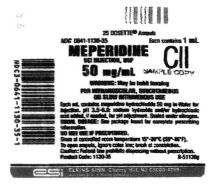 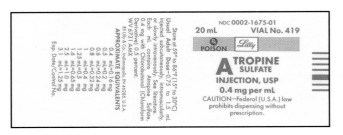

    a. How many milliliters of meperidine and how many milliliters of atropine would you administer? _____

    b. Explain how the two drugs would be mixed. _____

19. Order: heparin 2500 units (U), SC, q6h.
Drug available:

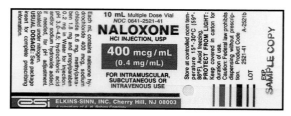

    a. Which heparin would you use? _____

    b. How many milliliters of heparin should the client receive? _____

20. Order: naloxone (Narcan) 0.5 mg, IM, STAT.
Drug available:

How many milliliters of naloxone should the client receive? _____

21. Order: NPH insulin 45 units and Humulin R (regular) 10 units.

    a. Explain the method for mixing the two insulins.

    _____

    b. Mark on the U 100/ml insulin syringe how much regular insulin and NPH insulin should be withdrawn.

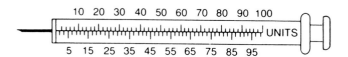

22. Order: vitamin B$_{12}$ 500 μg, IM, 3 × a week.
Drug available:

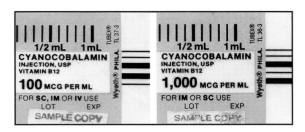

   a. Which cyanocobalamin would you select? Why?

   _____

   b. How many milliliters would you give? _____

23. Order: morphine gr ⅙, IM, STAT.
Drug available:

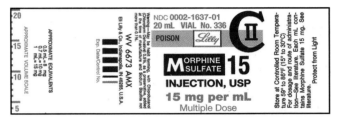

How many milliliters of morphine would you administer? _____

Note: Change grains to milligrams. Use conversion table if needed.

24. Order: phytonadione (AquaMEPHYTON) 5 mg, IM, STAT.
Drug available:

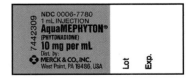

How many milliliters of AquaMEPHYTON would you administer? _____

25. Order: ranitidine HCl (Zantac) 35 mg, IM, q8h.
Drug available:

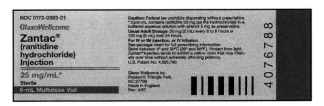

How many milliliters of Zantac should the client receive? _____

26. Order: tobramycin (Nebcin) 3 mg/kg/day, IM, in three divided doses.
Patient weighs 145 pounds.
Drug available:

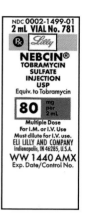

a. How many kilograms does the patient weigh? _____

b. How many milligrams of Nebcin should the client receive per day?

_____

c. How many milligrams of Nebcin should the client receive per dose?

_____

d. How many milliliters of Nebcin would you administer per dose?

_____

27. Order: bethanechol Cl (Urecholine) 2.5 mg, SC, STAT and may repeat in 1 hour.
Drug available:

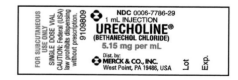

How many milliliters of Urecholine would you give? _____

28. Order: cefamandole (Mandol) 500 mg, IM, q12h.
Drug available:

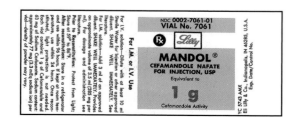

    a. How much diluent would you mix with the Mandol powder? (See label for mixing.) _____

    b. How many milliliters should be given? _____

29. Order: cefazolin (Ancef) 0.25 g, IM, q12h.
Mixing: Add 2.0 ml of diluent = 2.2 ml drug solution.
Drug available:

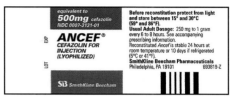

Note: Change grams to milligrams; drug label is in milligrams.
How many milliliters of Ancef should the client receive per dose? _____

30. Order: oxacillin sodium 150 mg, IM, q6h.
Drug available:

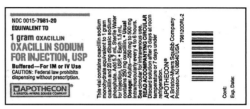

    a. Label states to add _____ ml of diluent to equal _____ ml per 250 mg.

    b. How many milliliters of oxacillin should the client receive per dose?

    _____

31. Order: ceftazidime (Fortaz) 750 mg, IM, q12h.
Add 2.5 ml of diluent = 3 ml of drug solution.
Drug available:

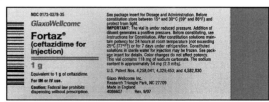

How many milliliters of ceftazidime would you administer per dose? _____

32. Order: gentamicin sulfate 4 mg/kg/day, IM, in three divided doses.
Client weighs 165 pounds.
Drug available: gentamicin 10 mg/ml and 40 mg/ml.

    a. How many kilograms does the client weigh? _____

    b. How many milligrams of gentamicin per day should the client receive?

    _____

   c. How many milligrams of gentamicin per dose? _____

   d. Which gentamicin bottle would you select? Explain.

   _____

   e. How many milliliters of gentamicin per dose should the client receive?

   _____

INTRAVENOUS

33. Order: 1000 ml of 5% dextrose/0.45% NaCl in 8 hours.
Available: 1 liter of 5% D/½ NSS; IV set labeled 10 gtt/ml.
How many drops per minute should the client receive?

_____

34. Order: 500 ml of D_5W in 2 hours.
Available: 500 ml of D_5W; IV set labeled 15 gtt/ml.
How many drops per minute should the client receive?

_____

35. Order: ticarcillin disodium (Ticar) 600 mg, IV q6h.
Available: Calibrated cylinder (Buretrol) set with drop factor 60 gtt/ml;
500 ml D_5W.
Drug available:

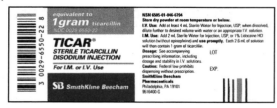

Instruction: Dilute drug in 60 ml of D_5W and infuse in 30 minutes.

   a. *Drug calculation:*

   _____

   b. *Flow rate calculation:*

   _____

36. Order: cefazolin (Kefzol) 500 mg, IV, q6h.
Available: Secondary set: drop factor 15 gtt/ml; 100 ml D_5W.
Add 2.5 ml of diluent to yield 3 ml of drug solution.
Drug available:

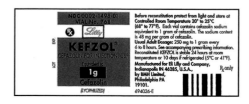

Instruction: Dilute drug in 100 ml D$_5$W and infuse in 45 minutes.

  a. *Drug calculation:*

_____

  b. *Flow rate calculation:*

_____

37. Order: chlorpromazine HCl (Thorazine) 50 mg, IV, to run for 4 hours.
Available: Secondary set: drop factor 15 gtt/ml; 500 ml of NSS (normal saline solution).
Drug available:

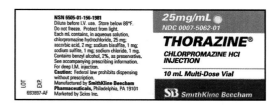

Instruction: Dilute Thorazine 50 mg in 500 ml of 0.9% NaCl (NSS) to run for 4 hours.

  a. *Drug calculation:*

_____

  b. *Flow rate calculation:*

_____

38. Order: cefepime HCl (Maxipime) 0.5 g, IV, q12h.
Available: Infusion pump.
Add 2.0 ml diluent = 2.5 ml.
Drug available:

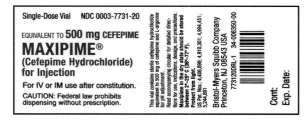

Instruction: Dilute in 50 ml of D$_5$W and infuse over 20 minutes.

  a. *Drug calculation:*

_____

  b. *Infusion pump rate:*

_____

39. Order: diltiazem (Cardizem) 10 mg/h, IV for 5 h.
Available: Infusion pump; 500 ml of D$_5$W.

Drug available:

NDC 0088-1790-32

CARDIZEM® Injectable
(diltiazem HCl Injection)   FOR DIRECT INTRAVENOUS BOLUS
                                    INJECTION AND CONTINUOUS
25 mg (5 mg/mL)   INTRAVENOUS INFUSION

Sterile 5-mL Vial

SINGLE-USE CONTAINER. DISCARD UNUSED PORTION. Mfd. for
Date Removed From Refrigeration_____   Hoechst Marion Roussel, Inc.
                                                   Kansas City, MO 64137 USA
Date To Be Discarded_____   50007742   C6

Instruction: Infuse diltiazem 10 mg/h over 5 hours.

a. *Drug calculation:*

_____

   (1) How many milligrams of Cardizem should the client receive over

      5 hours? _____

   (2) How many milliliters of Cardizem should be mixed in the 500 ml of

      D_5W? _____

b. *Infusion pump rate:*

_____

40. Order: ifosfamide (Ifex) 1.2 $g/m^2/d$ for 5 consecutive days.
    Client: Weight: 150 pounds; Height: 70 inches = 1.98 m^2.
    Available: Infusion pump; 5% dextrose solution.
    Add 20 ml of diluent to 1 g of Ifex.
    Drug available:

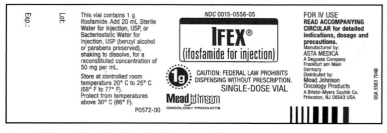

Instruction: Dilute Ifex in 50 ml of D_5W; infuse over 30 minutes.

a. *Drug calculation:*

_____

   How many grams or milligrams of Ifex should the client receive?

_____

b. How much diluent would you add to 2.4 g of Ifex?

_____

c. *Infusion pump rate:*

_____

PEDIATRICS

41. Child with cardiac disorder.
Order: Lanoxin pediatric elixir 0.5 mg, po, qd.
Drug available: Lanoxin 0.05 mg/ml.
Child's age and weight: 3 years, 15 kg.
Pediatric dose range: 0.040–0.060 mg/kg.

a. Is this drug dose within the safe range? _____

b. How many milliliters would you administer? _____

42. Child with high fever.
Order: ibuprofen (Motrin) 0.1 g, prn temperature >102°F.
Child's age and weight: 3 years, 15 kg.
Pediatric dose range: 100 mg, q6-8h, not to exceed 400 mg/day.
Drug available:

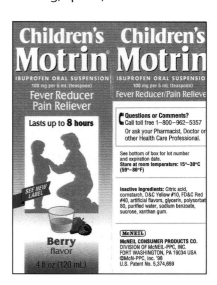

a. Is this drug dose within the safe range? _____

b. How many milliliters should the child receive per dose? _____

43. Child with strep throat.
Order: penicillin V potassium (Veetids) 400,000 units, po, q6h.
Child's age and weight: 8 years, 53 pounds.
Pediatric dose range: 25,000-90,000 units/kg/day in three to six divided doses.
Drug available:

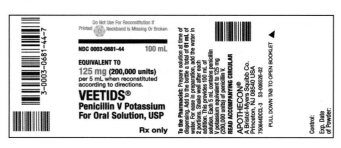

    a. Is the drug dose within the safe range? _____

    b. How many milliliters of penicillin V would you give? _____

44. Child with otitis media.
Order: amoxicillin (Amoxil) 250 mg, po, q6h.
Child's age and weight: 5 years, 19 kg.
Pediatric dose range: 20-40 mg/kg/day in three divided doses.
Drug available:

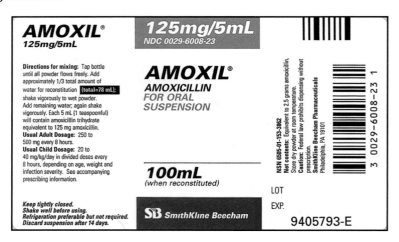

    a. Is the drug dose within the safe range? _____

    b. How many milliliters would you give? _____

45. Child with asthma.
Order: theophylline elixir 100 mg, po, q6h.
Child's age and weight: 7 years, 22 kg.
Pediatric dose: 400 mg/24 h in four doses.
Drug available: theophylline elixir 80 mg/15 ml.

    a. Is the drug dose within the safe range? _____

    b. How many milliliters would you give? _____

46. Child with pruritus.
Order: diphenhydramine HCl (Benadryl) 25 mg, po, tid.
Child's age and weight: 2 years, 16 kg.
Pediatric dose: 5 mg/kg/day.
Drug available: Benadryl 12.5 mg/5 ml.

    a. Is the drug dose within the safe range? _____

    b. How many milliliters would you give? _____

47. Child with a lower respiratory tract infection.
Order: cefaclor (Ceclor) 100 mg, q8h.
Child's age and weight: 4 years, 44 pounds.
Pediatric dose range: 20-40 mg/kg/day in three divided doses.

Drug available:

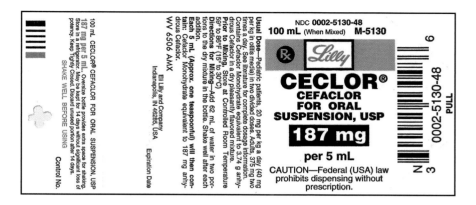

a. How many kilograms does the child weigh? _____

b. Is the drug dose within the safe range? _____

c. How many milliliters should the child receive? _____

48. Child with severe systemic infection.
Order: tobramycin (Nebcin) 15 mg, IV, q8h.
Child's age and weight: 18 months, 10 kg.
Pediatric dose range: 3-5 mg/kg/day in three divided doses.
Drug available:

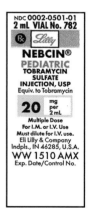

a. Is the drug dose within the safe range? _____

b. How many milliliters of tobramycin would you give? _____

49. Child with a severe central nervous system (CNS) infection.
Order: ceftazidime (Fortaz) 250 mg, IV, q6h.
Child's age and weight: 6 years, 27 kg.
Pediatric dose range: 30-50 mg/kg/day in three divided doses.

Add 2.0 ml of diluent = 2.4 ml of drug solution.
Drug available:

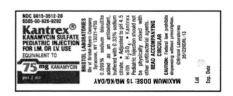

  a. Is the drug dose within the safe range? _____

  b. How many milliliters of Fortaz would be given? _____

50. Child with a severe respiratory tract infection.
Order: kanamycin (Kantrex) 60 mg, IV, q8h.
Child's age and weight: 1 year, 26 pounds.
Pediatric dose range: 15 mg/kg/day, q8-12h.
Drug available:

  a. How many milligrams of kanamycin will the child receive per day? Per

    dose? _____

  b. How many milliliters of kanamycin will the child receive per dose?

    _____

  c. Is the drug dose within the safe range? _____

A "Comprehensive Post-test" is available on the CD-ROM.

ANSWERS

Oral Preparations

  1. **a.** The Adalat CC, 60 container.
    b. For 90 mg, remove 1 tablet from the 30-mg container and 1 tablet from the 60-mg container.
  2. ½ tablet
  3. **a.** hs means hour of sleep, or at bedtime.
    b. 2 tablets of Pravachol.
  4. Nitrostat 0.3 mg (use conversion table as needed)

5. **a.** grain ¼ = 15 mg
   b. 2 tablets
6. **a.** 0.5 gram = 500 mg
   b. 2 tablets
7. **a.** 600 to 650 mg = gr x
   b. 325-mg bottle
   c. 2 tablets from the 325-mg bottle
8. **a.** 0.2 g = 200 mg
   b. 2 tablets
9. **a.** Compazine 5 mg/5 ml; Compazine 5 mg/ml is for injection.
   b. 10 ml
10. **a.** Select 250 mg/5 ml bottle. However, either bottle could be used; 125 mg/5 ml = 20 ml.
    b. 1 gram; 1000 mg
    c. 500 mg = 10 ml
11. **a.** Either 187 mg/5 ml or 375 mg/5 ml.
    b. With (preferred) 187 mg/5 ml bottle:

$$\frac{250 \text{ mg}}{187 \text{ mg}} \times 5 \text{ ml} = \frac{1250}{187} = 6.67 \text{ or } 7 \text{ ml per dose}$$

With the 375 mg/5 ml 3.3 ml per dose.

12. **a.** Zocor 20 mg bottle. Either bottle; however, with the 10-mg Zocor bottle, more tablets would be taken (Zocor 10-mg bottle = 4 tablets).
    b. 2 tablets (Zocor 20-mg bottle)
13. **a.** 150 pounds = 68 kg
    b. 0.75 × 68 = 51 mg or 50 mg
    c. Select 25-mg capsule bottle. Two capsules.
14. **a.** 5 mg × 70 kg = 350-mg loading dose
    b. Select the 150 mg/15 ml bottle.
    c. 35 ml theophylline
15. **a.** 10 ml = 100 mg Colace
    b. *Known mOsm (3900)* × Volume of drug (10 ml) = $\frac{39{,}000}{500}$ = 78 ml drug solution and water
       desired mOsm (500)
       78 ml of drug solution and water − 10 ml of drug solution
       = 68 ml of water to dilute the osmolality of the drug

Injectables

16. ½ ml or 0.5 ml

$$\text{BF: } \frac{D}{H} \times V = \frac{\overset{1}{\cancel{25} \text{ mg}}}{\underset{2}{\cancel{50} \text{ mg}}} \times 1 \text{ ml} = \frac{1}{2} \text{ ml}$$

RP: H : V :: D :X
  50 mg : 1 ml :: 25 mg : X
       50 X = 25
          X = $\frac{25}{50}$ = ½ ml

DA: no conversion factor needed

$$ml = \frac{1\ ml\ \times\ \overset{1}{\cancel{25}}\ \cancel{mg}}{\underset{2}{\cancel{50}}\ \cancel{mg}\ \times\ \ \ 1} = \frac{1}{2}\ ml$$

17. 1 ml

18. a. Meperidine 0.8 ml; atropine 1.25 ml

    b. (1) draw 1.25 ml of air and insert into the atropine bottle

        (2) withdraw 1.25 ml of atropine and 0.8 ml of meperidine from the ampule.

19. a. Could use either vial, U 5000/ml or U 10,000/ml

    b. 0.5 ml from the U 5000 vial or 0.25 ml from the U 10,000 vial.

20. 1.25 ml of Naloxone.

21. a. Withdraw the regular Humulin insulin first and then the NPH insulin.

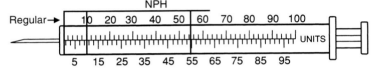

    b. Total of 55 units of regular and NPH insulin (10 units regular, 45 units NPH).

22. a. Select 1000 mcg/ml. If you chose the 100 mcg/ml cartridge, you would need 5 cartridges to give 500 μg (mcg).

    b. $\frac{1}{2}$ ml or 0.5 ml

23. grain $\frac{1}{6}$ = 10 mg (use conversion table as needed)

    0.66 ml or 0.7 ml

24. $\frac{1}{2}$ ml or 0.5 ml

25. 1.4 ml

26. a. 145 ÷ 2.2 = 65.9 kg or 66 kg

    b. 3 mg × 66 kg = 198 mg/day

    c. 198 ÷ 3 = 66 mg per dose

    d. BF: $\dfrac{66\ mg}{80} \times 2\ ml = \dfrac{132}{80}$ = 1.65 or 1.7 ml per dose **or**

        DA: $ml = \dfrac{2\ ml\ \times\ 66\ \cancel{mg}}{80\ \cancel{mg}\ \times\ \ \ 1} = \dfrac{132}{80}$ = 1.7 ml per dose

27. 0.5 ml

28. a. Add 3 ml diluent = 3.5 ml drug solution; 1 g = 1000 mg.

    b. $\dfrac{500\ mg}{1000\ mg} \times 3.5\ ml = \dfrac{1750}{1000}$ = 1.75 ml or 1.8 ml per dose

29. 0.25 g = 250 mg

    BF: $\dfrac{250\ mg}{500} \times 2.2\ ml = \dfrac{550}{500}$ = 1.1 ml per dose   **or**

    RP: H : V :: D :X

      500 mg : 2.2 = 250 : X

          500 X = 550

              X = $\dfrac{550}{500}$ = 1.1 ml

30. **a.** Add 5.7 ml diluent = 6.0 ml per 1 gram of oxacillin; 250 mg = 1.5 ml
    b. 0.9 ml per dose
31. 2.25 ml Fortaz
32. **a.** 165 lb ÷ 2.2 = 75 kg
    b. 4 mg × 75 kg = 300 mg/day
    c. 100 mg per dose
    d. Select 40 mg/ml bottle of gentamicin sulfate. (Normally less than 3 ml IM, should be given at one site.)
    e. 2.5 ml of gentamicin per dose

Intravenous

33. 125 ml per hour
$$\frac{125 \text{ ml} \times 10 \text{ gtt/min}}{60 \text{ min/hr}} = \frac{1250}{60} = 20.8 \text{ gtt/min or } 21 \text{ gtt/min}$$

34. 62-63 gtt/min
35. Add 2.0 ml diluent = 2.6 ml drug solution; 1 g = 1000 mg.
    a. $\dfrac{600 \text{ mg}}{1000 \text{ mg}} \times 2.6 \text{ ml} = \dfrac{15.6}{10} = 1.56 \text{ ml or } 1.6 \text{ ml Ticar per dose}$

    b. $\dfrac{\text{Amount of solution} \times \text{gtt/ml}}{\text{Minutes}} = \dfrac{60 \text{ mg} \times \overset{2}{60} \text{ gtt/ml}}{\underset{1}{30} \text{ minutes}} = 120 \text{ gtt/min}$

36. **a.** 1.5 ml

    b. $\dfrac{100 \text{ ml} \times \overset{1}{15} \text{ gtt/ml}}{\underset{3}{45} \text{ min}} = \dfrac{100}{3} = 33.3 \text{ or } 33 \text{ gtt/min}$

37. **a.** Add 2 ml Thorazine to 500 ml. For 4 hours: 500 ml ÷ 4 = 125 ml per hour.

    b. $\dfrac{125 \text{ ml} \times \overset{1}{15} \text{ gtt/ml}}{\underset{4}{60} \text{ min/1 h}} = \dfrac{125}{4} = 31 \text{ gtt/min for 4 hours}$

38. **a.** 0.5 g = 500 mg; add 2.0 ml of diluent = 2.5 ml of drug solution; 500 mg = 2.5 ml

    b. Amount of solution ÷ $\dfrac{\text{Min to admin}}{60 \text{ min/h}}$ = ml/hr

    2.5 ml drug + 50 ml ÷ $\dfrac{20 \text{ min}}{60 \text{ min/h}}$ = 52.5 ml × $\dfrac{\overset{3}{60}}{\underset{1}{20}}$ = 157.5 ml/hr

    Set pump to deliver in 20 minutes.

39. **a.** 10 mg/h × 5 h = 50 mg Cardizem
    b. $\dfrac{50 \text{ mg}}{5} \times 1 \text{ ml} = 10 \text{ ml Cardizem to add to } 500 \text{ ml}$

    c. 10 ml drug solution + 500 ml ÷ $\dfrac{300 \text{ min}}{60 \text{ min/hr}}$ = 510 ml × $\dfrac{\overset{1}{60} \text{ min}}{\underset{5}{300} \text{ min (5 h)}}$ = $\dfrac{510}{5}$ = 102 ml/hr

40. a. 1.2 g $\times$ 1.98 m^2 = 2.37 g or 2.4 g or 2400 mg

  b. 2.4 g $\times$ 20 ml/1 g = 48 ml diluent added to Ifex vials to yield 54 ml of drug solution

  c. 54 ml of drug solution + 50 ml $\div \dfrac{30 \text{ min}}{60 \text{ min}}$ = 104 ml $\times \dfrac{\overset{2}{\cancel{60} \text{ min}}}{\underset{1}{\cancel{30} \text{ min}}}$ = 208 ml/hr

  Set pump to deliver in 30 minutes.

Pediatrics

41. a. Drug dose is within safe range.

  b. 10 ml

42. a. Drug dose is within safe range.

  b. 5 ml or 1

43. a. Drug dose is within safe range; 53 pounds $\div$ 2.2 = 24 kg. 25,000 $\times$ 24 = 600,000 units; 90,000 $\times$ 24 = 2,160,000 units/day. Child receives 400,000 units $\times$ 4 (q6h) = 1,600,000 units/day.

  b. U 400,000 = 10 ml per dose

44. a. No; the drug dose is *NOT* within safe range. Do *NOT* give. Contact the physician or health care provider.

  Dosage parameters: 380 to 760 mg/day

  Order 250 mg $\times$ 4 (q6h) = 1000 mg/day; *not safe; exceeds parameters*

  b. Would not give medication.

45. a. Drug dose is within safe range.

  b. 18.75 ml or 19 ml theophylline elixir.

46. a. Drug dose is within safe range.

  5 mg $\times$ 16 kg = 80 mg; child receives 25 mg $\times$ 3 (tid) = 75 mg; *SAFE*

  b. 10 ml

47. a. 44 lb $\div$ 2.2 = 20 kg

  b. Drug dose is less than pediatric drug range. Check with the health care provider.

  20 mg $\times$ 20 kg = 400 mg/day; 40 mg $\times$ 20 kg = 800 mg/day.

  Child to receive 100 mg $\times$ 3 (q8h) = 300 mg/day; less than 400-800 mg/day.

  c. 2.67 ml or 2.7 ml per dose = 100 mg

48. a. Drug dose is within safe range.

  3 mg $\times$ 10 kg = 30 mg/day; 5 mg $\times$ 10 kg = 50 mg/day.

  Child to receive 15 mg $\times$ 3 (q8h) = 45 mg/day.

  b. 1.5 ml per dose

49. a. Drug dose is within the safe range.

  30 mg $\times$ 27 kg = 810 mg/day; 50 mg $\times$ 27 kg = 1350 mg/day.

  Child to receive 250 mg $\times$ 4 (q6h) = 1000 mg/day.

  b. 1.2 ml per dose

50. a. 180 mg/d; 60 mg/dose

  b. $\dfrac{60}{75} \times 2$ ml = $\dfrac{120}{75}$ = 1.6 ml per dose

  c. Drug dose is within safe range.

  Child's weight: 26 lb $\div$ 2.2 = 11.8 or 12 kg

  15 mg $\times$ 12 kg = 180 mg/day; child to receive 180 mg/day or 60 mg per dose.

References

Axton, S.E., & Fugate, T. (1987). A Protocol for Pediatric IV Meds. *American Journal of Nursing, 7,* 943-945.

Barnhart, E.R. (1998). *Physician's Desk Reference* (52nd ed.). Oradell, NJ: Medical Economics.

Briars, G.L., & Bailey, B.J. (1994). Surface Area Estimation: Pocket Calculator vs. Nomogram. *Archives of Disease in Childhood, 70,* 246-247.

Colangelo, A. (1987). Drug Preparation Techniques for IV Drug Delivery Systems. *American Journal of Hospital Pharmacy, 44,* 2550-2553.

Daniels, J.M., & Smith, L.M. (1990). *Clinical Calculations* (2nd ed.). Albany, NY: Delmar Publishers.

Deglin, J.H. (1988). *Dosage Calculations Manual.* Springhouse, PA: Springhouse.

Deglin, J.H., Vallerand, A.H., & Russin, M.M. (1991). *Davis's Drug Guide for Nurses* (2nd ed.). Philadelphia: F.A. Davis.

Department of Veterans Affairs, Veterans Health Administration. (January 2002). *Bar Code Medication Administration, Version 2, Training Manual.* Washington, DC: Authors.

Edmunds, M.W. (1991). *Introduction to Clinical Pharmacology.* St. Louis: Mosby.

Estoup, M. (1994). Approaches and Limitations to Medication Delivery in Patients with Enteral Feeding Tubes. *Critical Care Nurse, 14,* 68-79.

Gahart, B., & Nazarento, A. (2003). *Intravenous Medications* (19th ed.). St. Louis: Mosby.

Gilman, A.G., Goodman, L.S., & Gilman, A. (Eds.). (1996). *Goodman and Gilman's The Pharmacological Basis of Therapeutics* (9th ed.). New York: Pergamon Press.

Gin, T., Chan, M.T., Chan, K.L., & Yen, P.M. (2002). Prolonged Neuromuscular Block after Rocuronium in Postpartum Patient. *Anesthesia-Analgesia, 94*(3), 686-689.

Gurney, H. (1996). Dose Calculation of Anticancer Drugs: A Review of Current Practice and Introduction of an Alternative. *Journal of Clinical Oncology, 14*(9), 590-611.

Gurney, H.P., Ackland, S., Gebski, V., & Farrell, G. (1998). Factors Affecting Epirubicin Pharmacokinetics and Toxicity: Evidence against Using Body-Surface Areas for Dose Calculation. *Journal of Clinical Oncology, 16,* 2299-2304.

Hodgson, B.B., & Kizior, R.J. (2000). *Saunders Nursing Drug Handbook 2000.* Philadelphia: Saunders.

Kalyn, A., Blatz, S., & Pinelli, M. (2000). A Comparison of Continuous Infusion and Intermittent Flushing Methods in Peripheral Intravenous Catheters in Neonates. *Journal of Intravenous Nursing, 23*(3), 146-153.

Katzung, B.G. (1992). *Basic and Clinical Pharmacology* (5th ed.). Norwalk, CT: Appleton & Lange.

Kee, J.L., & Hayes, E.R. (2003). *Pharmacology: A Nursing Process Approach* (4th ed.). Philadelphia: Saunders.

Kee, J.L., & Paulanka, J.B. (1998). *Fluids and Electrolytes with Clinical Applications* (6th ed.). Albany, NY: Delmar Publishers.

Krupp, K., & Heximer, B. (1998). The Flow. *Nursing '98, 4,* 54-55.

Lack, J.A., & Stuart-Taylor, M.E. (1997). Calculation of Drug Dosage and Body Surface Area of Children. *British Journal of Anaesthesia, 78,* 601-605.

Lacy, C., et al. (1990-2000). *Drug Information Handbook* (7th ed.). Cleveland: Lexi-Corp, Inc.

Lilley, L.L., & Guanci, R. (1994). Getting Back to Basics. *American Journal of Nursing, 9,* 15-16.

Loan, T., Magnuson, B., & Williams, S. (1998). Debunking Six Myths About Enteral Feeding. *Nursing '98, 8,* 43-48.

Merenstein, G., & Gardner, S. (1998). *Handbook of Neonatal Intensive Care* (4th ed.). St. Louis: Mosby.

Miyagawa, C.I. (1993). Drug-Nutrient Interactions in Critically Ill Patients. *Critical Care Nurse, 13,* 69-87.

Oyama, A. (2000). Intravenous Line Management and Prevention of Catheter-Related Infections in America. *Journal of Intravenous Nursing, 23*(3), 170-175.

Phillips, L. (1997). *Manual of IV Therapeutics.* Philadelphia: F.A. Davis.

Piecoro, J.J. (1987). Development of an Institutional IV Drug Delivery Policy. *American Journal of Hospital Pharmacy, 44,* 2557-2559.

Rapp, R.P. (1987). Considering Product Features and Costs in Selecting a System for Intermittent IV Drug Delivery. *American Journal of Hospital Pharmacy, 44,* 2533-2538.

Ratain, M.J. (1998). Body-Surface Area as a Basis for Dosing of Anticancer Agents: Science, Myth, or Habit? *Journal of Clinical Oncology, 16*(7), 2297-2298.

Reilly, K.M. (1987). Problems in Administration Techniques and Dose Measurement that Influence Accuracy of IV Drug Delivery. *American Journal of Hospital Pharmacy, 44,* 2545-2550.

Rimar, J.M. (1987). Guidelines for the Intravenous Administration of Medications Used in Pediatrics. *Maternal Child Nursing, 12,* 322-340.

Savinetti-Rose, B., & Bolmer, L. (1997). Understanding Continuous Subcutaneous Insulin Infusion Therapy. *American Journal of Nursing, 97,* 42-49.

Skokal, W. (1997). Infusion Pump Update. *RN, 60,* 35-38.

Spratto, G., & Woods, A. (2003). *PDR Nurse's Drug Handbook.* Albany, NY: Delmar Publishers.

Terry, J., Baranowski, L., Lonsway, R., & Hedrick, C. (1995). *Intravenous Therapy: Clinical Principles and Practice.* Philadelphia: Saunders.

Vallerand, A.H., & Deglin, J.H. (1991). *Nurse's Guide for IV Medications.* Philadelphia: F.A. Davis.

Volumetric Infusion Pump Manual. (1999). Alaris Medical Systems, San Diego, California.

Weyant, H. (1984). Utilization of an Intravenous Drug Guide. *Focus on Critical Care, 2,* 58-62.

Wong, D.L., Hockenberry-Eaton, M., Wilson, D., Winkelstein, M.L., Ahmann, E., & DiVito-Thomas, P.A. (1999). *Whaley & Wong's Nursing Care of Infants and Children* (6th ed). St. Louis: Mosby.

Wyeth Laboratories. (1988). *Intramuscular Injections.* Philadelphia: Author.

Zenk, K.E. (1987). Intravenous Drug Delivery in Infants with Limited IV Access and Fluid Restriction. *American Journal of Hospital Pharmacy, 44,* 2542-2545.

Guidelines for Administration of Medications

OUTLINE

GENERAL DRUG ADMINISTRATION
ORAL MEDICATIONS
INJECTABLE MEDICATIONS
INTRAVENOUS FLOW AND MEDICATIONS

GENERAL DRUG ADMINISTRATION

1. Check medication order against doctor's orders, MAR (i.e., medication administration record), medicine card (if available), and/or other methods, such as computerized records.
2. Check label of drug container three times.
3. Check drug label for expiration date of *all* drugs. Return drugs that are outdated to the pharmacy.
4. Identify the patient by identification bracelet and by asking patient his or her name.
5. Stay with the patient until the medication is taken.
6. Give medications last to patients who need more assistance.
7. Report any drug error immediately to the head nurse and physician. An incident report must be made.
8. Record drug given, including the name of the drug, dosage, date, time, and your initials.
9. Record drugs soon after they are given, especially STAT medications. Also indicate on the drug sheet if the drug was not given.
10. Record the amount of fluid taken orally with medication if client's intake (I) and output (O) are being recorded.
11. Be aware that nurses have the right to question drug orders. Physicians are responsible for medication order, dosage, and route of drug administration. Nurses are responsible for administering medications.
12. Administer drug within 30 minutes of its prescribed time (30 minutes before or 30 minutes after prescribed time).
13. Do not guess when preparing medications. Check the order sheet if the drug order is not clear. Call the pharmacist, physician, and/or nursing supervisor if in doubt.
14. Do not give drugs poured by others.
15. Do not leave drug tray or cart out of your sight.
16. Know that patients have the right to refuse medication. If possible, ascertain why a patient refuses the medication. Report refusal to take medications.
17. Check if patient states that he or she has an allergy to a drug or a drug group.
18. Know the five *rights:* right drug, right dose, right route, right time, and right client.

ORAL MEDICATIONS

1. Wash hands before preparing oral medications.
2. Pour tablet or capsule into drug container's cap (top) and *not* into your hand. Drugs prepared for unit dose can be opened at the time of administration in the patient's room. Discard drugs that are dropped on the floor.
3. Pour liquids on a flat surface at eye level with your thumbnail at medicine cup line indicating the desired amount.
4. Do not mix liquids with tablets or liquids with liquids in the same container. Tablets and capsules can be put in the same container *except* for oral narcotics, digoxin, and PRN and STAT medications.

5. Do not pour drugs from containers with labels that are difficult to read.
6. Do not return poured medication to its container. Properly discard poured medication if not used.
7. Do not transfer medication from one container to another.
8. Pour liquid medications from the side opposite the bottle's label to avoid spilling medicine on the label.
9. Dilute liquid medications that irritate gastric mucosa, e.g., potassium products, or that could discolor or damage tooth enamel, e.g., SSKI (saturated solution of potassium iodide), or have client take the drug with meals.
10. Offer ice chips before administering bad-tasting medications in order to numb the client's taste buds.
11. Assist the patient into upright position when administering oral medications. Stay with the patient until medication is taken.
12. Give at least 50 to 100 ml of oral fluids with medications unless the patient has a fluid restriction. Doing so helps to ensure that medication reaches the stomach.
13. For patients having difficulty in swallowing or for patients receiving nutrients through a nasogastric or gastric tube, crush tablets (*not* spansules) and dissolve in juice or applesauce for oral ingestion or in water for tube administration. Give oral medication in small amounts to prevent choking. For the patient who has difficulty swallowing, gently stroke the throat in a downward motion to enhance swallowing.
14. For drugs given by oral syringe, direct the syringe across the tongue and toward the side of the mouth.
15. If a patient or a child spits out *all* of the liquid medication, repeat the dose. If a patient or a child spits out more than one half of the liquid medication, repeat one half of the dose. If the patient or child spits out less than one half of the liquid medication or if there is a question regarding repeating the dose, the physician must be notified and another route of administration must be chosen.

INJECTABLE MEDICATIONS

1. Wash hands before preparing injectable medications.
2. Select the proper syringe and needle size for the type of medication to be administered.
3. Assess the amount of subcutaneous fat at the injection site before choosing the needle length for an intramuscular injection.
4. Select the injection site according to the drug.
5. Check for drug compatibility before mixing drugs in the same syringe.
6. Check the expiration date on the drug label before preparing medication. If in doubt, check with the pharmacist.
7. Check the label on the drug container to determine method(s) for drug administration, e.g., intravenous (IV), intramuscular (IM), subcutaneous (SC).
8. Do not give parenteral medications that are cloudy, are discolored, or have precipitated.
9. Aspirate the plunger before injecting medication. If blood returns, *stop*, withdraw the needle, and prepare a new solution. Check the policy of your institution.

10. Do not massage the injection site if using the Z-track method, intradermal injection, heparin, or any anticoagulant solution.
11. Do not administer injections into inflamed and edematous tissues or into lesion (moles, birthmarks, scar tissue) sites.
12. Recognize that individuals experiencing edema, shock, or poor circulation have a very slow tissue absorption rate with intramuscular injection.
13. Discard liquid drugs into the sink or toilet, *not* into the trash can.
14. Discard needles safely into the proper container.
15. Refrigerate unused reconstituted powdered medication in a vial. Write date, time, and your initials on the vial.
16. Discard unused solution in ampules. After they are opened, ampules cannot be used again.
17. Do not administer IM medications subcutaneously. Poor medication absorption and sloughing of the subcutaneous tissue could occur.

INTRAVENOUS FLOW AND MEDICATIONS

1. Wash hands before changing IV fluids and tubing and before preparing IV drugs.
2. Use aseptic technique when inserting IV catheters and changing IV tubing and bags. Be able to recognize symptoms of septicemia, such as chills, fever, and tachycardia.
3. Select appropriate IV tubing sets for continuous IV infusion. For IV fluids to be infused in 10 hours or *more, use* a microdrip set (60 gtt/min); for IV fluids to be infused in 10 hours or *less, use* a macrodrip set (10, 15, 20 gtt/min).
4. Add IV drugs such as vitamins and potassium chloride to the IV fluid before connecting the IV fluid container to the IV tubing. Invert the IV bag or bottle several times to ensure drug distribution. If the IV fluid is running and IV medication needs to be added, temporarily stop the flow of IV fluid by clamping the tubing, invert the IV bag or bottle several times, then unclamp the tubing and maintain the ordered IV flow rate.
5. Check for patency of the IV catheter (heparin lock) before administering drugs by injecting 2 ml of saline solution. Flush IV line with 15 ml of saline solution to empty the IV line of drug solution, if necessary.
6. Use the proper diluent to reconstitute a powdered drug, and use the proper IV solution for infusion. Drug labels and drug information inserts usually indicate the types of diluents to use.
7. Record on the vial containing unused drug the date of reconstitution and your initials.
8. Monitor all IV flow rates (conventional tubing or IV pumps) hourly as needed. IV flow rates can be altered by the client's position or by a kink in the tubing.
9. Check for air bubbles in the IV tubing. Remove air from the tubing by clamping below the air bubbles and aspirating with a syringe, or use the method indicated by your institution.
10. Assess for allergic reactions to the IV drug. If reactions are seen, stop the flow of IV drug immediately.

11. Avoid administering drugs rapidly in IV solutions. Speed shock could occur as a result of drug concentration and accumulation. Symptoms of speed shock include tachycardia, syncope, and drop in blood pressure.

12. Observe the infusion site for signs and symptoms of infiltration, such as swelling, coolness, and pain. If these signs and symptoms are observed, discontinue IV infusion and restart at another site.

13. Assess for signs and symptoms of phlebitis, such as redness, warmth, swelling, and pain. Redness may be seen above the infusion site along the vein.

14. Do not forcefully irrigate IV catheters. A clot could be dislodged from the catheter site and become an embolus.

15. Avoid using leg veins, elbow (antecubital) sites, and affected limbs for IV therapy.

16. Change the IV site every 3 days or as indicated. Certain IV catheters, such as polyethylene catheters, can cause phlebitis.

17. Change IV tubing every 72 to 96 hours, and change IV bags every 24 hours.

18. Apply cold compresses, followed later by warm compresses, to any hematoma site, according to the physician's orders.

Nomograms

OUTLINE

BODY SURFACE AREA (BSA) NOMOGRAM FOR ADULTS
WEST NOMOGRAM FOR INFANTS AND CHILDREN

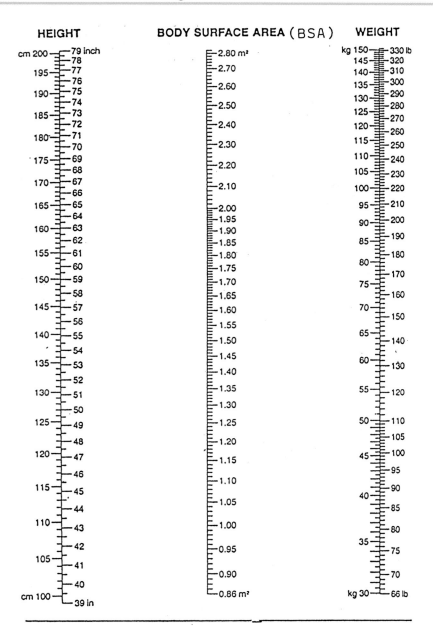

HEIGHT

BODY SURFACE AREA (BSA)

WEIGHT

Body surface area (BSA) nomogram for adults. *Directions:* (1) Find height; (2) Find weight; (3) Draw a straight line connecting the height and weight. Where the line intersects on the BSA column is the body surface area (m^2). (From Deglin, J.H., Vallerand, A.H., and Russin, M.M. [1991]. *Davis's Drug Guide for Nurses* [2nd ed.]. Philadelphia: F.A. Davis, p. 1218. Used with permission from Lentner C. [ed.]. [1981]. *Geigy Scientific Tables.* [8th ed.] Vol. 1. Basel, Switzerland: Ciba-Geigy, pp. 226-227.)

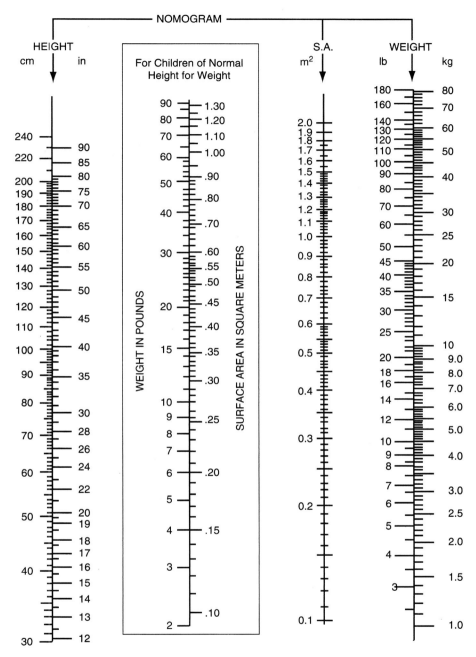

West nomogram for infants and children. *Directions:* (1) Find height; (2) Find weight; (3) Draw a straight line connecting the height and weight. Where the line intersects on the SA column is the body surface area (m²). (Modified from data of E. Boyd and C.D. West. In Behrman, R.E., Kliegman, R.M., and Jenson, H.B. [2000]. *Nelson Textbook of Pediatrics* [16th ed.]. Philadelphia: W.B. Saunders.)

Index

A

Abbreviations, 62-64, inside front cover
  drug form, 62t
  drug measurements, 62t
  practice problems, 64
    answers, 65
  route of drug administration, 63t
  time of drug administration, 63t
Alternative methods for drug administration, 67-78
  ear drops, 74, 75
  eye drops, 73
  eye ointment, 73,74
  inhalation, 69-71
    metered-dose inhaler, 69, 70
    metered-dose inhaler with spacer, 70
    nasal inhaler, 70, 71
  nasal drops, 71, 72
  nasal spray, 71, 72
  pharyngeal lozenge, 76
  pharyngeal mouthwash, 75
  pharyngeal spray, 75
  rectal suppository, 77
  topical preparations, 76, 77
    creams and ointments, 76, 77
    lotion, 76
  transdermal patch, 68
  vaginal preparations, 78
    cream, 78
    ointment, 78
    suppository, 78
Ampules, 148
Angles of injection, 154
Apothecary system, 25-28
  abbreviations, 26t
  conversion within, 26, 27

Apothecary system (*Continued*)
  practice problems, 27, 28
    answers, 31
  summary practice problems, 31, 32
    answers, 32
Arabic system, 3

B

Bar code, 56, 57t
  reader, 57t
Basic formula, 80-82
Basic math, 1-16
  answers, 11, 12, 16
  post-math test, 13-16
BSA, 99-103, 238, 239
Body surface area (BSA), 99-103, 238, 239
  practice problems, 104-106
  square root, 100, 105, 106
Body weight, 98, 99, 103, 104, 235-237
  practice problems, 103, 104

C

Calculating drugs in solution, 260, 261
  micrograms per milliliter, 261
  milligrams per milliliter, 261
  units per milliliter, 260
Calculation, of intravenous flow rate, 202, 204, 205, 212
Calculations of orals, 114-130, 139-144
  liquids, 118-120
  sublingual tablets, 120, 121
  tablets, 114-118
Capsules, 114-118
Carpuject syringe, 153
Cartridge syringes, 152, 153
Central venous access sites, 193
Charting medications, 57, 58
  medication record, 58t

Page numbers followed by "t" refer to tables.

Clark's rule, 250

Commercial drug solutions, osmolalities of, 137t

Community, 312-326
  calculating solution from ratio and percentage, 316, 317
  guidelines for home solutions, 318, 319
  home infusion devices, 321t
  home infusion therapy, 320-322
  household to metric conversion, 313t
  metric to household conversion, 312
    practice problems, 312-314
      answers, 322
    preparing solution of desired concentration, 314-316
      practice problems, 316
        answers, 323, 324
    preparing weaker solution from stronger solution, 317, 318
      practice problems, 319, 320
        answers, 324-326

Computer-based medication administration, 55, 56
  medication screen, 55t, 56t

Continuous intravenous (IV) administration, 199-207
  calculation of flow rate, 201, 202
  intravenous sets, 200, 200t
  mixing drugs for, 203
  practice problems, 206, 207
    answers, 223, 224
  safety considerations, 203
  type of solutions, 204t

Conversion in metric and apothecary systems by weight, 35-37
  equivalents, 35t
  grains and milligrams, 36
  grams and grains, 35, 36
  practice problems, 37
    answers, 40
  ratio and proportion, 36, 37
  summary practice problems, 41-43
    answers, 43, 44

Conversion in metric, apothecary, and household systems by volume, 38-40
  equivalents, 35t
  liters and ounces, 38
  milliliters and drops, 38, 39
  ounces and milliliters, 38

Conversion in metric, apothecary, and household systems by volume (Continued)
  practice problems, 39, 40
    answers, 40
  ratio and proportion, 38, 39
  summary practice problems, 42
    answers, 43, 44

Conversion of metric and apothecary tables, 86t

Cream, 76, 77

Critical care, 260-292
  basic fractional formula, 269, 270
    practice problems, 270, 271
      answers, 286-290
  calculating concentration of solution, 260-262
    practice problems, 261, 262
      answers, 277-279
  calculating infusion rate for concentration and volume per unit of time, 263-265
    practice problems, 266, 267
      answers, 279-286
  calculating infusion rate of drugs for specific body weight per unit of time, 267-269
  calculating units per milliliter, 260, 261
  pediatric. See *Pediatric critical care.*
  titration of infusion, 271-274
    practice problems, 274-276
      answers, 290, 291
  total amount of drug infused over time, 276
    practice problems, 276
      answers, 291, 292

D

Decimals, 7-9, 12
  dividing, 8, 9
  fractions, 8
  multiplying, 8
  practice problems, 9, 12

Dimensional analysis, 86-88
  practice problems (additional), 92-94
    answers, 96

Direct intravenous injections, 194-199
  practice problems, 197-199
    answers, 221-223

Dividing fractions, 6

Drug administration, alternative methods for. See *Alternative methods for drug administration.*
  five rights in, 59-62

Drug administration, alternative methods for
   (Continued)
   guidelines for, 354-357
   pediatrics. See *Pediatric drug administration.*
Drug differentiation, 50-52
Drug distribution, 58, 59
   methods, 59t
Drug dosage, pediatric from adult, 249
Drug labels, interpretation of, 46-50
   practice problems, 48-50
      answers, 64
Drug orders, 52-55
   patient orders, 53t
   practice problems, 53, 54
      answers, 65
   prescription pad, 53t
   types of, 54t
Drug reconstitution, powdered, 168, 169
Drug solution, 166-168
   commercial, osmolalities of, 137t

E
Ear drops, 74, 75
Electronic intravenous delivery devices,
   209-216
   calculating flow rates, 212-216
   flow rate for infusion, 211
   IV delivery pumps, 209, 210
      patient-controlled analgesia (PCA),
         210, 211
      syringe pumps, 210, 211
   practice problems, 217-221
      answers, 225-227
Enteral medications, 136-139
   calculation for dilution, 136-139
   osmolalities of commercial drug
      solutions, 137t
   practice problems, 139
      answers, 144, 145
Enteral nutrition, 131-136, 144
   calculation (percent), 134, 135
   common enteral formulations, 131
   enteral infusion pump, 133
   gastrointestinal tubes, 132
   practice problems, 136
      answers, 144
   type of solutions, 131t
Eye drops, 74, 75
Eye ointment, 73, 74

F
Five rights in drug administration, 59-62
   checklist, 60t
Fractional equation, 84, 85
Fractions, 4-7
   decimal, 6
   dividing, 6
   improper, 5
   mixed, 5
   multiplying, 5, 6
   practice problems, 6, 7
   proper, 5
Fried's rule, 250

G
Gastrointestinal enteral feeding tubes, 132
Guidelines for drug administration, 354-357
   general drug administration, 354
   injectable medications, 355, 356
   intravenous flow and medications,
      356, 357
   oral medications, 354, 355

H
Home infusion therapy, 320-322
Household system, 28-31
   conversion within, 28, 29
   practice problems, 30
      answers, 31
   summary practice problems, 32
      answers, 32
   units of measurements, 28t

I
Infusion devices, 194, 209-211
Infusion, titration of, 271-274
   total, over time, 276
Inhalation, 69, 70
   metered-dose inhaler, 69, 70
   metered-dose inhaler with spacer, 70
   nasal inhaler, 70, 71
Injectable preparations and types, 148-154
   ampules, 148
   angles of injection, 154
   needle size and length, 152-154, 153t
   parts of needle, 153
   parts of syringe, 149
   practice problems, 155
      answers, 183

Injectable preparations and types *(Continued)*
  syringes, 149-153
    cartridge, 152, 153
    five milliliter, 149, 150
    insulin, 151, 152
    three milliliter, 149, 150
    tuberculin, 151
  vials, 138
Injections, 154-183
  insulin, 159, 164
  intradermal, 154, 155
  intramuscular, 165-183
  subcutaneous, 154-158
Insulin injections, 159-165
  insulin pump, 164, 165
  insulin syringe and insulin bottle, 159
  intranasal, 163, 164
  jet injectors, 164
  mixing insulins, 161, 162
  pen injectors, 163
  practice problems, 151, 152
    answers, 184, 185
  types of insulin, 159-161
Insulin pump, 164, 165
Insulin syringe, 151, 152, 159
Intermittent infusion devices, 209
Intermittent intravenous (IV) administration,
    208, 209, 212-221, 224-227
  calculating flow rate, 212-216
  practice problems, 216-221
    answers, 224-227
  secondary intravenous sets, 208, 209
Interpreting drug labels, 46-50
  practice problems, 48-50
    answers, 64, 65
Intradermal injections, 154, 155
Intramuscular injection administration, 165-190
  drug solution, 166-168
  mixing injectable drugs, 170-173
  powdered drug reconstitution, 168, 169
  practice problems, 173-183
    answers, 185-190
  sites (injection), 166, 167t
Intramuscular injection sites, 166, 167t
  deltoid, 166
  dorsogluteal, 166
  vastus lateralis, 166
  ventrogluteal, 166
Intranasal insulin, 163, 164

Intravenous access sites, 192-195
  central venous access sites, 193
  flushing venous access devices, 195t
  intermittent infusion devices, 194
Intravenous (IV) administration, 194-227
  access sites for, 192-195
  continuous. See *Continuous intravenous (IV)
    administration.*
  direct intravenous, 194-199
  electronic IV delivery devices, 209-211
  intermittent. See *Intermittent intravenous (IV)
    administration.*
  methods of calculation, 202, 204, 205, 212
  needleless infusion devices, 194
Intravenous delivery devices, electronic. See
    Electronic intravenous delivery devices.
Intravenous flow rate, 202, 204, 212
Intravenous injection, direct, 194-199
Intravenous sets, 200, 201
  secondary. See *Secondary intravenous sets.*
Intravenous solutions, 204
  types, 204t
IV push, 194-199

J
Jet injector insulin, 163

L
Labor and delivery, 302-310
  factors influencing IV fluid and drug
    management, 302
  intravenous fluid bolus, 306-308
  intravenous loading dose, 304-306
  summary practice problems, 308, 309
    answers, 309, 310
  titration of medication, 302-304
Liquid drugs, 118-120
Lozenge (pharyngeal), 76

M
Metered-dose inhaler, 69-70
Metered-dose inhaler with spacer, 70
Methods of calculation for individualized drug
    dosing, 97-109
  body surface area (BSA), 99-103
  body weight, 98, 99
  nomograms, 101, 102
  summary practice problems, 103-106
    answers, 106-109

Methods of drug calculations, 80-96
  basic formula, 80-82
  dimensional analysis, 86-88
  fractional equation, 84, 85
  metric and apothecary conversions, 86t
  ratio and proportion, 82-84
  summary practice problems, 88-94
    answers, 94-96
Methods of drug distribution, 58, 59t
Metric and apothecary conversions, 86t, inside
    front cover
Metric, apothecary, and household
    equivalents, 34-44, 35t
Metric system, 20-25
  abbreviations, 21t
  conversion within, 22-24
  practice problems, 24, 25
    answers, 30
  prefixes, 20, 21t
  summary practice problems, 31, 32
    answers, 32
  units of measurement, 21t
Military time, 50, 51
Milliequivalents, 34
Mixing drugs, for intramuscular
    administration, 170-173
Mixing insulins, 161, 162
Mouthwash, pharyngeal, 75
Multiplying fractions, 5, 6

N
Nasal drops, 71, 72
Nasal inhaler, 70, 71
Nasal spray, 71, 72
Needles, 150, 153, 155, 153t
  parts of, 153
  practice problems, 155
    answers, 183
  SafetyGlide, 150
  size and length of, 153t
Nomograms, adult, 101, 360
  child, 102, 239, 361
Number systems, 2, 3
Nutrition, enteral, 131-136

O
Oral medications, 114-130, 139-144
  capsules, 114-118
  liquids, 118-120

Oral medications (Continued)
  practice problems, 121-130
    answers, 139-144
  sublingual tablets, 120, 121
  tablets, 114-118
Osmolalities, of commercial drug
    solutions, 137t

P
Patch, transdermal, 68
Patient-controlled analgesia (PCA), 210, 211
PCA, 210, 211
Pediatric critical care, 294-300
  calculating accuracy of dilution parameters,
    294-296
  factors influencing intravenous
    administration, 294
  summary practice problems, 297
    answers, 298-300
Pediatric drug administration, 232-258
  age rules, 250
    Fried's rule, 250
    Young's rule, 250
  body weight rule, 250
    Clark's rule, 250
  drug calculations, 234-239
    body surface area (BSA), 238, 239
    body weight, 235-237
  intramuscular injections, 233, 243, 244
    guidelines for, 233t
  intravenous, 233, 234, 244-249
    guidelines for IV therapy, 234t
  measuring devices, 232
  neonates, 248, 249, 258
  nomogram, 239t
  orals, 232, 240-249
  pediatric dosage from adult dosage, 249
  practice problems, 240-249
    answers, 250-258
Pediatric dosage from adult dosage, 249
Pediatric drug calculations, 232-258
  body surface area (BSA), 238, 239
  body weight, 235-237
Percentage, 11, 12
  practice problems, 11, 12
Percents, 34
Pharyngeal lozenge, 76
Pharyngeal mouthwash, 75
Pharyngeal spray, 75

Post-test (orals, injectables, intravenous, pediatrics), 329-346
  answers, 346-350
Preparing a solution of a desired concentration, 314-316
Preparing a weaker solution from stronger solution, 317-320

R
Ratio and proportion, 10, 36, 37, 82-84
  practice problems, 10, 11, 12
Rectal suppository, 77, 78
References, 351, 352
Rights, "5", 59-62
  checklist, 60t
  right client, 59
  right dose, 60, 61
  right drug, 59
  right route, 61, 62
  right time, 61
Roman numerals, 3, 4

S
Secondary intravenous sets, 208, 209, 212
  controllers, 209-211
    syringe pump, 210-211
    volumetric infusion pump, 209, 210
  drug calculations with secondary sets, 212
  patient-controlled analgesics (PCA), 210, 211
  without controllers, 209
    Buretrol, 209
    secondary sets, 209
Sites for IM injections, 166, 167t
Subcutaneous injections, 154-158
  calculation for, 156, 157
  practice problems, 157, 158
    answers,183, 184
Sublingual tablets, 120-121
Suppository, rectal, 77
Suppository, vaginal, 78

Syringe pumps, 210-211
Syringe(s), 148-153
  five milliliter, 150
  insulin, 151, 152
  prefilled cartridge and syringe, 152, 153
  three milliliter, 149, 150
  tuberculin, 151

T
Tablets, 114-118
  sublingual, 120, 121
Three milliliter syringe, 149, 150
Titration of infusion, critical care, 271-274
Titration of medications, labor and delivery, 302-304
Topical preparations, 76, 77
  creams and ointments, 76, 77
  lotion, 76
Total amount of drug infused over time, critical care, 276
Transdermal patch, 68
Tuberculin syringe, 151
Tubex syringe, 153
Types of insulins, 159-161

U
Units, 34

V
Vaginal cream, 78
Vaginal ointment, 78
Vaginal suppository, 78
Vials, 148

W
West nomograms, for children, 102, 239, 361

Y
Young's rule, 250

NOTES

NOTES

NOTES

NOTES

NOTES

NOTES

NOTES

NOTES

NOTES

NOTES